IMMUNOLOGY
IMMUNOPATHOLOGY
and IMMUNITY

IMMUNOLOGY IMMUNOPATHOLOGY and IMMUNITY

STEWART SELL, M.D.

Professor, Department of Pathology,
School of Medicine, University of California at San Diego, La Jolla, California

Medical Department

Harper & Row, Publishers

Hagerstown, Maryland

New York, Evanston, San Francisco, London

Library of Congress Cataloging in Publication Data

Sell, Stewart.
  Immunology, immunopathology, and immunity.

  Includes bibliographical references.
  1. Immunology. 2. Immunopathology. 3. Immunity.
I. Title. [DNLM: 1. Immunity. 2. Immunologic diseases.
QW504 S467i]
RC585.S44 1975 616.07'9 75-4934
ISBN 0-06-142371-8

Contents

I.   IMMUNOLOGY

II.   IMMUNOPATHOLOGY

III. IMMUNITY

Preface to the Second Edition

The enthusiastic reception of the first edition of IMMUNOLOGY, IMMUNOPATHOLOGY and IMMUNITY was of course, quite gratifying. Most reviewers, associates and students who commented on the text gave it high grades. This response encouraged both the publishers and me to undertake a necessary revision and in a large part sustained us during this tedious, but thankfully, sometimes stimulating task.

In this second edition, I have attempted to clarify some statements, to incorporate considerable new information and to include many new reference citations without disturbing the basic organization or diminishing the readability of the text. I am indebted to a number of reviewers, both official and unofficial, who have pointed out some shortcomings of the first edition and hope that these have been corrected in the second.

Considerable new material has been added in subject areas where advances in understanding have occurred since publication of the first edition. These subjects include cellular interactions in induction of antibody formation; genetics of the control of immune responses; the role of suppressor cells in tolerance and other immunologic reactions; cell-mediated killing of target cells; the relationship between HL-A antigens and mixed lymphocyte reactions and their role in predicting survival of organ grafts; the role of viral infections in certain immune-mediated diseases; transfer therapy of immune deficiency diseases; and the role of immune reactions in oncogenesis and immunotherapy of cancer. In addition, more details of hemolytic diseases, anaphylactic reactions, collagen diseases and immune-mediated skin eruptions are included.

The number of reference citations is more than double that in the first edition. As before, specific citation of references is given in the text so that the reader can check the original source for a given statement. This particular feature makes this text most useful for those who wish an introduction to immunology, immunopathology and immunity and also wish to be able to find more specific information in the literature.

A number of faculty at UCSD have helped by reviewing various segments of the text and I would like to express my gratitude for their always constructive, if not always kind, criticisms and suggestions. These include Harry Bluestein, Ken Brown, Richard Dutton, Robert Hamburger, Peter Lampert, John Mendelsohn, Douglas Redelman, and Park Trefts. A particular thanks must be given to Carol Prewitt, without whom the final accomplishment of a reasonable manuscript would have been impossible; to the artists, Mark Poler, Chuck Scott, Laurie Newell and Steve Coon, who spent long hours at the drawing board; to my fellow laboratory workers for excusing my unavailability at critical times, and last but not least, to my wife and family who have managed to put up with my preoccupation with immunology and my absent-mindedness to practical matters.

Preface to the First Edition

Frequently I have been asked by medical and biology students to recommend a text that covers both basic immunology and immunopathology. At best, I could recommend a basic text for immunology and individual chapters in several books for immunopathology—admitting that still, certain fundamental areas would remain uncovered. I could not identify a single text that encompasses the material that I thought important in a manner palatable to a beginner in the field.

In general, medical or pathology texts present immune reactions according to individual diseases or organ systems; they therefore lack a coherent mechanistic organization. Other texts, usually multiauthored, provide excellent reference sources but are too large and detailed and lack the organization necessary to be of general use for students unfamiliar with immunologic principles. My goal in writing this book is to give an organized, concise, yet meaningful presentation of immunology, immunopathology, and immunity, stressing their interrelationships. This book is intended for biology and medical students, house officers, and faculty who wish an introduction to the role played by immune mechanisms in disease.

In order to present both the protective and destructive mechanisms of the mammalian immune system, the text is divided into three parts: Immunology, Immunopathology, and Immunity. The first part, Immunology, presents the basic principles of the induction and expression of specific immune reactions. Aspects of immunology important for the understanding of immunopathologic mechanisms are emphasized. This provides an introduction for the second and major part of the book, Immunopathology. In this section, I have organized the fundamentals of how immune reactions cause tissue damage and disease in order to stress a classification based on immune mechanisms. The last part, Immunity, covers the role of immune reactions in protecting against infection and cancer. Detailed coverage is provided in areas of current interest, such as tissue transplantation and tumor immunity; the more classical topics receive a simplified treatment.

These exciting fields, especially the role that immune reactions play in producing disease, were brought to life for me by a number of teachers, in particular the excellent lectures and notes of Frank J. Dixon and Byron H. Waksman. I am indebted to them and to P.G.H. Gell for providing so much insight into immunological phenomena. In addition, I would like to thank: Richard N. Baney, for several careful readings that contributed to the clarity of presentation; Robert H. Fennell, Jr., for his continued enthusiastic support; William O. Weigle, for his discussions of tolerance; H.T. Wepsic, for his perspective on tumor immunology; the many investigators who gave me permission to reproduce their data or figures; the secretaries and artists both in Pittsburgh and LaJolla who translated my writing into legible typescript and my drawings into understandable figures; and the medical students who made constructive criticisms of my teaching.

Glossary of Terms

ABC	antigen-binding capacity
ALS	antilymphatic serum
ATP	adenosine triphosphate
B cell	bone marrow-derived cells (antibody-forming cell precursors)
BCG	bacillus Calmette-Guérin
BGG	bovine gammaglobulin
BSA	bovine serum albumin
BSA*	radiolabeled BSA
CBH	cutaneous basophil hypersensitivity
CEA	carcinoembryonic antigen
CGD	chronic granulomatous disease
Con A	concanavalin A; a plant mitogen
Cyclic Amp	cyclic adenosine 3′,5′-monophosphate
Cyclic Gmp	cyclic guanosine 3′,5′-monophosphate
DH	delayed hypersensitivity
DL	Donath-Landsteiner antibody
DNA	deoxyribonucleic acid
DNCB	dinitrochlorobenzene
DNP	dinitrophenol
DPT	combination injection for immunization against diphtheria, pertussis, tetanus
EAC	sheep cells coated with antibody and complement
EAT	experimental allergic thyroiditis
GA (GT)	copolymer of L-glutamic acid and L-tyrosine
GL	copolymer of L-glutamic acid and L-alanine
HL-A	histocompatible lymphocytes-antigens
H-PLL	hapten-poly-L-lysine conjugate
Ia	Ir gene-controlled antigen
Ig	immunoglobulins; five classes: IgA, IgG, IgM, IgD, IgE
Ir	immune response (gene)

IrE	immune response (gene) to ragweed
KLH	keyhole limpet hemocyanin
LATS	long-acting thyroid stimulator
LCM	lymphocytic choriomeningitis
LE	lupus erythematosus
LPS	bacterial lipopolysaccharide
M	macrophages
MLR	mixed lymphocyte reaction
MW	molecular weight
OT	old tuberculin
PHA	phytohemagglutinin
PLS	passive leukocyte-sensitizing activity
PPD	purified protein derivative
Ragg	rheumatoid agglutinators
RAST	radioallergoabsorbent test
RNA	ribonucleic acid
SLE	systemic lupus erythematosus
SNagg	serum normal agglutinators
Ss-Slp	genetic locus within the H_2 complex of mice controlling concentration and allotypic variation of a serum alphaglobulin
SSPE	subacute sclerosing panencephalitis
T cell	thymus-derived lymphocytes (helper cells)
TDM	thymus-derived mediator
Tla	thymus leukemia antigen
TPI	*Trepenoma pallidum* immobilization
TSTA	tumor-specific transplantation antigen

IMMUNOLOGY
IMMUNOPATHOLOGY
and IMMUNITY

I

Immunology

INTRODUCTION

Immunity has come to mean a specific protective response to a noxious agent or organism as the result of a previous exposure to it. The protection is specific in the sense that it is restricted to the agent or antigenically related agents to which the individual was previously exposed. The protection is mediated through the production of specifically modified serum proteins (antibodies) or specifically altered cells (sensitized cells) that have the capacity to recognize, react with, and neutralize the offending agent (antigen).

The terms immunity and allergy have been used interchangeably for manifestations of immune reactions, and because of this both words have lost preciseness of meaning. Immunity should be restricted to the protective manifestations of immune reactions. Von Pirquet originally defined allergy as "altered reactivity" due to a previous exposure to an agent without consideration of the effect of the altered reactivity upon the reacting individual. For the sake of clarity, allergy should now be reserved for instances in which the altered reactivity is deleterious rather than beneficial. However, in practice it is difficult to restrict the use of these terms (i.e., autoimmune is commonly used when autoallergic is preferrable). Hypersensitivity is also used for circumstances in which an allergic reaction causes tissue damage or an undesirable symptom. However, hypersensitivity is frequently applied to nonallergic as well as allergic reactions, and restriction of this term to allergic reactions is not practical. Immunopathology is the study of the tissue alterations that result from allergic reactions.

The induction and expression of immune reactivity are the subjects of the first part of this text. The mechanisms and effects of immune reactions in the production of tissue lesions and disease (allergic reactions) are the subjects of Part II. The role of these mechanisms in protection against disease (immunity), the effects of the lack of such protective mechanisms (immune deficiency diseases) and the relationship of immune mechanisms to cancer are the subjects of the third part of this text.

1

1

Antigenicity and Immunization

In all types of immune or allergic reactions an individual acquires specific information (learns) from contact with an antigen without the mediation of the nervous system. The essence of an immune or allergic response is the capacity to recognize an antigen.

ANTIGENS AND IMMUNOGENS

Any attempt to define an antigen with a simple statement is bound to ignore several known properties of antigens. Nevertheless, an antigen is classically defined as a molecular species capable of inducing an immune response and of reacting specifically with the products (antibody, sensitized cells) manufactured as a consequence of the immune response. The ability of material to induce an immune response is referred to as immunogenicity, and such a material may be called an immunogen. The ability of a material to react with the products of an immune response is referred to as antigenicity, and therefore such a material is an antigen. Antibodies join to antigen by noncovalent bonding of sites which can be juxtaposed because of a physical "lock and key" relationship. (See Chapter 6.) Antibodies are present in the serum component of whole blood (blood without fibrin and cells) and serum containing antibody is designated antiserum.

COMPLETE AND INCOMPLETE ANTIGENS

A complete antigen is one that can both induce an immune response and react with the products of that response. An incomplete antigen (hapten) is a chemically active substance of low molecular weight that is unable to induce an immune response by itself but can, by combining with larger molecules (carrier or "Schlepper"), become immunogenic. A complete antigen is both an immunogen and an antigen, while an incomplete antigen is not an immunogen, but is an antigen. For example, a chemically highly active small molecule such as dinitrophenol (an incomplete antigen) may combine with the host's protein (to form a complete antigen) so that sensitization occurs. An individual thus sensitized reacts with the dinitrophenol upon second contact with it (see Contact Allergy, Chapter 14).

PHYSICAL PROPERTIES OF ANTIGENS

The size, shape, rigidity, location of determinants, and tertiary structure have been shown to affect antigenicity (5,9).

Size

Complete antigens (immunogens) usually have a high molecular weight. Naturally occurring immunogens may have a fairly low molecular weight, such as ribonuclease (MW 14,000), insulin (MW 6,000), and angiotensin (MW 1,031). The artificial antigen N-acetyl-L-tyrosine$_3$ (MW only 450) has apparently evoked an immune response in some guinea pigs (9), but one cannot rule out the possibility that such a small molecule may combine with host protein so that the actual immunogen is a complex composed of the small molecule (hapten) and the host protein (carrier).

The sites of antigens that react with antibody are smaller than those that induce antibody formation. Kabat (4) has reviewed the size and characteristics of areas of antigen that react with antibody (antigenic determinants). This information is obtained by determining the ability of a given compound of low molecular weight to inhibit the reaction of antibody with the complete antigen of which the small compound is only a part. Antibodies to dextran polysaccharide are inhibited by six unit saccharides (MW 990), and antibodies to polypeptides are inhibited by four to five amino acid oligopeptides (MW 650). Homopolymers of amino acids are not usually immunogenic, but will function as haptens if added to carrier molecules such as a serum protein. Poly-L-lysine is not immunogenic, but the attachment of a dinitrophenyl group to poly-L-lysine may establish immunogenicity. DNP-L-lysine$_7$ is immunogenic, but DNP-L-lysine$_6$ is not. L-Lysine$_5$ inhibits the reaction of anti-L-lysine antibody with poly-L-lysine$_7$. Therefore a larger molecule is usually required to induce an immune response than is necessary to react completely with antibody.

Shape

The shape of a determinant is important, as certain components, such as the DNP in DNP-L-lysine, give form to a molecule that is evidently not found in the homologous polymer. Copolymers of two amino acids are immunogenic for some species, while polymers of three or four amino acids are required for other species. The presence of more than one amino acid in a polymer results in a configuration not available in the polymer of a single amino acid. The location of a structure within a determinant may also be important. In some cases antibody can be demonstrated to bind more strongly with certain structures within a determinant than with other structures. For instance, in determining the binding of antibody to D-alanine-glycine-ε-aminocaproic acid, it was found that the terminal alanine was responsible for most of the antibody binding. In this case, the D-alanine group is termed the immunodominant part of the determinant (4,9).

Rigidity

The role of rigidity and location of determinants in antigenicity is exemplified by the work of Sela (9) in regard to the alteration in immunogenicity and antigenicity of gelatin by the addition of poly-L-tyrosine to a gelatin backbone. Gelatin, which may have a very high molecular weight, is almost completely nonimmunogenic. Addition of 1% tyrosine increases the immunogenicity and antigenicity of gelatin, and the specificity of antibody produced is directed toward the gelatin. Addition of the tyrosine evidently makes the gelatine structure more stable or rigid. Addition of 3–10% tyrosine to gelatin results in the production of antibody with specificity directed toward the tyrosine, i.e., all the antibody activity can be removed by poly-L-tyrosine and none by gelatin.

Determinant Location

Sela also demonstrated that if the tyrosine is buried inside the tyrosine-gelatin molecule, it does not function as an antigen, but if the tyrosine is placed on the surface of the molecule it is recognized (9). This finding, along with the observations that new determinants may be exposed by partial denaturation of proteins, indicates that important antigenic determinants may be secluded inside large molecules and may be exposed by unfolding of the molecule. Denaturation of a protein generally decreases or destroys its immunogenicity and antigenicity. However, partial denaturation may result in exposure of different molecular configurations owing to alteration of the tertiary structure of the molecule, with the creation of new antigenic determinants.

Tertiary Structures

The tertiary structure of proteins (spatial folding) is important in determining the specificity of an antibody response. Antibodies produced to the A chains of insulin do not react with the natural molecule (11). Reduction and reoxidation of ribonuclease under controlled conditions produce a mixture of protein molecules different in third dimensional structure only. Some antisera to native ribonuclease are unreactive to these denatured molecules; other antisera to the native molecule do react with the denatured forms (6). These results indicate that the tertiary structure of immunogens is recognized by the immunologically reacting systems. Therefore no significant breakdown of the immunogen can occur before it is recognized by the specifically reactive cells. If catabolism did occur, the tertiary structure of the immunogen would be destroyed.

Catabolism

The optical activity of synthetic antigens has suggested that the ability to catabolize or break down the antigen is important for the induction of an immune response. Thus, L-amino acid heteropolymers are catabolizable and are immunogenic, while D-amino acid heteropolymers are not catabolizable and are poorly immunogenic (5). However, pneumococcal polysaccharides are not digested by mice, but are highly immunogenic in mice. The inability of D-amino acids to function as immunogens is not due to an inability of the reacting animal to recognize D-amino acids as foreign, since copolymers of L- and D-amino acids are immunogenic and some of the antibody formed reacts specifically with D-amino acid polymers. The immunogenicity of D-amino acid polymers is dependent upon dose in mice and rabbits. The response to D-isomers exhibits a strong maximum at about 1 μg per mouse, but that to L-isomers is largely independent of dose. Therefore, the failure to detect responses to the poorly catabolized D-isomers may be due to selection of the wrong immunizing dose. Antibody formed to poorly catabolized immunogens may be difficult to demonstrate because of blocking or binding of the antibody formed with the noncatabolized antigen still present in the serum (see Felton's Immune Paralysis, Chapter 7).

IMMUNIZATION

Immunogenicity is determined not only by the nature of the antigen, but also by characteristics of the responding animal and the manner in which the antigen is presented to the responding animal. The contact of immunogens and responding individuals may occur by natural exposure to organisms, chemical components or other immunogens in the environment, or may be artifically induced by controlled immunization. The following factors are involved in any controlled immunization and the detection of a subsequent immune response: 1) the source of the antigen, 2) the preparation of the antigen, 3) the form in which the antigen is given, 4) the route of immunization or anatomic location of initial contact, 5) the dose of antigen, 6) the time between the immunizing event and the testing for antibody or sensitized cells, 7) the number of immunizations given (primary or secondary response), 8) the type of test procedure employed, 9) the genetic makeup of the responding animal, 10) the condition of the responding animal, and 11) the presence of bacterial products in the immunizing mixture. Given such a number of variables, some generalizations may be made, but in practice each immunizing situation must be individually evaluated. Therefore, for the results of laboratory tests to be satisfactorily evaluated, the conditions under which an antiserum or population of sensitized cells is obtained must be thoroughly described.

Immunization is performed clinically to induce a protective reaction, as in vaccination with polioviruses or diphtheria toxoid (see Chapter 18). Experimental immunization may be performed to explore immune reactions or to produce an antiserum that might be used as an immunochemical reagent. The purposes for which a given immunization is done determine to a large extent how it is done.

Source of Antigen

The source of antigen depends upon the purpose of the immunization. For protective immune responses, individuals may be immunized with killed infectious agents or with nontoxic extracts (see Chapter 18). In experimental situations an individual may be immunized with the serum proteins or tissues of another individual of the same or a different species, or with artificially synthesized materials such as polypeptides.

Preparation of Antigen

The final preparation of an antigen used for immunization depends upon the degree of specificity desired. For example, immunization of a rabbit with whole rat spleen produces an antiserum that reacts with various cell populations in the spleen (erythrocytes, lymphocytes, macrophages) and with as many as 30 different plasma proteins. By careful removal of the cellular elements or by immunization with rat serum (defibrinated rat plasma), a rabbit antiserum that reacts with rat serum proteins may be obtained (rabbit anti-whole-rat serum). By fractionation of the rat serum, an antigen preparation may be obtained that contains only one serum protein. Further fractionation of an antigenic molecule may be accomplished by breaking the molecule into smaller units, and an antiserum that reacts with only part of the molecule may be obtained.

Forms in Which Antigen Is Given

The form in which an antigen is administered also may vary. A serum protein may be administered in soluble form. It may be precipitated with alum to obtain a greater antibody response. An intense mononuclear infiltration at the site of injection is induced by injection of antigen incorporated into an emulsion with Freund's adjuvant (paraffin oil and "aquaphor") (1) to which mycobacteria may be also added (complete Freund's adjuvant). This greatly enhances the immune response (see below). Many other variations may be employed to modify the nature and extent of the immune response.

Route of Immunization

The routes of immunization include intradermal, subcutaneous, intramuscular, intraperitoneal, intravascular and intracranial injection, as well as injection into any organ. In addition, immunization may be accomplished by ingestion, inhalation, skin application, rectal infusion or intratracheal infusion. The type of immune response elicited depends upon the route used. Those routes which lead to distribution in vascular spaces generally lead to the formation of humoral antibodies, while those routes that lead to focal deposition in peripheral lymphoid tissue (intradermal injection or application on the skin surface) lead to the development of cellular sensitivity. Inoculation into organs of external secretion such as salivary glands, breast or nasal mucosa may result in the production of antibodies of a different class of immunoglobulins (IgA) than would be found following intramuscular injection (IgG). (For a discussion of immunoglobulin classes of antibody see Chapter 5.)

Dose of Antigen

The amount of antigen given is extremely important, as too little or too much may result in a loss of immune responsiveness (see Chapter 7). A few milligrams of any antigen is usually enough to induce an immune response. Much smaller amounts may actually be more effective, depending on the nature of the antigen. If a specific antiserum is desired, relatively small amounts of the antigen preparation should be used. If large amounts are used, trace contamination with undesirable antigens may result in the production of an antiserum with multiple specificities.

Interval Between Immunization and Testing

Antibody may be detected within a few hours following immunization, if very sensitive detection techniques are used. However, in most controlled immunizations circulating antibody does not appear in significant amount until 7–10 days following immunization. The immunoglobulin class of antibody produced also may change with time. Early antibody tends to be of the IgM class, while later antibodies are of the IgG class (10). Also, late antibodies may bind more strongly to antigens than early antibodies (see Affinity and Avidity, Chapter 6). Usually after 3–5 weeks the amount of antibody produced starts to decline so that later blood analyses give lower titers of antibody.

Number of Immunizations Given

The amount of antibody formed after a second injection of a given antigen (secondary, or memory response) usually is much greater than that formed after one injection (primary response). If a high-titered antiserum is desired, a series of injections is commonly given. However, after three or more injections, the titer of antibody may be less than after only two injections. The antibody formed after a second injection of antigen (booster) tends to be of the IgG class and more avid (binds more strongly to antigen) than the antibody formed after one injection, which may be of the IgM class. Each blood analysis of an immunized animal may yield antibody in different titer, of different avidity, and perhaps of different specificity. Each blood sample must be separately tested to ensure that results obtained with different bleedings can be compared.

Type of Test Procedure Employed

The tests used for detection of antibody differ markedly in their ability to measure antibody activity (see Table 6–1). If a bactericidal or phage neutralization test is used, extremely small amounts of antibody may be detected within a few hours of immunization. If the double diffusion-in-agar technique utilizing a soluble protein antigen is used, a million times as much antibody may be needed for detection to occur. In some situations antibody may be detected in vivo (by skin test or systemic anaphylaxis), while in vitro test are negative. The procedures used for detection of antibody are discussed in more detail in Chapter 6. Whether antibody is found following immunization may well depend upon the test used for detection.

Genetic Make-Up of the Responding Animal

The ability to produce an immune response and the type of response produced to some antigens are under genetic control. This subject is discussed on page 52.

Condition of the Responding Animal

A wide variety of factors may affect immune responses. For best results young, healthy adult animals should be used. Very young or very old animals may not react well to a given antigen. Diseases, immunosuppressive agents, and diet may alter immune reactivity. Further discussion of the factors influencing the immune response may be found in Chapter 18.

Presence of Bacterial Products in Immunizing Mixture

Bacteria or bacterial products added to a known specific antigen such as serum albumin may greatly increase the subsequent production of antibodies to the albumin (7). The mechanism of action of agents that produce such an increased immune response is unknown, but it is believed that they nonspecifically cause a recruitment of more specific antibody-forming cells.

ANTIGENIC SPECIFICITY

The antibody molecules formed after immunization may demonstrate a variety of antigen-binding specificities. If the inducing antigenic specificity is limited to a small chemical group, the specificity of antibody binding may be exquisitely specific; if the immunogen is a large molecule, a large number of overlapping antigen-binding specificities may be represented in the antibody formed (see Chapter 6).

Chemical Structures

The antigenic specificity of an immunogen may be so exact that it is directly related to a chemically definable structure, and the specificity of the resulting antibody may be used to determine, in part, the chemical structure of unknown molecules. Heidelberger (2) related the specificity of antibody to pneumococcal polysaccharide Type SII to D-glucose joined in 1,4,6-linkages. He reacted anti-SII antisera against glycogens, glycogen limit dextran, and amylopectins, all of which contained 1,4,6-linkages, and all cross-reacted with the anti-SII antisera. The chemical structures of some unknowns were then predicted by the finding that these unknowns reacted with the anti-SII sera, and direct chemical analysis later verified the presence of 1,4,6-linkages in the unknowns.

Functional Specificity

Serum proteins with different functional activities have different antigenic specificities. The albumin, α-globulins, and immunoglobulins of a given species do not possess antigenic specificities in common. Rabbit antihuman albumin does not react with human immunoglobulins, and vice versa. However, the albumins of different species may contain common determinants. Rabbit antihuman albumin may react with bovine albumin. Thus, serum proteins that perform similar functions in different species may share antigenic specificities.

Species Specificity

Rabbit antihuman albumin reacts more strongly with human albumin than with the albumin of any other species. Human albumin and other human serum proteins contain antigenic specificities unique for humans.

Allospecificity

Some individuals of a given species possess antigenic specificities not shared with other individuals of the same species. These specificities depend upon small structural differences and are best exemplified by ABO blood group specificities. Within the human species, the red blood cells of some individuals have antigenic specificities in common, while the red blood cells of other individuals have different antigenic specificities. The same is true of serum proteins (immunoglobulins, β-lipoproteins) and solid tissues. The older terminology of blood group specificities referred to differences between individuals as isospecificities; the more recent terminology introduced to cover solid tissue transplantation antigens employs the term allospecificities. The attempt to identify and classify allospecific antigens in solid tissues is an important advance in human tissue transplantation (see Graft Rejection, Chapter 14).

Heterogenic Specificity

In some cases, for unknown reasons, an identical antigenic specificity is present in the tissues of different species (3). The classic example is the Forssman antigen. Anti-Forssman antibody is produced by injecting sheep red blood cells into rabbits. The resulting antiserum reacts with sheep cells, goat cells, guinea pig tissue, human type A red cells, certain bacteria, plants, and other animal or fish tissues. There is no phylogenetic or functional relation for this antigenic specificity, and it appears due to some accidental chemical similarity. A similar relation exists between certain organisms. For instance, the Weil-Felix test depends upon the fact that antiserum against *Rickettsia* reacts also with *Proteus* OX-19.

Organ Specificity

The same organs of different species share some common antigenic specificities. Thus, the thyroid antigens of one species are shared by the thyroid of another species; the adrenal or brain of one species shares specificity with the adrenal or brain of another species.

ANTIGEN PREVALENCE

The antigens that an individual reacts with naturally are usually provided by contact with other organisms (bacteria, viruses, fungi). Experimental or therapeutic procedures provide opportunity for contact with other potential antigens, such as artificially produced macromolecules (drugs), serum proteins, blood cells or tissues (grafts) from other individuals of the same species or of other species. A given animal does not usually muster an immune response to his own tissues, although his own tissues contain many potential antigens for other genetically different individuals in the same species and even greater numbers of potential antigens for individuals of other species. An individual may react against his own tissues (autoallergic reaction) if they are rendered antigenic by physical (heat, necrosis) or infectious processes, or if they combine with incomplete antigens (see Autoallergic Diseases, Chapter 14).

REFERENCES

1. Freund J: The mode of action of immunologic adjuvants. Adv Turberc Res 7:130, 1956
2. Heidelberger M: Lectures in Immunochemistry. New York, Academic Press, 1956
3. Jenkin CR: Heterophile antigens and their significance in the host-parasite relationship. Adv Immunol 3:351, 1963
4. Kabat EA: The nature of an antigenic determinant. J Immunol 97:1, 1966
5. Mauer PH: Use of synthetic polymers of amino acids to study the basis of antigenicity. Prog Allergy 8:1, 1964
6. Mills JA, Haber E: The effect on antigenic specificity of changes in the molecular structure of ribonuclease. J Immunol 91:536, 1963
7. Munoz J: Effect of bacteria and bacterial products on antibody responses. Adv Immunol 4:397, 1964
8. Schlossman SF, Herman J, Yaron A: Antigen recognition: In vitro studies on the specificity of the cellular immune response. J Exp Med 129:1031, 1969
9. Sela M: Immunological studies with synthetic polypeptides. Adv Immunol 5:30, 1969
10. Uhr JW: The heterogeneity of the immune response. Science 145:457, 1964
11. Yagi Y, Maier P, Pressman D: Antibodies against the component polypeptide chains of bovine insulin. Science 147:617, 1965

ADDITIONAL READING

Landsteiner K: The Specificity of Serological Reactions. New York, Dover Publications, 1962

Kabat EA: Structural Concepts in Immunology and Immunochemistry. New York, Holt, Rinehart and Winston, 1968

2

Leukocytes

Immune responses require the active participation of living cells. The cells involved in immune responses belong to a class termed leukocytes, or white cells (Fig. 2–1). These cells take part in various inflammatory reactions, both of immune and of nonimmune nature (2). They may be found in large numbers in certain organs (lymphoid organs), in smaller numbers in the stroma of many organs, and in the blood. The term white cells is applied because the leukocytes of the blood sediment in a thin, white layer between the erythrocytes (red blood cells) and the plasma when unclotted blood is allowed to stand for a certain period of time. This layer of white blood cells is called the buffy coat. Some white cells are present in both blood and tissue, while others are normally found only in tissue. The cells of the leukocyte series (discussed below) are lymphocytes, plasma cells, macrophages, polymorphonuclear leukocytes and blast cells (14).

LYMPHOCYTES

The lymphocyte is a small, round cell found in the peripheral blood, lymph nodes, spleen, thymus, tonsils, appendix and many other tissues (6,14). In smears of peripheral blood, lymphocytes appear slightly larger (7–8 μ) in diameter than erythrocytes and make up 20–45% of the total white blood cell count of normal man. A typical lymphocyte (Fig. 2–2) has very little cytoplasm and consists mostly of a spherical nucleus with prominent nuclear chromatin. Although difficult to see in the light microscope, there is usually a deep cleft of the cytoplasm extending into the nucleus. The narrow rim of cytoplasm contains scattered ribosomes as well as a few ribosomal aggregates, but is virtually devoid of endoplasmic reticulum (that cytoplasmic structure associated with protein secretion) or other organelles. The lymphocyte plays a prominent role in delayed hypersensitivity. Once believed to be a short-lived "end" cell, it is now known to survive for months or even years and to recirculate from lymph nodes to lymph and blood (6). The lymphocyte may be responsible for the primary recognition of antigen and is an immunologically specific effector cell (6). It is possible that the lymphocyte produces antibody-like

ERYTHROCYTE 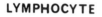 7.7

LYMPHOCYTE 7-8

NEUTROPHIL 9-12

EOSINOPHIL 10-14

PLASMA CELL 9-12

MAST CELL 18-24

MACROPHAGE 12-20

BLAST CELL 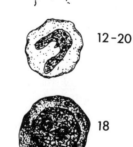 18

Fig. 2–1. Leukocytes. Composite drawing indicating relative size (microns) and morphology of cells involved in immune reactions and in nonimmune inflammatory reactions. The erythrocyte is included for size reference, since it is the most easily identified cell in blood smears and in many tissue sections.

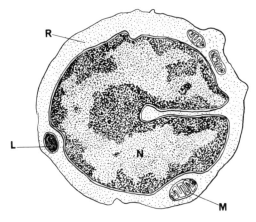

Fig. 2–2. **Lymphocyte.**   Cell is composed mainly of nucleus, with a paucity of cytoplasmic elements. Narrow rim of cytoplasm contains scattered ribosomes, a few membrane-limited bodies (lysosomes), and a few mitochondria. L, lysosome; M, mitochondria; N, nucleus; R, ribosomes.

Fig. 2–3. **Plasma cell.**   Cell is composed of abundant cytoplasm containing mostly laminated endoplasmic reticulum and a few other cytoplasmic organelles. Note polar location of nucleus and its cartwheel appearance produced by condensation of chromatin along nuclear membrane. ER, endoplasmic reticulum; G, Golgi apparatus; M, mitochondria; N, nucleus.

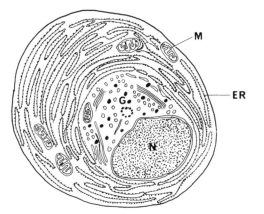

immunoglobulin molecules that remain fixed to the lymphocyte and serve as receptor sites for reaction with antigen (9). Considerable experimental evidence implicates the lymphocyte as the carrier of immunologic information. Immunologically competent cell and memory cell are functional terms which have been applied, but the histologic type or types of cells responsible for these functions is not established, although most investigators incriminate the lymphocyte. The developmental relation between the lymphocyte and some other cell types of the leukocyte series (plasma cell, macrophage) is uncertain, although the presence of morphologic intermediates (lymphocytoid plasma cell) has suggested to some workers that the plasma cell and the macrophage may arise from a common lymphocyte-like precursor (4,7). However, a direct developmental relation between the lymphocyte and other cell types has not been demonstrated.

PLASMA CELLS

The plasma cell (Fig. 2–3) is a small, round or oval cell (9–12 μ in diameter), with a small, compact, dense nucleus located at one pole (4). Aggregations of chromatin along the nuclear envelope give rise to the characteristic "cartwheel" appearance of the plasma cell nucleus. The cytoplasm is dominated by rough endoplasmic reticulum organized in concentric laminae. Large Golgi complexes are also present. Membrane-bounded amorphous densities (Russell bodies) believed to contain stored immunoglobulins may be observed in more mature plasma cells. Mitochondria and scattered ribosomes are seen in the cytoplasm. The characteristic laminated endoplasmic reticulum in the cytoplasm of the plasma cell is found in other cells in which protein secretion is a major function (e.g., pancreatic acinar cells). Both in vivo observations and in vitro determinations of protein production and content indicate that the production of immunoglobulins (antibody) for secretion is the primary function of the plasma cell. The Golgi apparatus of the plasma cell may play an active role in the secretion of immunoglobulins. Plasma cells are prominent in the lymph nodes, spleen and sites of chronic inflammation. An increase in the number of plasma cells occurs in lymphoid organs draining the site of antigen injection during the induction of antibody formation (13).

MACROPHAGES

The blood macrophage (monocyte), the primary phagocytic cell, is the largest of the lymphoid cells normally found in the peripheral blood (11). It ranges from 12–15 μ in diameter, and constitutes 3–8% of the normal leukocyte count. The nucleus is centrally located and usually has a bilobed reniform shape with considerable peripheral condensation of nuclear chromatin (Fig. 2–4). The cytoplasm contains a large variety of organelles, including endoplasmic reticulum, a Golgi complex, mitochondria, free and aggregated ribosomes, and various membrane-limited phagocytic vacuoles (lysosomes, dense bodies, myelin figures, microbodies).

The tissue macrophage (histiocyte) is similar in appearance, but larger (15–18 μ in diameter) and may contain more cytoplasmic vacuoles than the monocyte. The blood and tissue macrophages are grouped together, on the basis of their phagocytic function, into the reticuloendothelial system. This system includes phagocytic cells in the blood, lymph nodes and spleen; the Kupffer cells of the liver; alveolar macrophages; peritoneal macrophages; some glial cells of the central nervous system; and many phagocytic cells in loose connective tissue (11). There is convincing evidence that blood macrophages migrate into tissues, where they become tissue macrophages.

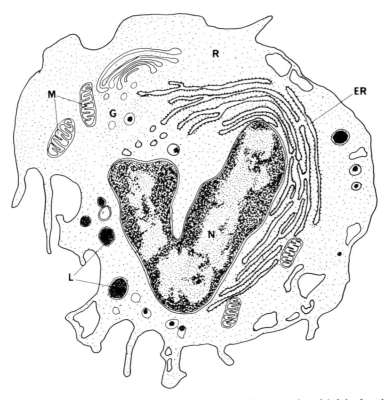

Fig. 2–4. Macrophage. Large nucleus is centrally located and bilobed or kidney-shaped. Cytoplasm is extensive and contains a wide variety of organelles. **ER**, endoplasmic reticulum; **G**, Golgi apparatus; **L**, lysosomes; **M**, mitochondria; **N**, nucleus; **R**, ribosomes.

Fig. 2–5. Neutrophil. Cytoplasm contains large numbers of membrane-limited bodies (lysosomes) that stain pale pink with usual staining agents. Nucleus is divided into round or oval lobes connected to one another by thin strands of nuclear material. **G**, Golgi apparatus; **L**, lysosomes; **M**, mitochondrion; **N**, nucleus; **R**, ribosomes.

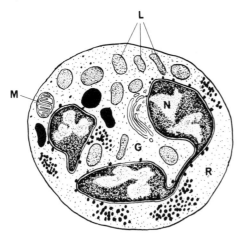

Properties of Macrophages

Macrophages play a prominent role in the later stages of the inflammatory response and may accumulate in large numbers in sites of inflammation (12). Although the migration of macrophages (both blood and tissue) into inflammatory sites is generally believed to be immunologically non-specific and the result of the poorly understood phenomenon of chemotaxis, it has been demonstrated that lymphocytes and macrophages interact in certain immune reactions. Macrophages obtained from normal animals migrate when cultured in vitro, but macrophages obtained from immunized animals do not migrate in vitro in the presence of the specific antigen. This effect is the result not of a direct action of the antigen upon the macrophages, but of the presence of lymphocytes in the cell population studied. Specifically sensitized lymphocytes have the ability to recognize and react with antigen. As a result of this reaction, substances are released from lymphocytes that affect macrophages. Upon incubation with antigen, lymphocytes obtained from sensitized animals release soluble factors that affect the behavior of macrophages. These factors may be important in the mechanism of production of delayed hypersensitivity reactions. Only a few specifically sensitized lymphocytes reacting with antigen in tissue can cause localization of large numbers of macrophages, which in turn are responsible for the lesions observed (see Chapter 14).

Phagocytosis

The primary function of the macrophage is phagocytosis. Following the intake of foreign material into the cell, the material may be digested by the action of enzymes present within the macrophage (3). The process of phagocytosis is discussed in Chapter 8. The uptake of antigens by macrophages which localize in the germinal centers of lymphoid organs is the first step in the processing of antigen leading to the production of circulating antibody (see Chapter 3). In such cases the antigen is not completely degraded by the macrophage, but becomes bound to macrophage RNA. The information required for a specific immune response then is passed on either by the RNA or by the RNA-antigen complex (5). At the present time, the macrophage is not believed to be the cell that recognizes antigen as foreign; the macrophage nonspecifically processes the antigen so that it becomes more palatable for a recognition cell (8). Macrophages are stimulated by a number of substances (paraffin oils, tubercle bacilli) to transform into the epithelioid and giant cells characteristic of granulomatous hypersensitivity (see Chapter 15).

POLYMORPHONUCLEAR LEUKOCYTES

Polymorphonuclear leukocytes (PMNs) are intermediate in size between lymphocytes and macrophages (9–12 μ in diameter) and are characterized by a multilobulated nucleus. They may be classified according to the staining characteristics of their prominent cytoplasmic granules into neutrophils, eosinophils, and basophils (1,10).

Neutrophils

Neutrophils have cytoplasmic granules that do not stain strongly red or blue with the usual dyes employed for staining smears of blood, but show only a pale pink coloration (10). Such cells make up from 50–75% of the leukocytes of the peripheral blood and may be found scattered diffusely in many tissues, although they are most frequently found in areas of acute inflammation or acute necrosis. Like the macrophage, the neutrophil is active in phagocytosis and has been named by some a microphage. The nucleus of the neutrophil, as of all the PMNs, is divided into round or oval lobes connected to one another by thin strands of nuclear material (Fig. 2–5). As with other leukocytes, there is condensation of chromatin at the periphery of the nucleus. The other outstanding feature of this type of cell is the large number of uniform membrane-delineated granules. The cytoplasm of a mature PMN contains few other cytoplasmic organelles, though most PMNs contain a few mitochondria, a little endoplasmic reticulum, and a small Golgi apparatus. Like some of the granules of the macrophage, the granules of the neutrophil contain a wide variety of hydrolytic enzymes. Neutrophils are rapidly migrating cells that appear quickly in areas of infection or tissue damage. They actively phagocytize cell debris or organisms and are responsible for the characteristic pathologic appearance of acute inflammation. The role of the neutrophil in acute inflammation is taken over by the macrophage in the chronic stage of inflammation. The appearance of neutrophils in areas of inflammation is believed to be nonspecific in the sense that these cells do not carry immune information.

Eosinophils

Eosinophils are similar in appearance to neutrophils except that they have prominent eosinophilic (red) granules that may contain rod-like crystalloid inclusions when viewed by electron microscopy (Fig. 2–6). These eosinophilic granules contain large amounts of hydrolytic enzymes (lysosomes). The granules differ from those of neutrophils in a high content of peroxidase, which is perhaps related to the crystalloid structure. The chemotactic response of eosinophils is basically identical to that of neutrophils, but eosinophils are found in unusually high numbers about antigen-antibody complexes and parasites. In spite of these associations, the function of eosinophils remains a mystery. Eosinophils make up from 2–4% of the circulating leukocytes.

Basophils

Basophils are PMNs with prominent blue-staining cytoplasmic granules. Basophils located in tissue are called mast cells and are found in loose (areolar) connective tissue (1). Blood basophils are rounded while mast cells are elongated or irregular. Blood basophils make up 0.5–1% of the peripheral leukocytes. Mast cell nuclei are round or oval, while circulating basophils have a lobulated form (polymorphonuclear). However, they, like the eosinophil, tend to have bilobed rather than multilobulated nuclei. The outstanding feature of basophils is the abundance of oval basophilic

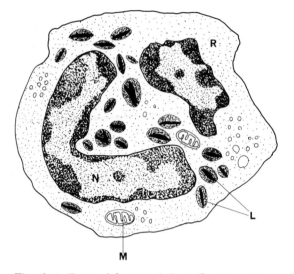

Fig. 2–6. Eosinophil. Morphologically the cell resembles the neutrophil, but prominent cytoplasmic membrane-limited bodies (lysosomes) stain red with usual staining agents and contain rod-like crystalloid structures when observed by electron microscopy. **L**, lysosomes; **M**, mitochondria; **N**, nucleus; **R**, ribosomes.

(blue) granules which have a finely granular or reticular ultrastructure. The predominance of granules overshadows other cytoplasmic structures, although mitochondria, endoplasmic reticulum, ribosomes and Golgi apparatus may be seen. Basophil granules contain heparin, histamine, serotonin (5-hydroxytryptamine) and a battery of hydrolytic enzymes. The presence of these pharmacologically active agents in mast cell granules and the prominence of mast cells in perivascular tissues suggest that the release of such agents would have a marked effect on the smooth muscle of arterioles and the permeability of capillaries. Indeed, release of these agents by mast cells is believed to be the mechanism responsible for the unleashing of anaphylactic or atopic allergic reactions (see Chapter 12).

BLAST CELLS

A well recognized feature of active immune responses is the presence of large, immature, "blast" cells (Fig. 2–7) (7). This cell has a large nucleus containing finely divided chromatin and prominent nucleoli. The cytoplasm is strongly basophilic and contains dense collections of free and aggregated ribosomes. A variety of other subcellular organelles may be found in the cytoplasm, including a Golgi apparatus, a varying amount of endoplasmic reticulum, and mitochondria. Blast cells are found in lymphoid organs draining sites of antigen injection and in active inflammatory lesions, particularly those of delayed hypersensitivity reactions; they may be induced in vitro in pure cultures of lymphocytes by certain mitogenic agents. It has been postulated that the blast cell is an intermediate cell between

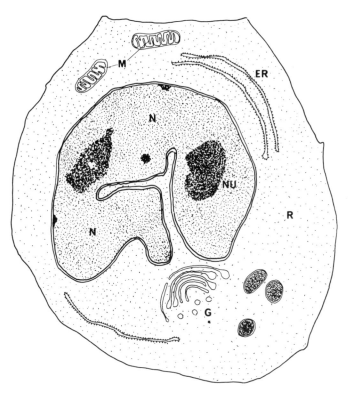

Fig. 2–7. Blast cell. Cell has large nucleus containing finely divided chromatin and prominent nucleoli. Cytoplasm stains blue with usual staining agents and contains dense collections of ribosomes as well as other organelles. ER, endoplasmic reticulum; G, Golgi apparatus; M, mitochondria; N, nucleus; NU, nucleolus; R, ribosomes.

the lymphocyte and the plasma cell (7). Thus, antigen-recognizing lymphocytes are stimulated by antigen to undergo transformation into blast cells that divide and differentiate into plasma cells. This theory is supported by indirect evidence that shows morphologic intermediates between lymphocytes and plasma cells, including blast cells with little or no endoplasmic reticulum (immunoblasts), blast cells with increasing amounts of endoplasmic reticulum (plasmablasts), and cells more typical of the plasma cell series with abundant laminated endoplasmic erticulum (preplasma cells) (7). There is a separate cell line for the production of specifically sensitized lymphocytes and for antibody-producing plasma cells. The precursor cell for a plasma cell is termed a B cell; that of a sensitized lymphocyte, a T cell (see Chapter 4). Although claims have been made that the human T cell is smooth and the B cell villous when examined by scanning electromicroscopically, such differences have not been observed using mouse T and B cells, and in fact may reflect reactions of the cells to the processing used prior to examination. It is impossible to identify clearly a T cell and a B cell by morphologic criteria, as both look like small lymphocytes.

REFERENCES

1. Benditt BP, Lagunoff D: The mast cell: Its structure and function. Prog Allergy 8:195, 1964
2. Braunsteiner R, Zuker-Franklin D (eds): The Physiology and Pathology of Leukocytes. New York, Grune & Stratton, 1962
3. Cohn ZA: The structure and functions of monocytes and macrophages. Adv Immunol 9:163, 1968
4. Feldman JD: Ultrastructure of immunological processes. Adv Immunol 4:175, 1964
5. Fishman M: Antibody formation in vitro. J Exp Med 114:837, 1961
6. Gowans, JL, McGregor DD: The immunological activities of lymphocytes. Prog Allergy 9:1, 1965
7. Movat HZ, Fernando MVP: The fine structure of lymphoid tissue during antibody formation. Exp Mol Pathol 4:155, 1965
8. Schwartz RS, Ryder RJW, Gottlieb BAA: Macrophages and antibody synthesis. Prog Allergy 14:81, 1970
9. Sell S, Asofsky R: Lymphocytes and immunoglobulins. Prog Allergy 12:86, 1968
10. Spicer SS, Hardin JH: Ultrastructure, cytochemistry, and function of neutrophil leukocyte granules. Lab Invest 20:488, 1969
11. Stuart AE: The Reticuloendothelial System. Edinburgh, Livingstone, 1970
12. Suter, E, Ramseier H: Cellular reactions in infection. Adv Immunol 4:117, 1964
13. Turk JL, Oort J: Germinal center activity in relation to delayed hypersensitivity. In Germinal Centers in Immune Responses. Cottier H, Odortchenko N, Schindler R, Congdon CC (eds). New York, Springer, 1967
14. Yoffey JM, Courtice FC: Lymphatics Lymph and the Lymphomyeloid Complex. New York, Academic Press, 1970

3

Lymphoid Tissue

The introduction of an immunogen into a responsive individual leads to extensive changes in the responding tissue. This response usually takes place in organs containing large numbers of the involved cells, i.e., lymphocytes, macrophages and plasma cells. These cells are known as lymphoid cells; organs containing them are called lymphoid organs (11). Other tissue sites, such as local areas of inflammation containing lymphoid cells, may also take part in an immune response.

THE LYMPHOID SYSTEM

Lymphoid tissue is found in the lymph nodes, the spleen, the thymus and certain organs associated with the gastrointestinal system (tonsils, Peyer's patches, appendix). The thymus and the gastrointestinal lymphoid organs are designated the central lymphoid system. The roles of these organs in the development of immune maturity (ontogeny) are presented in Chapter 18. The lymph nodes and the spleen are called peripheral lymphoid organs.

STRUCTURE OF LYMPHOID ORGANS

All lymphoid organs have similarities in structure. The organ is encapsulated by collagenous connective tissue and divided into lobules by strands of connective tissue (trabeculae). It is supplied with blood by a single artery and is drained by both veins and lymphatics. The artery enters through an indentation in the capsule (the hilus) and extends into the organ in the trabeculae. Smaller arteries and arterioles extend from the trabeculae into the parenchyma of the organ. Venous drainage begins in the parenchyma and flows out through veins in the trabeculae to the major draining vein, which exits at the hilus. The arrangement of the lymphatic drainage both to the organ (afferent) and from the organ (efferent) is different for each set of organs and will be described separately. The parenchyma is divided into two areas—the cortex and the medulla. The cortex lies between the capsule and the medulla and contains tightly packed lymphoid cells. This is the area of proliferation of lymphoid cells. Lymphoid

21

cell proliferation may occur either in bands of tightly packed lymphoid cells or in ball-like clusters called germinal centers. The appearance of the cortex depends upon immune responses to antigens and will be discussed after descriptions of the normal organs. The medulla occupies the center of the organ and contains a supporting structure of reticular phagocytic cells. The medulla generally appears to function as a collecting and draining area for cells or products of cells produced in the cortex.

Lymph Nodes (Fig. 3–1)

Lymph nodes are located in areas of lymphatic drainage in the body and serve as filters for tissue fluid in lymphatic vessels. The lymphatic vessels are a network of thin-walled vascular channels that serve to collect fluid and cells which have escaped from the circulation and to channel any foreign materials gaining access into the body and return them, via the lymph node filter system, to the circulation. The lymph node cortex contains tightly packed nodules of lymphocytes (primary follicles), more loosely arranged nodules surrounded by a rim of tightly packed lymphoid cells (secondary follicles or germinal centers), and strips of tightly packed lymphoid cells lying between germinal centers (paracortical areas) which extend irregularly into the medulla. Thymectomy of neonatal animals leads to a depletion of lymphoid cells in the paracortical zones, therefore the paracortical zone has become known as a thymus dependent area (3,4). On the other hand, depletion of the primary follicles and germinal centers occurs in birds upon removal of an organ known as the Bursa of Fabricius. The follicular areas are therefore termed *Bursa dependent* (4). The interrelationship of various lymphoid organs during development is discussed in detail in Chapter 18. The medulla consists of a network of draining sinusoids formed by a meshwork of phagocytic reticular cells. Afferent lymphatic vessels drain into a subcortical sinus; lymphatic sinusoids drain through the cortex around follicles and paracortical areas into the extensive sinusoidal network of the medulla. The medullary sinuses drain into efferent lymphatics, which empty into the main efferent lymphatic vessel, which exits through the hilus. The arteries divide into capillaries in the cortex. These capillaries drain into veins in the cortex, so that the cortex is supplied with circulating blood in a conventional manner, while the medulla is mainly supplied with lymph fluid by afferent and efferent lymphatics.

Spleen (Fig. 3–2)

The spleen is comprised primarily of sinusoids. The splenic lymphoid follicles are not demarcated into a cortical area as in the lymph node, but are scattered through the sinusoids. The lymphoid follicles are called white pulp, and the sinusoidal area, which usually contains large numbers of red blood cells, is called red pulp because of the color seen on gross examination of the freshly cut organ. The lymphoid follicles may be primary or secondary. A collection of densely packed lymphocytes surrounding the central arteriole corresponds to the paracortical zone of the lymph node. The spleen contains no lymphatic vessels. Blood enters through arteries running in trabeculae. The arteries branch and extend into the red pulp.

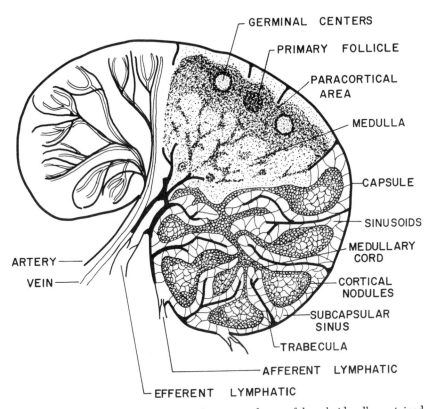

GERMINAL CENTERS

PRIMARY FOLLICLE

PARACORTICAL AREA

MEDULLA

CAPSULE

SINUSOIDS

MEDULLARY CORD

ARTERY

VEIN

CORTICAL NODULES

SUBCAPSULAR SINUS

TRABECULA

AFFERENT LYMPHATIC

EFFERENT LYMPHATIC

Fig. 3–1. Normal lymph node. Nodes are made up of lymphoid cells contained in meshwork of reticular fibers surrounded by connective tissue capsule. Most lymph nodes are bean shaped, with an indented area known as hilus. Cortex (outer layer) contains densely packed lymphoid cells and includes germinal centers responsible for production of antibody-synthesizing plasma cells and paracortical areas where lymphocytes are produced. Medulla (central area) consists of sinusoidal channels maintained by reticular cells. Columns of lymphoid cells (medullary cords) extend into medulla from cortex, and other lymphoid cells are found both in medullary sinusoids and between sinusoids in areas containing reticular macrophages (for further details of sinusoidal structure, see Fig. 3–2). Afferent lymphatics drain through cortex around germinal centers into medullary sinusoids. Medullary sinusoids drain into efferent lymphatics and are collected by main efferent lymphatic which drains from hilus. Main artery divides into capillaries supplying cortex. These capillaries drain into veins which follow trabeculae and exit at hilus. (Modified from Bloom W, Fawcett DW: A Textbook of Histology. 9th ed. Philadelphia, Saunders, 1969)

The white pulp is positioned as a sleeve around the smaller arterioles which continue out of the white pulp and supply the red pulp either by direct connections with the medullary sinusoids or by drainage into the intersinusoidal reticular tissue. The sinusoids have a basic structure similar to that of the lymph node, but drain into branches of the splenic vein and *not* into efferent lymphatics. There are four types of phagocytic macrophage-like cells in the spleen: 1) cells lying free in the sinusoids,

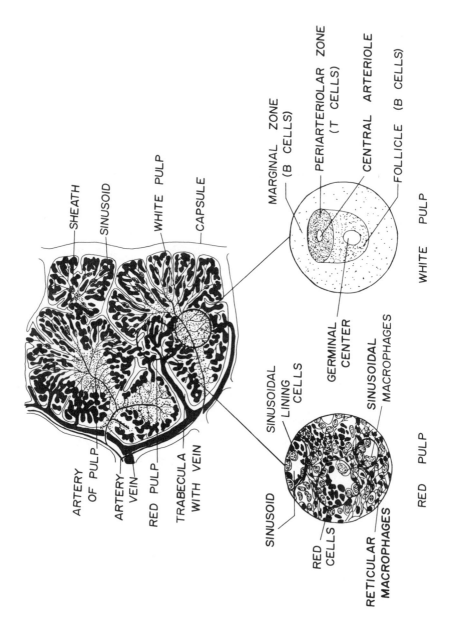

SHEATH

SINUSOID

WHITE PULP

CAPSULE

ARTERY OF PULP

ARTERY VEIN

RED PULP

TRABECULA WITH VEIN

MARGINAL ZONE (B CELLS)

PERIARTERIOLAR ZONE (T CELLS)

CENTRAL ARTERIOLE

FOLLICLE (B CELLS)

GERMINAL CENTER

SINUSOIDAL MACROPHAGES

WHITE PULP

SINUSOIDAL LINING CELLS

SINUSOID

RED CELLS

RETICULAR MACROPHAGES

RED PULP

2) fixed sinusoid-lining cells, 3) reticular cells lying between sinusoids which form a meshwork of reticular fibers, and 4) cells found in areas surrounding the white pulp and sometimes within the white pulp.

Thymus (Fig. 3–3)

The thymus contains a cortical area of packed lymphoid cells, a medulla, a fibrous capsule, prominent trabeculae which divide the organ into lobules, and a hilus with entering arteries and draining veins and lymphatics (6,7). The thymus differs from the lymph nodes and the spleen in three important features: 1) Normally, there are no lymphoid follicles. The cortex consists of packed small lymphocytes and many proliferating cells in the lymphocyte series. 2) The reticular stroma is mainly of epithelial origin (third brachial pouch), not mesodermal, although some mesodermal reticular cells may be present. The medulla contains remnants of epithelial islands which appear as concentric rings of eosinophilic tissue known as Hassall's corpuscles. 3) The medulla does not contain sinusoids but is an epithelial reticular network in which are found large numbers of lymphocytes. The cortex can be differentiated from the medulla because the lymphocytes are much more closely packed in the cortex. There are no afferent lymphatics in the thymus. The drainage of the thymus has not been well characterized; most drainage appears to occur through the vein, although significant lymphatic drainage has been claimed by some observers. The cortex is an area of active proliferation, with complete turnover of cells believed to occur every 3 or 4 days. The primary function of the normal adult thymus is the production of thymic lymphocytes (thymocytes). However only about 1% of the lymphocytes produced ever leaves the thymus, the other 99% are destroyed locally (3,4). The thymus is important for the development of immune resistance of the cellular type (see Chapter 20) and for normal maturation of the paracortical areas of the lymph node and of the periarteriolar collection of lymphocytes in the white pulp of the spleen. This maturation may be mediated by a soluble factor produced by the thymus (thymosin) (see page 38).

Fig. 3–2. Normal splenic lobule. Spleen is composed of network of sinusoidal channels filled mainly with red blood cells (red pulp). Cords of lymphoid cells are located around small arteries (white pulp). Germinal centers may form in white pulp and are associated with production of plasma cells. Lymphocytes are also produced in white pulp in areas around or away from germinal centers. There are no lymphatic vessels. Blood enters through arteries which may empty directly into splenic sinusoids or into reticular area between sinusoids. Sinusoids are drained by veins which exit via trabecular veins to large vein which leaves spleen at hilus. A zone of densely packed lymphocytes surrounding central arteriole contain T cells (thymus dependent area) while B cells are found surrounding the germinal center (1). (Modified from Bloom W, Fawcett DW: A Textbook of Histology. 9th ed. Philadelphia, Saunders, 1969, also Goldschneider I, McGregor DD: J Exp Med 127:155, 1968)

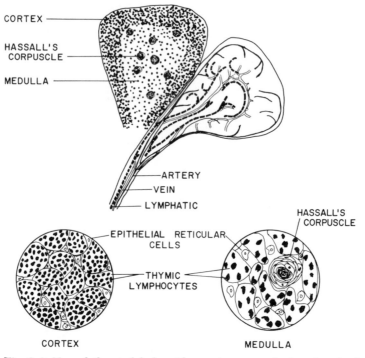

CORTEX

HASSALL'S
CORPUSCLE

MEDULLA

ARTERY
VEIN
LYMPHATIC

HASSALL'S
CORPUSCLE

EPITHELIAL RETICULAR
CELLS

THYMIC
LYMPHOCYTES

CORTEX

MEDULLA

Fig. 3–3. Normal thymic lobule. Thymus is composed of meshwork of epithelial reticular cells with densely packed lymphocytes and lymphocyte precursors in cortex and less densely packed lymphocytes in medulla. Plasma cells are rarely identifiable; cortex normally contains no germinal centers. Medulla contains remnants of epithelial islands (Hassall's corpuscles), which appear as laminated circular whirls sometimes surrounding dense central areas. Cortex is supplied by branches of thymic artery, drained by branches of thymic vein. Drainage of medulla is not well defined, but appears to occur by both veins and lymphatics. There are no sinusoids or afferent lymphatics.

Gastrointestinal Lymphoid Tissue

Local collections of lymphoid tissue underlie the submucosa of many areas of the gastrointestinal tract. In some areas the collections become large enough to be identified individually. These areas are the tonsils (lingual, palatine, pharyngeal, and tubal; (Fig. 3–4); the appendix (Fig. 3–5); and Peyer's patches (Fig. 3–6). The lymphoid tissue of these organs contains mainly lymphoid follicles (primary or secondary), with little or no medullary element; however, careful evaluation of the structure of the Peyer's patches of experimental animals reveals thymus-dependent interfollicular areas and domes of lymphoid tissue that might serve as a site for lymphoid cell (see Chapter 4) cooperation (Fig. 3–7). The overlying mucosa is characteristic of each location; lingual tonsil, stratified squamous; palatine tonsil, stratified squamous; pharyngeal tonsil, pseudostratified columnar; tubal tonsil, pseudostratified columnar; appendix, columnar goblet cells (crypts of Lieberkühn); Peyer's patches, intestinal villi. The tonsils form a ring

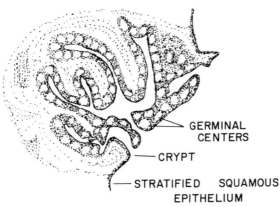

GERMINAL
CENTERS

CRYPT

STRATIFIED SQUAMOUS
EPITHELIUM

Fig. 3–4. Tonsil. Tonsils are composed of closely packed layer of germinal centers underlying epithelium. There are no afferent lymphatics, and efferent lymphatics are poorly defined. Overlying epithelium is characteristic of area where tonsil is located (see Gastrointestinal Lymphoid Tissue). Lymphoid cells produced by tonsil appear within overlying epithelium and are believed to emigrate into crypts. (Modified from Bloom W, Fawcett DW: A Textbook of Histology. 9th ed. Philadelphia, Saunders, 1969)

Fig. 3–5. Appendix. Appendicular lymphoid tissue is composed of a layer of germinal centers underlying mucosa. Mucosa consists of crypts of goblet cells characteristic of this part of intestine. Many cells produced in appendix appear to be discharged into lumen. Afferent lymphatics drain around germinal centers from origin in crypts; efferent lymphatics drain from germinal centers. (Modified from Bloom W, Fawcett DW: A Textbook of Histology. 9th ed. Philadelphia, Saunders, 1969)

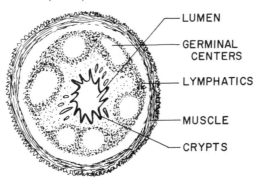

LUMEN

GERMINAL
CENTERS

LYMPHATICS

MUSCLE

CRYPTS

of lymphatic tissue at the base of the tongue and pharynx (Waldeyer's tonsillar ring). The gastrointestinal lymphoid tissue is believed necessary for development of the antibody-forming organs (germinal centers, plasma cells; see Chapter 20). It is thought to play a primary role in immunity to infectious agents entering the body through the mouth and has been shown to synthesize more immunoglobulin A (present in gastrointestinal secretions) than the peripheral lymph nodes. The basic structure is that of a focal collection of germinal centers (cortex). Three different areas

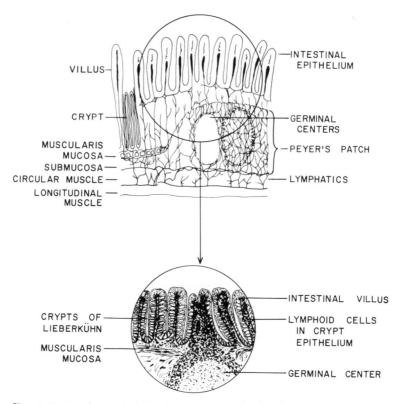

VILLUS

INTESTINAL EPITHELIUM

CRYPT

GERMINAL CENTERS

MUSCULARIS MUCOSA

PEYER'S PATCH

SUBMUCOSA
CIRCULAR MUSCLE
LONGITUDINAL MUSCLE

LYMPHATICS

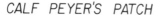

INTESTINAL VILLUS

CRYPTS OF LIEBERKÜHN

LYMPHOID CELLS IN CRYPT EPITHELIUM

MUSCULARIS MUCOSA

GERMINAL CENTER

Fig. 3–6. Peyer's patch. Peyer's patches are focal collections of germinal centers found mainly in submucosa of ileum. Afferent lymphatics drain from intestinal villi, around germinal centers, and into efferent lymphatics which drain into thoracic duct. Lymphoid cells can be seen extending through overlying mucosa and are believed to enter intestinal lumen. (Modified from Bloom W, Fawcett DW: A Textbook of Histology. 9th ed. Philadelphia, Saunders, 1969)

Fig. 3–7. Morphology of Peyer's patches. Three basic elements of lymphoid tissue are present in the Peyer's patches of experimental animals as illustrated here for the calf: the dome, the follicle and the interfollicular thymus dependent areas. The dome–follicle complex contains mainly B cells. Domes appear early in life and are believed to be the site of origin of B cells; the follicles serve as an "amplification site" for proliferation of B cells. It is also possible that some T cells migrate from the thymus dependent areas to the lateral margins of the dome, thus providing an anatomic site for T–B cell cooperation. (From Waksman BH: J Immunol 111:878, 1973)

CALF PEYER'S PATCH

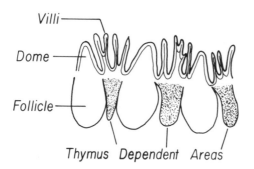

Villi

Dome

Follicle

Thymus Dependent Areas

of lymphoid tissues may be identified in Peyer's patches (Fig. 3–7): the dome, the follicle and the thymus-dependent area (9), so that the gastrointestinal lymphoid tissue contains the same morphologic elements as lymph node and spleen. There is production of both immunoglobulin antibody and lymphoid cells by the gastrointestinal lymphoid tissue. These are delivered to the systemic circulation by draining lymphatics, but many of the proteins and cells produced are secreted into the gastrointestinal lumen.

Bone Marrow

The stem cells of all the blood elements are located in the bone marrow, including the precursors of lymphoid cells. These stem cells and their progeny are organized into islands of cells located in fatty tissue (Fig. 3–8). In the bone marrow the cell types are admixed so that precursors of red blood cells (erythroblasts), macrophages, platelets (megakaryocytes), polymorphonuclear leukocytes (myeloblasts) and lymphocytes (lymphoblasts) may be seen in one microscopic field. It is impossible to differentiate the stem cells for one cell line from those of another cell line by morphologic appearance alone. However, stem cells are usually surrounded by more mature cells of the same cell line so that a given stem cell may be identified by the company it keeps. In normal bone marrow the myelocytic series makes up approximately 60% of the cellular elements, the erythrocytic, 20–30%. Lymphocytes, monocytes, reticular cells, plasma cells and megakaryocytes constitute only 10–20%. Lymphocytes make up 5–15% of the cells of the normal adult marrow and 20–30% of a child's marrow. Normally, lymphocytes are mixed diffusely with the other cellular elements, but focal collections of lymphocytes may be seen in the marrow of elderly individuals. Plasma cells normally constitute less than 1% of the marrow cells. Circulating blood enters via arteries which enter through the periostium and pass through the compact bone in small canals. The marrow is drained by venous sinuses that collect mature blood elements for distribution into the peripheral blood. The mechanism whereby the mature cells escape into the bloodstream while immature ones are held back is not known.

Bone marrow lymphocytes are not usually able to react with, or respond to, antigen. Marrow lymphocytes circulate from the marrow to other lymphoid organs and differentiate into lymphocytes capable of immune function (for more details of the ontogeny of immune cells, see Chapter 19). Thus, the marrow is believed to be the organ of origin of the stem cells of the immune system. Cells originating in the marrow populate the thymus where they may differeniate into T cells while marrow cells which populate the gastrointestinal lymphoid tissue differentiate into B cells (see Chapter 4 for a description of T and B cells). An intriguing observation is that in the human, naturally occurring tumors of plasma cells that produce immunoglobulin (multiple myeloma) essentially always arise in the bone marrow; extramedullary multiple myeloma is exceedingly rare. This suggests that the precursors of plasma cells with malignant potential are located exclusively in the marrow.

In vitro studies of bone marrow after fractionation of the cells suggest that some immunologically reactive cells may be present in the bone marrow and are able to respond to antigenic stimulation. The contribution

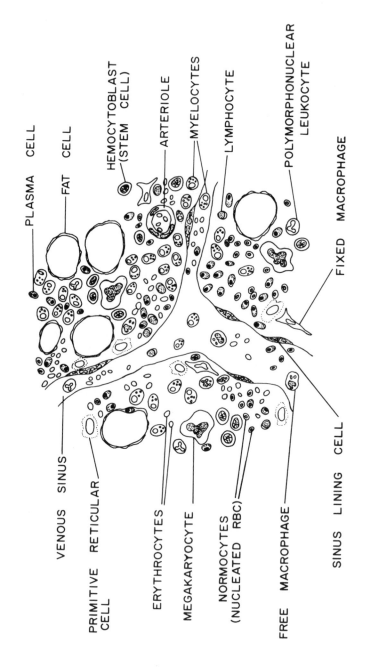

PLASMA CELL

FAT CELL

HEMOCYTOBLAST (STEM CELL)

ARTERIOLE

MYELOCYTES

LYMPHOCYTE

POLYMORPHONUCLEAR LEUKOCYTE

FIXED MACROPHAGE

VENOUS SINUS

PRIMITIVE RETICULAR CELL

ERYTHROCYTES

MEGAKARYOCYTE

NORMOCYTES (NUCLEATED RBC)

FREE MACROPHAGE

SINUS LINING CELL

of bone marrow cells to the immune response of the normal whole animal remains undefined.

EFFECT OF ANTIGENS UPON LYMPHOID TISSUE

The normal structure of the lymphoid organs depends upon antigenic contact. In germ-free animals, which have little antigenic contact, the lymphoid organs contain fewer primary or secondary follicles and have sparse paracortical areas; the serum immunoglobulin levels may be only one-tenth those of conventional animals (6). The medullary areas contain sinusoids relatively depleted of mononuclear cells, with both sinusoidal and intersinusoidal areas filled with red blood cells or lymph fluid. If antigen is introduced, there is a marked increase in cortical follicles and paracortical tissue, and the serum immunoglobulin may increase to almost normal levels (6).

The morphologic changes that occur in lymphoid tissue depend upon the type of immune response that is stimulated. Two general types of immune responses with characteristic changes in lymphoid tissue have been recognized: stimulation of humoral antibody or of specifically sensitized cells (delayed hypersensitivity).

ANTIBODY PRODUCTION

A diagrammatic representation of the immune response leading to antibody formation is shown in Figure 3–9. Upon contact with a responsive individual, both radiolabeled antigens that stimulate the production of circulating antibody, as well as nonantigens, are taken up mostly by the phagocytic cells (macrophages) of the medullary areas of lymph nodes and spleen, but also by dendritic macrophages in the cortex or white pulp (5). Dendritic macrophages are elongated, spindle-shaped cells with cytoplasmic extensions that are in close association with the lymphocytes of the cortex or white pulp (10). Localization of labeled antigen by dendritic macrophages does not necessarily determine that an immune response will occur, as nonantigens may undergo similar localization in certain circumstances. Within a few days after immunization, progenitors of antibody-forming cells are released into the circulation and are disseminated to other lymph nodes and the spleen. Lymphoid follicles form around the dendritic macrophages containing the antigen.

The precursors of antibody-forming cells possess cell surface antibody receptors which permit them to recognize and respond to the stimulating

Fig. 3–8. Bone marrow. The bone marrow consists of an admixture of cells producing blood cells, fat cells, supporting stroma and vessels. Blood enters through afferent arterioles and exits, enriched in blood cells, from veins draining marrow sinuses. Most of the blood-forming cell lines are myelocytic (polymorphonuclear leukocytes) and erythrocytic (red blood cells). These cell types tend to be organized into small groups. Scattered megakaryocytes, monocytes, reticular cells, lymphocytes and plasma cells are also present.

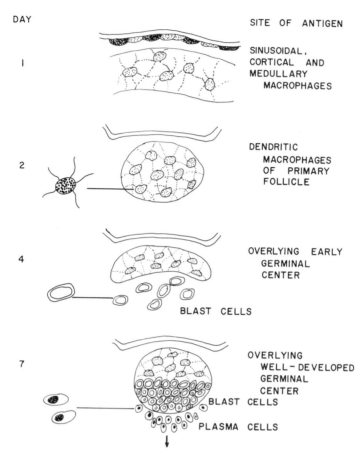

DAY

SITE OF ANTIGEN

1

SINUSOIDAL,
CORTICAL AND
MEDULLARY
    MACROPHAGES

2

DENDRITIC
    MACROPHAGES
    OF PRIMARY
    FOLLICLE

4

OVERLYING EARLY
    GERMINAL
    CENTER

BLAST CELLS

7

OVERLYING
    WELL-DEVELOPED
    GERMINAL
    CENTER
BLAST CELLS
PLASMA CELLS

Fig. 3–9. Germinal center formation. Localization of labeled antigen in lymph node following immunization demonstrates distribution in both medullary and cortical macrophages. Antigen first appears in lining cells of subcortical sinus. On day 2, dendritic macrophages are heavily labeled. They are scattered through cortex, but tend to occur in primary follicles. By day 4, blast cells can be identified underlying the antigen-containing cells. These cells increase in number until typical germinal center (secondary follicle) is formed, with antigen-containing cells overlying area of active proliferation in crescent-shaped arc. By day 7, plasma cells appear deep to germinal center. These cells then migrate into medullary cords. [Modified from Nossal GJV, et al. (5)]

antigen (see below). The role of the macrophage in the induction of antibody formation is the subject of much debate (see Chapter 4). Cell proliferation (2) leads to development of a nodule of cells that pushes the antigen-containing macrophages to the periphery overlying the center of proliferation (5).

Five to seven days after immunization, plasma cells appear below the germinal center and migrate into the medullary cords where they produce and secrete immunoglobulin antibody which is released into the medullary sinusoids. Plasma cells may be observed in large numbers in the adjacent medullary cords or red pulp for at least 10 weeks after immunization (5). The dendrite macrophages do not make antibody, but interact with cells in the lymphoid series (immunologically competent cells) that are capable of responding (3). The function of different lymphoid cells in the induction of immune responses is discussed in Chapter 4.

DELAYED HYPERSENSITIVITY

The morphologic changes occurring in a lymph node during the development of specifically sensitized cells (delayed hypersensitivity) are different from those occurring during the production of circulating antibody (Fig. 3–10). During the development of delayed hypersensitivity, the morphologic changes in the lymph node occur not in the follicles or germinal centers, but in the other areas of the lymph node cortex containing tightly packed lymphocytes (the paracortical area) (8). Here, a few days after contact

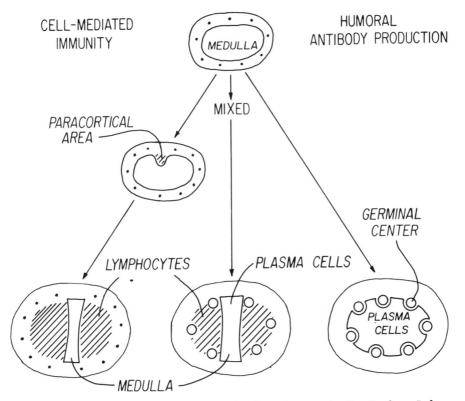

Fig. 3–10. Morphologic response of lymph node to antigenic stimulus. Induction of essentially pure delayed hypersensitivity reaction leads to proliferation of lymphocytes in paracortical zone. Induction of pure humoral antibody formation results in germinal center formation and appearance of plasma cells in medullary cords. Immunization with most antigens produces both changes with enlargement of paracortical zones and production of germinal centers. [Modified from Turk JL, Oort J (8)]

with an antigen, large pyroninophilic immature blast cells and mitotic figures (dividing cells) may be recognized. A temporary increase in the number of small lymphocytes occurs in this area 2–5 days after immunization. It is likely that these are the specifically sensitized cells that are rapidly released into the draining lymph and disseminated throughout the body.

It is not clear how antigen is recognized during the development of delayed sensitivity. There is evidence that competent lymphocytes possess antibody-like receptor mechanisms that react with antigenic determinants (7). This recognition may actually occur at a site distant from the lymph node where the sensitizing antigen is located, as in the skin. The reacting lymphocyte returns to the lymph node, lodges in the paracortical area, and undergoes rapid replication resulting in the formation of large numbers of sensitized cells that can now recognize and react with the sensitizing antigen.

REFERENCES

1. Goldschneider I, McGregor DD: Anatomical distribution of T and B lymphocytes in the rat. Development of lymphocyte specific antisera. J Exp Med 138:1433–1465, 1973
2. Makinodan T, Albright JF: Proliferative and differentiative manifestations of cellular immune potential. Prog Allergy 10:1, 1967
3. Metcalf D: The thymus: Its role in immune responses, leukemia development, and carcinogenesis. In Rentchnick P (ed). Recent Results in Cancer Research. Vol. 5. New York, Springer, 1966
4. Miller, JRAP, Osoba D: Current concepts of the immunological function of the thymus. Physiol Rev 47:437, 1967
5. Nossal GJV, Ada GL, Austin CM: Antigens in immunity. IV Cellular localization of ¹²⁵I-labeled flagella in lymph nodes. Aust J Exp Biol Med Sci 42:311, 1964
6. Sell S: Development of restrictions in the expression of immunoglobulin specificities by lymphoid cells. Transplant Rev 5:19, 1970
7. Sell S, Asofsky R: Lymphocytes and immunoglobulins. Prog Allergy 12:86, 1968
8. Turk JL, Oort J: Germinal center activity in relation to delayed hypersensitivity. In Germinal Centers in Immune Responses. Cottier H, Odortchenko N, Schindler R, Congdon CC (eds). New York, Springer, 1967, p. 311
9. Waksman BH: The homing pattern of thymus-derived lymphocytes in calf and neonatal mouse Peyer's Patches. J Immunol 111:878, 1973
10. White RG: Functional recognition of immunologically competent cells by means of fluorescent antibody technique. In The Immunologically Competent Cell. Wolstenholme GEW, Knight J (eds). London, Churchill, 1963
11. Yoffey JM, Courtice FC: Lymphatics, Lymph and the Lymphomyeloid Complex. New York, Academic Press, 1970

4

The Immune Response

FUNCTIONAL POPULATIONS OF LYMPHOID CELLS

The function of different lymphoid cell types in the induction of immune responses has been the subject of extensive investigation, both in vivo and in vitro. At least three cell lines are required for maximal antibody production to most antigens—T cells, B cells and macrophages (17,22,62,84,90,94). (A simple presentation of this concept is provided in Fig. 4-1.) Experiments in mice demonstrate that mixtures of "thymus-derived cells" (T cells) and lymphoid cells from the bone marrow (B cells) are synergistic when tested for the ability to produce antibody in irradiated recipients [passive transfer (17,90)] or when stimulated in vitro (22,94). Both populations as well as macrophages are present in the spleen, as spleen cells alone yield optimal responses in vitro.

ORIGIN OF T CELLS AND B CELLS

T cells and B cells both arise from a common precursor stem cell in the bone marrow and develop in the thymus (T cells) and gastrointestinal lymphoid organs (B cells) respectively (see Chapter 19). In other lymphoid tissue most, if not all, of the lymphocytes present are committed to a given cell line due to maturation events. When lymphocytes are examined by conventional or electron microscopy, it is impossible to differentiate T cells from B cells. Cells with the morphologic features of lymphocytes may have the ability to become plasma cells, sensitized lymphocytes or macrophages (96). However, it is likely that any one lymphoid cell outside the bone marrow has the ability to differentiate into only one of these cell types, i.e., it is precommitted to becoming a T cell, a B cell or a macrophage, and is not multipotent.

T CELLS

The term *T cell* has been applied to the thymus-derived lymphocyte which originates in the thymus from stem cells arising in the bone marrow

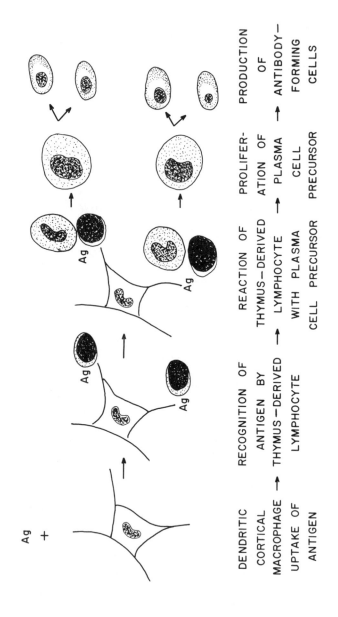

DENDRITIC   RECOGNITION OF   REACTION OF   PROLIFER-   PRODUCTION
CORTICAL   ANTIGEN BY   THYMUS—DERIVED   ATION OF   OF
MACROPHAGE → THYMUS—DERIVED → LYMPHOCYTE → PLASMA → ANTIBODY—
UPTAKE OF   LYMPHOCYTE   WITH PLASMA   CELL   FORMING
ANTIGEN   CELL PRECURSOR   PRECURSOR   CELLS

and circulating to the thymus from which point they are released into the circulation to localize in thymus-dependent areas of the other lymphoid organs (28,86,102). Passively transferred thymus-derived cells are identified either by chromosomal markers or by the presence of specific identifying antigens. The antigens used to identify thymus cells are basically strain-related differentiation markers (alloantigens) present only on T cells such as the thy antigen of mouse T cells. Anti-thy serum is produced by immunizing a strain of mouse that does not have the given thy antigen with thymus cells from mice that do (7,109). The presence of thy antigen on lymphocytes may be identified by immunofluorescent or immunoelectron microscopic labeling or by specific killing of lymphocytes by anti-thy sera. Another class of antigens specific for mouse thymus cells may be revealed by immunizing other species (such as rabbit) with mouse brain. The resulting anti-mouse brain serum will demonstrate specificity for mouse T cells (39). Using antithymus sera and cytotoxicity tests, T cell-associated antigen is found on approximately 90% of thymus lymphocytes but only on a subpopulation of lymphocytes (T cells) in peripheral tissues (109–111). Approximately 65–85% of lymph node cells and 30–50% of spleen cells contain thymus antigens. These percentages are greatly reduced in thymectomized or anti-lymphocyte treated mice (111).

Subpopulations of T Cells

The capacity of T cells to mediate many apparently diverse immune phenomena has been documented, and investigations of the mechanisms of these reactions have identified functional subpopulations of T cells. Antigenic stimulation induces T cell proliferation and also differentiation resulting in the production of large numbers of specifically sensitized lymphocytes that mediate delayed hypersensitivity reactions. More than one of these populations is required to obtain the full expression of T cell-mediated reactions (13,141). The mechanism of this T cell–T cell cooperation is poorly understood. In the mouse one population of T cells has a higher concentration of surface thy antigen, homes to the spleen and has a short half-life; a second population has a lower thy concentration, homes to the lymph node and has a longer half-life. It is believed that the first population (T_1) evolves into the second population (T_2) as a result of maturation (86,110). This maturation process may require antigen-specific stimulation to drive cells from T_1 to T_2. Some T cell populations not only

Fig. 4–1. Cellular interactions in induction of antibody formation. Antigen is localized by dendritic macrophage. Specific recognition of antigen requires second cell type, thymus-derived lymphocyte (T cell) which is produced in thymus and migrates to peripheral lymphoid tissue, where it comes in contact with antigen. Thymus-derived lymphocyte presents antigen in some way to precursor of plasma cell (B cell) which is then stimulated to divide and differentiate into antibody-producing plasma cell. For further discussion of T and B cell interaction, see Figs. 4–2 through 4–4.

do *not* enhance antibody production, but actually suppress immune responses. These "suppressor" T cells are believed to play an important role in the control of immune responses (59). (See Tolerance, Chapter 7)

Thymus Factors

T cell maturation may depend upon the presence of a soluble product of the thymus, i.e., thymosin (38), or thymic humoral factors (142). Animals rendered immunologically deficient following surgical removal of the thymus (see Chapter 19) may be restored to full immunologic function by transplantation of thymus tissue within a diffusion chamber that does not permit emigration of living cells (86,137). In addition, the lives of neonatally thymectomized female mice are prolonged in pregnancy, presumably due to the production by the fetal thymus glands of a thymic factor that crosses the placenta and functions to restore partially the immune capacity of the mothers (86,137). Extracts from the thymus provide conflicting results in regard to restoration of the immune capacity of thymectomized animals (38,86,137,142). However, some factors which are claimed to restore immune reactivity have been partially characterized (38,142). Thy negative cells from nude mice (149) can be converted from thy antigen negative to thy antigen positive upon incubation in vitro with thymus (65) extracts. Thus cells lacking thymus marker antigen may be converted to cells with thymus markers upon incubation with extracts of the thymus. These extracts do not themselves contain thy antigen, thereby eliminating simple cytophilic acquisition.

B CELLS

B cells arise in the bone marrow and differentiate in the bursa of Fabricius of birds or in the gastrointestinal tract or fetal liver of other animals (18a). Those in mice contain readily detectable surface immunoglobulin, while T cells either do not have surface immunoglobulin or it is present in amounts not easily detectable by immunofluorescence (43,44,92,108). When tissue sections are tested by fluorescent antiimmunoglobulin sera, 10–20% of lymph node, 25–35% of spleen and 1–2% of thymus cells of the mouse contain surface immunoglobulin (43,44,108,109,111), suggesting that the lymphoid cells in these organs that do not contain thy antigen have surface immunoglobulin (108). The differences in T cells and B cells as described in the mouse are presented in simplified form in Table 4–1. B cells are the precursors of plasma cells so that following antigenic stimulation they are induced both to proliferate and to differentiate into antibody-secreting plasma cells.

HUMAN T AND B CELLS

In the human, lymphoid cells believed to be analogous to mouse T cells form rosettes with normal sheep erythrocytes (55,93,150); B cells do not—but they will form rosettes with sheep cells coated with antibody and complement [EAC] (4,67,83) due to receptor sites for the third com-

TABLE 4-1
Some Properties of Mouse T and B Lymphocytes

	T cells	B cells
	Thymus	Gastrointestinal lymphoid tissue
Surface markers		
Ig	Scarce	Plentiful
Thy	+	−
TL[a]	+	−
Ly[b]	+	−
PC[b]	−	+
H₂[c]	+	+
Fc receptor[d]	−	+
C receptor[d]	−	+
Frequency (%)		
Blood	85	15
Lymph node	85	15
Spleen	65	35
Bone marrow	Rare	Many
Thymus	90	2–3
Functions		
Secretion of Ab	−	+
Helper effect	+	−
CMI[e] effector cell	+	±
Stimulator for MLR[f]	−	+
Reactor in MLR	+	−
Inactivation by		
X irradiation	+	++++
Corticosteroids	+	++
Antilymphocyte serum[g]	++++	+
Tissue distribution	Interfollicular (T dependent) zones	Follicles around germinal centers
Mitogen responses[h]		
Soluble con A	+	−
Insoluble con A	+	+
PHA	+	+
PWM	+	+
PPD	−	+
LPS	−	+

[a] *TL*: Thymus–leukemia antigen, present in some mouse strains, but absent in others (7). *Ly*, antigen present on thymus cells and circulating lymphocytes (T cells); specificities are strain-specific (7).

[b] *Pc* antigen is specific for plasma cell membrane antigen. (Niederhuber JE, Möller E: Antigenic markers on mouse lymphoid cells: The presence of MBLA on antibody-forming cells and antigen-building cells. Cell Immunol 3:559, 1972; Takahashi T, Old LJ, Boyse EA: Surface alloantigens of plasma cells. J Exp Med 131:1325, 1970; Takahashi T, Carswell EA, Thorebecke GJ: Surface antigens of immunocompetent cells. I. Effect of O and PC. 1. Alloantisera on the ability of spleen cells to transfer immune reaction. J Exp Med 132:1181, 1970)

[c] *H₂*: histocompatibility antigens (see page 228).

[d] *Fc*: The Fc fragment of immunoglobulin, C-complement (4,93). Basten A, Miller JFAP, Sprent J, Pye J: A receptor for antibody on lymphocytes. I. Method of detection and functional significance. J Exp Med 135:610, 1972; Möller G: Effect of B cell mitogen on lymphocyte subpopulations possessing C¹3 and Fc receptors. J Exp Med 139:969, 1974

[e] Cell-mediated immunity (see page 209).

[f] Mixed lymphocyte reaction (see page 228).

[g] Antilymphocytic serum may be made specific for T or B cells depending on the cell source of antigen used for immunization and the adsorptions used for removing crossreacting specificities.

[h] *Con A*–concanavalin A, *LPS*–bacterial lipopolysaccharide, *PHA*—phytohemagglutin, *PWM*—pokeweed mitogen, *PPD*–purified protein derivative. PPD is a B cell mitogen for normal mouse cells; but may be a T cell mitogen in mice immunized to react to PPD (91).

ponent of complement. A rosette is identified microscopically as a lymphocyte surrounded by red blood cells—usually one central nucleated lymphocyte with four or more red cells attached to its surface. In addition, some
human lymphocytes (thought to be B cells) contain surface immunoglobulin, as detected by immunofluorescence or by rosettes whose red cells are
coated with Ig but not complement (93). These techniques have been
used to characterize human lymphoid cell populations; 80–100% of human
thymus cells form rosettes with unsensitized sheep red blood cells and
no rosettes with EAC.

Spleen, peripheral blood and lymph nodes contain approximately 20–30%
B cells and 60–75% T cells by these criteria (114,129). Lymphomas may
consist of either T cells or B cells (14) whereas acute lymphoblastic leukemia cells are usually T cells (14,47,114,148a), and chronic lymphatic leukemia cells are B cells in most cases (4,47,150,151). The blood of patients
with a peculiar skin rash (erythroderma) may contain atypical lymphocytes.
This condition is known as Sézary's syndrome. The Sézary cell has characteristics of T lymphocytes (148a) and is usually larger than most peripheral
blood lymphocytes, has a convoluted nuclear structure and may be a type
of immature T cell. The number of T cells is decreased in some patients
with cancer (151) and in patients with lepromatous leprosy (33).

T AND B CELL RECEPTORS FOR ANTIGEN

Both T cells and B cells have cell surface receptors that recognize
and react with antigen. The receptor for the B cell is immunoglobulin
(92). The immunoglobulin product of the plasma cells produced as a result
of stimulation of B cells reflects the antigenic binding specificity of the
original B cell receptor (103). The receptor for the T cell has not yet
been clearly identified. While many studies have identified immunoglobulin
on T cells, the results of others have been negative in this regard (92).
However, both T cells and B cells may be activated through reaction with
cell surface receptors (91).

Specific immunoglobulin classes may be associated with lymphocytes.
IgD has been found on a high proportion of human lymphocytes (116);
monomeric IgM has been identified on the surface of mouse T cells, and
several different immunoglobulin classes have been identified on mouse
human B cells (92). A receptor for T cells may be B_2-microglobulin (93a).
B_2-microglobulin is an 11,000-MW protein fragment found on the surface
of lymphocytes in association with histocompatibility antigens. It has an
amino acid sequence similar to the Fc portion of IgGl (93a,135). Although
B_2M might serve as a recognition site for T and B cell interaction or
for some regulatory molecule, it is not likely to be a receptor for antigen
since antigen recognition is not associated with the Fc portion of IgG
molecules (see page 70). It is more likely that T cells of most species contain only that portion of the Ig molecule required for antigen recognition—
the V_H regions—and not the constant regions (see Chapter 5), making it difficult to identify immunoglobulins as such on the surface of the T cell.
However, the actual recognition unit of the antigen receptor of T and B
cells (123) is probably the same.

CELLULAR INTERACTIONS IN THE INDUCTION OF ANTIBODY FORMATION

The interaction of T cells, B cells and macrophages in the inductive phase of humoral antibody formation may be summarized as follows: The T cell recognizes immunogenic determinants, i.e., carrier molecules; B cells recognize smaller determinants, i.e., haptens (18,22,89,140), while the macrophage is an accessory cell required for maximal response. As discussed in Chapter 1, carriers are molecules that can both induce an immune response (immunogenic) and react with the products of the response (antigenic), while haptens cannot induce an immune response (see page 2). If haptens are coupled to immunogenic carriers, antibody that reacts with the hapten will be produced. Thus, haptens require carriers to be immunogenic. A population of T cells may be "carrier primed" by immunization of an animal with uncomplexed carrier (see Fig. 4–2). This effect was first noted in vivo when it was shown that rabbits primed with dinitrophenol (DNP) hapten coupled to bovine gamma globulin carrier (DNP-BGG) would produce a secondary antibody response to DNP only if the boosting antigen contained DNP coupled to the same carrier as used for immunization (101). When carrier-primed T cells are mixed with virgin B cells in vitro and exposed to the carrier complexed to hapten, the B cells produce a much more rapid and increased antibody production to the hapten than is produced by the virgin B cells in the absence of primed T cells. Antibody produced by mixtures of thymus-derived cells (T cells) and bone marrow-derived cells (B cells) is made by the B cells (18,22). The specificity of the T cell receptor is for the carrier and is similar to that required for the elicitation of delayed hypersensitivity reactions (35); that of the B cells is for the hapten and is essentially identical to that of circulating immunoglobulin antibody (18,103,140).

Mitchison's demonstration of cellular cooperation in induction of antibody formation and the carrier effect (89,90) is illustrated in Figs. 4–2 and 4–3. Two different populations of primed lymphoid cells (T and B cells) were transferred into irradiated recipients and antibody response of recipients of different cell combinations tested (90). One donor population consisted of spleen cells from an irradiated mouse injected with thymus cells from a syngeneic donor. These thymus-derived spleen cells were taken after immunization of the donor with bovine serum albumin (BSA) which will be the carrier in immunization of the third mouse. The second donor cell population consisted of spleen cells from mice immunized with NIP (4-hydroxy-5-iodo-3-nitrophenacetyl) hapten conjugated to chicken gamma globulin as carrier (NIP–CGG). Aliquots of each of these cell populations were treated with antitheta serum and complement to remove T-dependent cells.

Mixtures of cells with and without antithy serum treatment were transferred into the third mouse one day following its irradiation. One day after cell transfer, this third mouse was immunized with NIP–BSA. Maximum antibody response was obtained with T-derived BSA-primed cells and NIP–CGG primed spleen cells (B cells). This stimulation only occurred

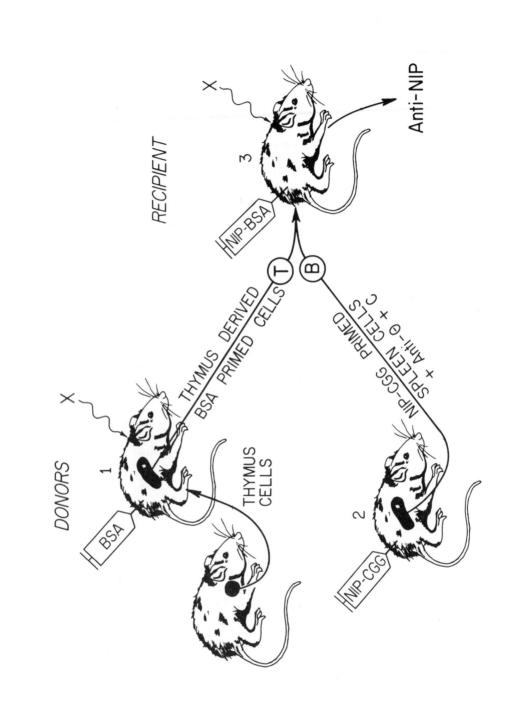

DONORS

RECIPIENT

BSA

1

THYMUS
CELLS

THYMUS DERIVED
BSA PRIMED CELLS

NIP-CGG
PRIMED
SPLEEN CELLS
+ Anti-θ + C

2

NIP-CGG

NIP-BSA

3

T

B

X

X

Anti-NIP

when NIP was coupled to BSA; uncoupled mixtures of NIP and BSA or NIP and CGG produced a very poor response. The contribution of NIP-CGG-primed spleen cells was not affected by treatment with antithy serum, and the contribution of BSA-primed T cells was abolished by this treatment. Using appropriate combinations of T and B cell donors, it was demonstrated by determining allotypic markers on the antibody product that the antibody formed was the product of the B cell. A schematic presentation of the results of this experiment is presented in Fig. 4–3.

MECHANISMS OF LYMPHOID CELL INTERACTIONS

Variations in the postulated ways that macrophages (M), thymus-derived cells (T) and bone marrow-derived cells (B) might interact in the inductive phase of antibody production are shown in Fig. 4–4. The reader should be advised that many of the postulated mechanisms of cellular cooperation in antibody induction are based on artificial in vitro systems and may play no part in events in vivo.

Four general classifications of cell interactions have been postulated:

I.   Macrophage processing of antigen for B cells
II. T cell–B cell interactions
III. Macrophage receptor transfer
IV. Macrophage–T cell–B cell interactions

I. Macrophage–B Cell Interactions

The theories that implicate macrophage processing of antigen do not necessarily require T cells. Additionally, those theories dealing with the transfer of specific information from macrophages to B cells imply that there may be no specific receptor on either. Macrophages may 1) concentrate or focus antigen so that a critical number of (? divalent) B cell receptors are stimulated (144), 2) produce a "super" antigen by attachment of part of its surface that serves to stimulate B cells that would not be stimulated by reaction with antigen alone (144), 3) transfer specific RNA with immunologic information after processing of antigen (32,40) and 4) transfer nonspecific RNA complexed with antigen that has the capacity to "turn on" B cells (40,119).

Fig. 4–2. **Mitchison's demonstration of T and B cell cooperation.** Mouse 1 is irradiated, given an injection of thymus cells from a syngeneic recipient and immunized with BSA carrier. The spleen of this mouse then contains BSA-primed T cells. Mouse 2 is immunized with NIP hapten complexed to CGG and the spleen cells treated with anti-thy (θ) + complement which kills T cells, producing NIP primed B cells. When mixtures of the BSA-primed T cells and NIP-primed B cells are transferred to mouse 3 after irradiation, immunization with NIP–BSA results in antibody production to NIP by the B cells which requires the function of the BSA carrier primed T cells (for details see text).

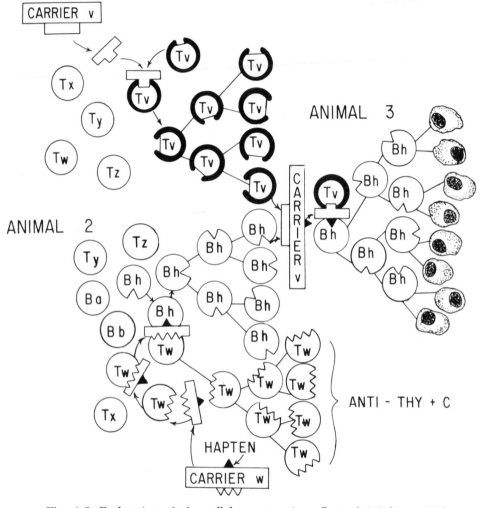

Fig. 4–3. Explanation of the cellular cooperation effect of Mitchison (90). Immunization of animal 1, the irradiated thymus reconstituted donor, with BSA (designated carrier V) results in a proliferation of thymus-derived cells that react with carrier V (carrier V-primed T cells, T_V). Immunization of animal 2 with hapten-carrier W conjugate produces a proliferation of T cells primed for carrier $W(T_W)$ and B cells specific for the hapten (Bh) through the action of T cells specific for carrier W. The T cells of animal 2 are removed by treatment of its spleen cells with anti-thy serum and complement. After irradiation animal 3 is given a mixture of B cells primed for the hapten and T cells primed for carrier V. Immunization of animal 3 with hapten coupled to carrier V results in an amplified antihapten antibody production due to the cooperation of B cells primed to hapten and T cells primed to carrier.

II. T Cell–B Cell Interactions (84,85)

The interaction of T and B cells might occur by 1) antigen concentration (89,90), the B cell being turned on by multiple interactions of antigen with divalent receptors, 2) a double signal from divalent Ag reaction and T–B cell surface interactions (8,60), 3) a double signal given by Ag receptor interaction and alteration in tertiary structure of the Ab–Ag complex in the presence of T and B cells, and 4) a double signal from Ag-receptor interaction and a thymus-derived mediator (TDM) (23). TDM may be produced by T cells after reaction with specific antigen or by an antigenically unrelated stimulus (allogenic effect) (58,117).

III. T Cell Receptor Transfer (29,31)

The transfer of receptors from T cells to macrophages upon contact with antigen and subsequent B cell stimulation by antigen on macrophages has been proposed. B cell stimulation under these circumstances may be by 1) antigen concentration by macrophages of T cell receptors containing antigen permitting reaction of the antigen with a critical number of B cell receptors, 2) a two-signal interaction produced by reaction of B cells with antigen on T cells and simultaneously on macrophages, 3) two signals arising from antigen reacting with the specific B cell receptor and the T cell receptor acquired by the macrophage, and 4) a combination of antigen reaction with B cell and a macrophage mediator. Reaction of the B cell receptor may be with antigen bound either to T cell receptor on the T cell or to T cell receptor acquired by the macrophage.

IV. Macrophage–T Cell–B Cell Interactions

For a maximal antibody response to some antigens in vitro, macrophages, T cells and B cells must be present (94,95). Macrophage–T cell–B cell interactions may take place with no specific antigen receptor on the macrophage but by nonspecific macrophage processing of, or focusing of, antigen and specific T cell–B cell receptor reactions (76,98). 1) The macrophage may focus antigen nonspecifically and serve to bring together T cells and B cells in the presence of concentrated antigens (144). Permissive signals may derive from B cell bound antigen concentrated by T cells or by the macrophage. 2) Reaction of B cell receptors with macrophage-concentrated antigen in the presence of T cells also reacting with macrophage-concentrated antigen may generate two signals, one from the reaction of the B cell receptor, the other from a T cell factor released after reaction of the T cell receptor (23). 3) The specific signal may come from reaction of the B cell receptor with T cell concentrated antigen and a macrophage factor (118) stimulated by reaction of the macrophage with antigen bound by the T cell. 4) Finally, the presence of antigen on macrophages and T and B cells may permit a variety of signals to be generated. Permissive B cell signals belong in general to specific signals generated by interaction of receptors with specific antigen and to nonspecific signals from macrophages, T cells or alterations in the form of the antigen by cell interactions (carrier generated signal).

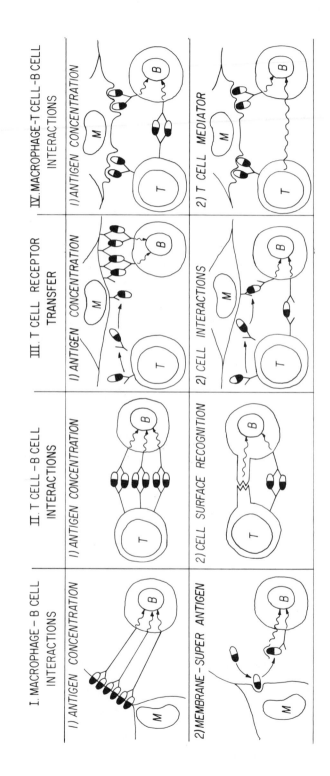

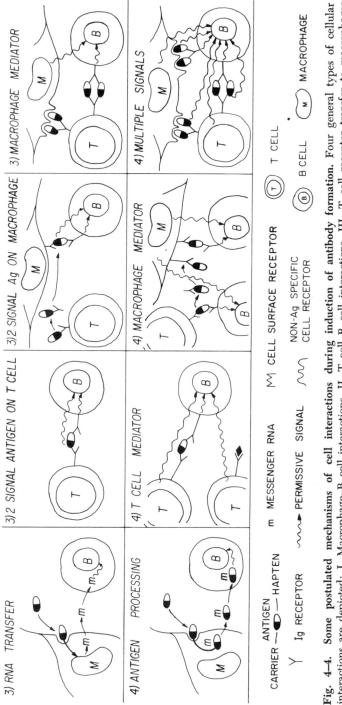

Fig. 4-4. Some postulated mechanisms of cell interactions during induction of antibody formation. Four general types of cellular interactions are depicted: I. Macrophage–B cell interactions. II. T cell–B cell interactions. III. T cell receptor transfer to macrophages with subsequent macrophage–B cell interactions, and IV. Macrophage–T cell–B cell interactions. Evidence for each of the above mechanisms has been obtained using in vitro culture systems. The most likely in vivo interactions include antigen processing of antigen by macrophages leading to T cell and B cell cooperation (see Fig. 4-1). The exact mechanism is not known, as indicated by the large number of possibilities postulated. (For details see text.)

The labels within the figure read:

3) RNA TRANSFER

4) ANTIGEN PROCESSING

3) 2 SIGNAL ANTIGEN ON T CELL

4) T CELL MEDIATOR

3) 2 SIGNAL Ag ON MACROPHAGE

4) MACROPHAGE MEDIATOR

3) MACROPHAGE MEDIATOR

4) MULTIPLE SIGNALS

CARRIER ━━ ANTIGEN   m MESSENGER RNA   ʍ CELL SURFACE RECEPTOR   Ⓣ T CELL

━━● HAPTEN   ∿∿➤ PERMISSIVE SIGNAL   NON-Ag SPECIFIC CELL RECEPTOR   Ⓑ B CELL

Y Ig RECEPTOR   ⬭ MACROPHAGE

The specific signal serves to select the B cell on the basis of its surface receptor. The nonspecific signal most likely serves to stimulate the cell to proliferation and differentiation. Subpopulations of B cells in different stages of differentiation may require different signals to maintain the response. In addition, different antigens may evoke different signals. The functional role of the above mechanisms during an in vivo increase response remain poorly defined.

There is evidence that in order for T and B cells to cooperate, they must be genetically compatible, indicating that the B cells may contain an "acceptor" molecule for a T cell product or for the T cell itself (60). In addition, the B cell must be genetically capable of responding to the carrier molecule even though the antibody produced by the B cell is to the hapten (61). This was found using the combination of two strains of mice, one a responder to the carrier and the other a nonresponder. The F_1 hybrid of these strains is a responder and is histocompatible with both parental strains (see Histocompatibility), which are responders to the hapten. The F_1 carrier-primed T cells were only able to cooperate with B cells from the parental strain responsive to the carrier for antihapten antibody formations. However, other evidence does not support the requirement of histocompatibility for T and B cell cooperation (79), and matching of Ir genes is believed to be required. A further discussion of the genetic control of immune responses and the role of gene products in cellular interactions is presented (see page 52).

In summary, the most likely cellular interactions in induction of antibody formation are as follows: An immunogen is first processed by a macrophage. The macrophage does not have a specific receptor for the antigen, although some macrophages may carry specific receptors transferred from T or B cells (cytophilic antibody). The macrophage in some way concentrates or processes the immunogen and facilitates T and B cell interactions. Although macrophage recognition of immunogen may not require specific recognition, there is an explicit requirement for compatibility between macrophages and T cells (113a,127a). B cells are activated by a combination of signals, one specific (reaction of B cells with antigen) and one antigenically nonspecific (cell surface interaction, macrophage or T cell mediation). Once the B cell is "turned on," it passes through a series of maturation divisions resulting in the appearance of antibody-producing plasma cells. Continued presence of antigen in some form is probably required to complete the proliferation–maturation phase.

B cells may be stimulated in the absence of macrophages or T cells through the use of "thymus-independent" antigens (30,91) or B cell mitogens (19). Thymus-independent antigens stimulate B cells directly, are usually polymeric (30) and bypass the two signal mechanisms required for thymus-dependent antigens. Such antigens may be able to provide stimulation of the specific antigenic receptor of the B cells as well as stimulate proliferation, i.e., be an immunogen and a mitogen (19,91).

LYMPHOID CELL INTERACTIONS IN VIVO

The anatomic locus of M, T and B cell interactions in vivo has not been clearly identified. The identification of T and B cells in lymphoid tissue using specific antisera indicates that T cells are absent in primary follicles but are present in secondary follicles (48). Thus, T and B cells may not be anatomically located in sites of immune responses but achieve juxtaposition during the induction of a primary antibody response. A special mechanism may exist to permit circulating T lymphocytes to lodge not only in thymus-dependent areas but also in a "thymus-dependent" corona around primary lymph node follicles or within splenic follicles (36,42,88,102), thus providing an anatomic focus for the interaction of T and B cells (18). Lymphoid cell interactions may occur dynamically during induction of a primary immune response as illustrated by the morphologic events that occur in the spleen leading to the production of the white pulp (Fig. 4–5). Labeled antigen localizes in dendritic macrophages (146) that lie along the penicilli arterioles. These macrophages migrate to the point of bifurcation of the arteriole where other lymphoid cells accumulate, leading to the production of a "germinal center" (147). By

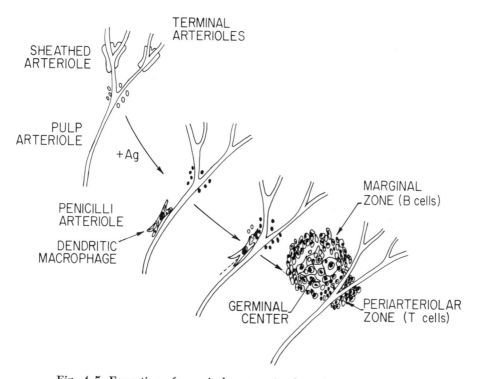

Fig. 4–5. Formation of germinal centers in the splenic white pulp following immunization. Penicilli arterioles of the spleen may be divided into three segments: the pulp arteriole, the sheathed arteriole and terminal arteriole. Injected antigen is taken up by dendritic macrophages located adjacent to penicilli arterioles and germinal centers formed at the bifurcation of the arteriole after migration of the periarteriolar macrophage. The antigen-localizing macrophage may serve as a nucleus about which T and B cells interact, resulting in formation of a mature germinal center. Antibody-secreting plasma cells are produced by proliferation and differentiation of B cells and may migrate into the cords of the splenic red pulp (129).

4 days after injection, antigen-containing macrophages may be observed in the periarteriolar sheath, and by 6 days in the germinal center. In fully developed splenic follicles several zones of lymphoid cells may be found (see Fig. 3–2) which correspond to the location of T and B cells. T cells are found in the periarteriolar zone while B cells are present in the marginal zone (36,37). It is not clear just how macrophages, T cells and B cells come together during the primary antibody response in vivo, but structures such as the white pulp of the spleen may permit cellular interactions to take place. The dendritic macrophages of lymphoid organs may act to bring together thymus-derived cells and bone marrow precursor cells, with proliferation of the bone marrow precursors resulting in the formation of germinal centers (99,146). In a mature lymph node germinal center, the dendritic macrophages are pushed into a cap overlying the germinal center while differentiating plasma cells migrate or are pushed downward into the medullary cords (99).

BLAST TRANSFORMATION

The addition of antigen to lymphocytes from sensitized individuals produces transformation of the lymphocytes in vitro (21,69,105), which results in enlargement of small lymphocytes into immature "blast" cells, with subsequent DNA synthesis and mitosis (78,145). Most of this antigen-specific transformation is thought to be due to stimulation of T cells (87,100), although B cells participate in antigen-induced stimulation in certain circumstances (26,63). This induction of proliferation in vitro is analogous to the effect of an immunogen in vivo (see page 31).

The addition of antisera to immunoglobulin or immunoglobulin allotypic specificities to lymphocytes of certain species may also lead to a marked stimulation of blast transformation (121,123). Antisera to rabbit immunoglobulins may stimulate as high as 90% of rabbit peripheral blood lymphocytes to transform into blast cells (121), which demonstrates that lymphocytes have surface immunoglobulin and that reaction of antibody with this surface Ig can activate the cells (214). However, only slight stimulation of the lymphocytes of other species is inducible with antiimmunoglobulin sera. It is not yet clear if the cells activated by anti-Ig in the rabbit are T cells or B cells or both, but it is probable they are T cells (126).

SPECIFICITY OF MITOGENIC AGENTS FOR T AND B CELLS

The addition of certain other agents (mitogens) to cultures of lymphocytes may also stimulate these cells to undergo division even though they are not sensitized to the agent (69,91). Many mitogens are derived from plants [i.e., lectins, such as concanavalin A from the Jack bean (Con A), phytohemagglutinin from the red kidney bean (PHA) and an extract of the root of pokeweed]; other sources include bacterial products (endotoxin, PPD of tubercle bacilli), metal ions and polynucleotides. Although mitogens may act as complete antigens if injected into an animal, the mechanism of their stimulation effect in vitro does not require antigenicity. Mitogens appear to bypass the mechanism whereby antigens activate a small subset of lymphocytes with specific antigen receptors because they stimulate a wide spectrum of antigen-sensitive cells.

The specificity of some of these mitogens is different for T cells than for B cells. B cells may only respond to Con A in insoluble form, while T cells respond to soluble Con A, but not to bacterial lipopolysaccharide (2,136) or PPD (97)–agents to which B cells respond well. Both T and B cells respond to phytohemagglutinin (2). Thus, the response of a given population of cells to these mitogens may be used to identify the type of cell (T or B) in the population, but caution must be taken in extrapolating results obtained with artificial cell populations to what may be expected with natural cell populations. Mitogen-activated B cells may differentiate and produce the immunoglobulins for which they are genetically programmed (2,91).

MECHANISM OF MITOGENIC ACTIVATION

Although the mechanism of mitogenic activation remains obscure, it is known that following mitogenic stimulation, surface receptors of some cells may be observed to "migrate" into a polar cap (106,139). This was thought to be the first step in mitogenic stimulation, but capping occurs on cells that are not stimulated to transform, and rabbit lymphocytes may be stimulated to divide without cap formation. The first event that occurs when antibodies to rabbit immunoglobulin are used to stimulate rabbit lymphocytes is endocytosis of surface immunoglobulin (73), and PHA induces endocytosis of PHA receptors on human peripheral blood lymphocytes. An almost immediate increase in membrane transport is observed in mitogen-stimulated cells (82,148) associated with an increased turnover of membrane phosphatidylinosital (75). Increased synthesis of other membrane components may be observed within 10–30 minutes of stimulation (112). Thus the initial event in stimulation almost certainly involves changes in the cell membrane, including a loss of the receptor by endocytosis or stripping, but the mechanism whereby these observed changes lead to the increased nucleic acid synthesis and mitosis is still unknown.

The role of cyclic nucleotides in lymphocyte stimulation has been studied in view of their role as a second messenger system for hormonally controlled cellular functions (56,113). Addition of mitogens leads to a decrease in cyclic AMP (cyclic 3′5′-Adenosine), and stimulation of lymphocytes can be significantly inhibited by agents which elevate intracellular cyclic AMP (81,130). On the other hand, the intracellular concentration of cyclic GMP (cyclic 3′5′-Guanosine) may rise 10- to 50-fold following mitogen stimulation (50). Therefore, cyclic cAMP may inhibit transformation while cyclic cGMP may be an active intracellular signal for induction of proliferation.

Whatever the sequence of stimulating events, the original stimulating mitogen must remain in contact with the reactive cells for an extended period before DNA synthesis begins. If the mitogen is removed prior to the initiation of DNA synthesis, the transformation process may be aborted and enlarging lymphocytes will revert back to small lymphocytes (122), therefore necessitating maintenance of the stimulating signal. It is unlikely, that transient events such as membrane surface modulation or cyclic nucleotide alterations are the irreversible signals initiating transformation. However, following these events protein synthesis, RNA synthesis and eventually DNA synthesis is stimulated, and the reactive cells undergo mitosis (16,125).

GENETIC CONTROL OF THE IMMUNE RESPONSE

One of the most active areas of immunologic investigation during the last few years has been in genetic control of certain immunologic responses (34,80).

GUINEA PIGS

The initial discovery that certain immune responses are under genetic control was made in the guinea pig as an inherited dominant trait appearing to be determined by a single autosomal gene (70). Approximately 40% of random-bred guinea pigs make an immune response to the antigenic complex of the hapten DNP conjugated to poly-L-lysine (H-PLL) (57). All of inbred strain 2 respond, while animals of inbred strain 13 respond very poorly. The responding animals demonstrate both antibody production and delayed hypersensitivity. The specificity of the response is directed to the carrier in the H-PLL system and the capacity to respond is referred to as due to the PLL gene (57). A number of experiments, including those involving passive transfer of cells from high responder to low responder animals (45), indicates that low responder animals do not have the full carrier recognition function required for induction of either antibody production or delayed hypersensitivity (34,80).

The presence of two separate genetic cistrons controlling responses to random copolymers of amino acids was demonstrated using inbred guinea pigs. A random copolymer of L-glutamic acid and L-alanine (GA) was immunogenic in strain 2 guinea pigs (but not in strain 13), whereas a copolymer of L-glutamic acid and L-tyrosine (GT) was immunogenic in strain 13 but not in strain 2. F_1 hybrids (2×13) responded to both GA and GT (5). Further observations demonstrated that the ability to respond was linked to the loci controlling the major histocompatibility locus; i.e., the cistrons responsible for immune responsiveness and those controlling the expression of tissue antigens responsible for tissue graft rejection (see Graft Rejection, p. 221) are located close together on the same chromosome (6). The close functional relationship of histocompatibility specificities and the immune response was further demonstrated by the finding that antisera to the histocompatibility antigens will inhibit a cellular reaction to antigens to which the response in controlled by the immune-response (Ir) gene (127). Among the possible explanations is the suggestion that the cellular receptor for antigen may be expressed on the cell surface of responsive cells in close approximation to the histocompatibility antigens.

MICE

Studies of the genetic control of immune responses in the mouse provide even more insight into the relationship of histocompatibility loci to Ir loci.

The H-2 Chromosomal Complex

The H-2 chromosomal area of the mouse includes genetic material controlling a complex set of genetic traits, the most important for the present discussion being the major transplantation antigens and the immune responses to a variety of antigens. The H-2 system can be studied in detail because of Snell's development of cogenic-resistant inbred strains, genetically identical, but differing only in H-2 (133). The H-2 complex controls the major histocompatibility antigens (H-2), the immune response (Ir), the concentrations of certain serum proteins (Ss-Slp) and the thymus leukemia antigen (Tla) (128). The genetic map for these properties is given in Fig. 4–6.

Histocompatibility H-2 Cistrons

The major histocompatibility antigens were once thought to be controlled by one locus, but are now known to be under the control of two loci, H-2K and H-2D. If tissue grafts are made between strains of mice that differ in these loci, a prompt immunologic rejection of the graft will take place (see Graft Rejection, p. 221). In addition, antibodies to the H-2 antigenic specificities will appear in the sera of animals that have rejected such grafts or have otherwise been immunized with H-2 antigens (134). These antigens, termed *serologically defined antigens*, are the antigens responsible for graft rejection and are controlled by the H-2D and H-2K loci (see Histocompatibility Matching, p. 229).

The Ir Region

The Ir region controls a number of immune responses and also may be divided into at least two loci. Ir-1A controls responses to synthetic polypeptides, i.e., antigens built on a backbone of poly-L-lysine (79). Ir-1B controls the response to lactic dehydrogenase and to certain myeloma protein antigens (128). The myeloma proteins of IgA and IgG (IgG2a) classes of mice contain different allotypic markers. When inbred strains are immunized for IgA allotypic markers, the immune responses are controlled by an Ir region different from Ir-1A (71). A subdivision of the Ir-1B locus

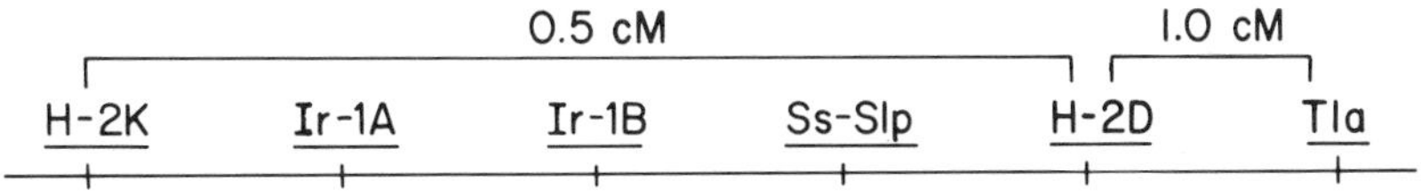

Fig. 4–6. Six genes are included in the H-2 complex: H-2K and H-2D, control cellular alloantigens responsible for histocompatibility; Tla, which controls thymus-specific antigens limited to normal thymocytes and certain leukemic cells; Ss-Slp, controlling the serum concentration of certain proteins; and Ir, the locus controlling the immune response. The length of the H-2 complex is defined as 1.5 centimorgans, based on the finding that recombination occurs between H-2K and Tla at a frequency of 1.5%. There could be a great many more loci in this complex that have not yet been identified (128).

is possible since responses to the IgG (IgG2a) allotypes were found to be genetically separate and distinct from responses to the IgA allotypes (72). Therefore, at least three, and most likely many more, Ir loci will be identified between the H-2K and Ss-Slp loci. Differences in the Ir region do not necessarily lead to skin graft rejection as do differences in the H-2 region (74).

Other immunologic responses involving lymphocyte reactivity are also controlled by the Ir region. Thus mixed lymphocyte reactions (3) (see p. 228) and graft-vs-host reactions (64) (see p. 236) are also controlled by the Ir region. The antigens responsible for these reactions have been grouped together as lymphocyte-activating determinants (20) while the H-2D and H-2K controlled antigens are termed serologically defined determinants (3). In addition, antisera to as many as 18 Ir region products have recently been produced (41). The antigens identified using such antisera are termed Ia antigens (51). A knowledge of the Ir region products is critical for advancing our understanding of immunologic phenomena.

Lymphocytes (T cells) sensitized to antigens on a target cell have the capacity to react with and kill target cells (see Cell-Mediated Immunity, p. 209). It has been reported that the ability of killer lymphocytes to be *induced* by exposure to target cell antigens depends upon differences in the Ir region products between the killer and target cell; however, *expression* of killing by sensitized lymphocytes requires differences in H-2D and/or H-2K (1). Thus a killer lymphocyte population may be activated by a mixed lymphocyte reaction induced by cells which differ at the Ir locus but which have identical H-2D and H-2K product. These sensitized cells will not kill the cells that induced the state of sensitization, but will kill target cells that differ in H-2D or H-2K (1). Further studies are needed to establish this interesting concept.

Cellular Defect in Low Responders

It is generally accepted that Ir function is selectively expressed by T cells, i.e., thymus-derived antigen-reactive lymphocytes, and not by B cells (34,79,80). Low responder animals to PLL will produce normal amounts of antibody to PLL if the PLL is complexed to an immunogenic carrier so that it functions as a hapten. Therefore, low responder animals have B cells that will recognize and produce antibody to PLL. In contrast, T cells of low responders require a separate carrier and are unable to process the PLL. The most elaborate data supporting the concept that the Ir locus is expressed in the T cell involves the use of tetraparental mice (79), which are created by fusing the eight-cell cleavage stage of two embryos of cogenic resistent strains of mice which differ only at the Ir and H loci. Some of these mice develop into immunologic chimeras, as demonstrated by sharing immunoglobulin allotypes of both the original strains used for fusion. When the immunoglobulin allotype of these mice was determined for the specific antibody to the test antigen, antibody of the low responder allotype was produced in a number of the animals. Thus, tetraparental mice made from these high responder and low responder mice contained two sets of T cells, high responder and low responder, and two sets of B cells—high responder making one immunoglobulin allotype and low responder making another. The finding of low responder allotypic markers in the antibody following immunization indicates that the low responder B cells were activated by the high responder T cells to produce the antibody to the test antigen, the T cells of the low responder being poorly functional (79). However, it must be pointed out at this time that these results are in conflict with those of Katz et al. (60) that state H-2 compatibility is required to obtain T–B cell cooperation (see page 48), as T–B cell cooperation is obtained by the tetraparental mice across an H-2 difference. A satisfactory explanation for this conflict is that it is the Ir products which must be the same, not the H-2 products.

The defect in T cell function in genetic low responder animals has not been clearly defined. A decrease in cells with receptors for antigen is not seen; low responder animals contain as many antigen-binding lymphocytes as high responder animals. T cells in low responder animals may not be able to carry out the function of cooperating with B cells after reacting with the antigen, but the nature of this functional loss is unknown. It is also possible that low responder animals contain an excessive number of antigen-specific suppressor T cells (see page 114).

MAN

The concept of genetic control of the immune response described for mice and guinea pigs appears to be valid for the human. For further discussion of the significance of human histocompatibility antigens, see Chapter 14.

THEORIES OF ANTIBODY FORMATION

The mechanism by which antigen initiates a specific immune response is unknown. Two types of mechanisms have been proposed—instructive and selective.

INSTRUCTIVE THEORIES

Instructive theories of antibody formation may be classified as *direct* or *indirect*. The *direct* theory states that antigen serves as a template upon which antibody molecules are folded to impose an antigen combining site (52,66). This theory was in vogue in the early part of the twentieth century and was supported by the findings of Pauling, who denatured antibody and then tried to recover activity by renaturation of the antibody (104). He was unable to do so in the absence of antigen. It is now known that the tertiary structure of antibody can be destroyed by breaking the disulfide bonds of the molecule, but when these bonds are rejoined, the antigen-binding activity of the antibody is restored even in the absence of antigen (49). The primary structure of a protein determines the tertiary structure (12,27,107), and therefore the antigen-binding specificity of an antibody must be dictated by the amino acid sequence of the antibody molecule.

The *indirect* template theory states that in some way the antigen affects the read-out of the genetic massage from DNA so that the sequence of amino acids incorporated is affected by the presence of antigen (9,52,120). There is no known example of such a mechanism.

The instructive theories imply that antigen is present in the antibody-forming cells to influence the production of antibody. The rate of antibody production per antibody-forming cell can be estimated at about 1,500 molecules per second. This requires a minimum of 100,000 production sites. When the distribution of trace-labeled antigen molecules is followed, the maximum number of antigen molecules per antibody-producing cell is estimated to be less than 10 (99). Therefore the amount of antigen present is insufficient to affect the production of antibody by this means. Most immunologists now agree that instructive theories are no longer tenable in light of our present knowledge of molecular biology.

SELECTIVE THEORIES

Selective theories state that the coding for antibody specificity is genetically determined and already present in the responding cell; contact of the cell with antigen serves to stimulate the expression of the preexisting potential (10,11,68). There are two variations of selective theories, *germ line* (15,46,53,132) and *somatic mutation* (10,11). The germ line selective theory postulates that invertebrates have a separate gene cistron for each polypeptide chain that has developed with evolution of the species. The somatic mutation theory postulates that the evolution of immune cells occurs within the lifetime of the individual by mutation or modulation of a much smaller number of inherited cistrons.

Germ Line Theories

In 1900 Ehrlich presented his side-chain theory in which he stated that all cells, not just lymphoid cells, had a variety of side chains (termed haptophores) that had evolved in the germ line. These side chains normally functioned as receptors for metabolites but also could react with antigens (24,25). As a result of reaction with antigen there was a compensatory synthesis of new side chains. This synthesis resulted in an excess of side chains so that many were released into the circulation and became detectable as antibodies.

In 1955 Jerne postulated the natural selection theory (54), which took into account some of the information that had accumulated over the preceding 50 years. Jerne postulated the production of specific receptor molecules by lymphoid cells at random. The number of antigenic specificities that these receptor molecules would recognize was finite and dictated by the genome of the individual. Receptor molecules were released from the cells (natural antibody), and antigen served to select the specific circulating receptors with which it reacted (natural selection). The receptor which had reacted with antigen was then carried back to the cell with the potential to produce antibody, and the antigen-receptor molecule complex in some way stimulated the cell to proliferate, differentiate and produce more receptor molecules (antibody). Szilard in 1960 postulated that there was a separate gene which coded for each antibody and that the complete array of genes required for all antibodies was present in each potentially reacting cell (138). Antigen served to induce cell differentiation, fix the specificity of the reacting cell, and stimulate production of antibody. Both Jerne and

Szilard said that the precursor of the antibody-producing cell was omnipotent and could recognize all immunogens.

Somatic Mutation

Burnet was the first to postulate the immune potential was the result of somatic mutation (10,11). He reasoned that the immune response to a specific antigen originated in a few omnipotent stem cells which were highly mutable. During somatic development individual precursor cells that had the capacity to respond to one or a very limited number of antigens were differentiated. Upon contact with the specific antigen these precursors were stimulated to proliferate, and the progeny constituted a clone of cells producing the specific antibody (clonal selection). Burnet's clonal selection theory stimulated a vast amount of important research. A number of workers have extended Burnet's theory and have implicated various genetic mechanisms as occurring during somatic development to explain the amino acid structure of immunoglobulins. However, somatic mutation on a random basis, as a means of creating the diversity needed for recognition by the individual of many different antigens, implies uncontrolled production of information with a high rate of nonsense mutations (wastage) (53). In addition, the existence of genetically controlled immune responses to specific antigens supports germ line development of at least some immune responses.

The most pressing questions to be explained by any theory are 1) how does an immunologically reactive cell recognize antigen? 2) How does this recognition stimulate antibody production? And 3) how does an individual develop the capacity to recognize so many different antigenic specificities (generation of diversity)?

It is now generally accepted that immunologically reactive cells recognize antigens by means of antibody or antibody-like molecules present on their surface (123). The process whereby this reaction of antigen with a reactive or precursor cell stimulates the cell to proliferate is unknown, although the ability of antigen to stimulate proliferation is well documented. Generation of diversity may occur by germ line evolution or by somatic mutation. It is still not clear whether each reactive cell has the capacity to react with many or all antigens (omnipotent) or is limited to recognition of one or very few antigens (restricted). It is known that each differentiated antibody-producing plasma cell is restricted to producing antibody of one specificity and immunoglobulin of one type, but the potential of the recognition cell or precursor cell is not clearly defined. It is possible that the recognition cell (?thymus-derived cell) may not be restricted and that the plasma cell precursor is restricted or that restriction may occur during differentiation of a given cell line (121).

IMMUNE MEMORY

Following stimulation by antigen, the responding lymphatic tissue undergoes proliferation and differentiation into plasma cells that synthesize and secrete antibody (humoral immunity) or into lymphocytes (specifically sensitized cells) that have the ability to react specifically with antigen (cellular immunity). In addition, a specific cell or cell line with a particular property of reacting upon second contact with the original antigen by a more rapid and increased proliferation and differentiation is also produced (memory cell). A second contact with the same or a closely related antigen stimulates a more rapid reaction, with the production of a greater specific immune response (77,99). This anamnestic, or secondary, response is believed due to the presence of the memory cells produced as a result of the preceding antigenic stimulation. Memory is expressed by both T and B cells. In certain situations where two antigens share some common antigenic determinants but also have determinants specific for each antigen, exposure to the related antigen (after previous exposure to the other antigen) results in an anamnestic response to the specific determinants of the first antigen even though the second antigen does not contain such determinants (original antigenic sin).

CONTROL OF ANTIBODY PRODUCTION

A feedback mechanism appears to control the production of antibody (115,131,143). Following primary or secondary immunization, there is a burst of antibody production that peaks in a few days. Serum antibody titers then fall off gradually owing to catabolism of the antibody formed. Further antibody formation occurs at a very low rate and may eventually be undetectable if no re-exposure to the antigen occurs. Regulatory mechanisms are all-important in controlling the size, nature and duration of an immune response. If the response were not controlled antigen stimulation of proliferation would lead to an overgrowth of body tissues similar to that seen with some lymphoid tumors, such as multiple myeloma, lymphoma or leukemia. Passively administered specific antibody can suppress the induction of an immune response to the specific antigen without affecting responses to other antigens. The mechanism of action of the specific antibody in this situation is unknown, but the observation supports the concept that specific antibody inhibits further production of antibody of the same specificity by a feedback control system. In addition, suppressor T cells (see Chapter 7) may serve to control the immune response.

REFERENCES

1. Alter BJ, Schendel DJ, Bach ML, Bach FH, Klein J, Stimfling JH: Cell-mediated lympholysis. Importance of serologically defined H-2 regions. J Exp Med 137:1303–1309, 1973
2. Andersson J, Sjöberg O, Möller G: Mitogens as probes for immunocyte activation and cellular cooperation. Transplant Rev 11:131–177, 1972
3. Bach FH, Widmer MB, Bach ML, Klein J: Serologically defined and lymphocyte defined components of the major histocompatibility complex in the mouse. J Exp Med 136:1430–1444, 1972
4. Bianco C, Patrick R, Nussenzweig V: A population of lymphocytes bearing a membrane receptor for antigen-antibody-complement complexes. J Exp Med 132:702–718, 1970
5. Bluestein HG, Green I, Benacerraf B: Specific immune response genes of the guinea

pig. I. Dominant genetic control of immune responsiveness to copolymers of L-glutamic acid and L-alamine and L-glutamic acid and L-tyrosine. J Exp Med 134:458, 1971

6. Bluestein HG, Green I, Benacerraf B: Specific immune response genes of the guinea pig. IV. Demonstration in random-bred guinea pigs that responsiveness to a copolymer of L-glutamic acid and L-tyrosine is predicated upon the possession of a distinct strain 13 histocompatibility specificity. J Exp Med 134:1538, 1971

7. Boyse EA, Old LJ: Some aspects of normal and abnormal cell surface genetics. Ann Rev Genetics 3:269–290, 1969

8. Bretcher PA, Cohn M: A theory of self–non self discrimination. Science 189:1042, 1970

9. Burnet FM: Enzyme, Antigen, and Virus. London, Cambridge University Press, 1956

10. Burnet FM: The clonal selection theory of acquired immunity. London, Cambridge University Press, 1959

11. Burnet FM: The integrity of the body: A discussion of modern immunological ideas. Cambridge, Mass, Harvard University Press, 1962

12. Canfield RE, Anfinsen CB: Concepts and experimental approaches in the determination of the primary structure of proteins. In The Proteins: Composition, Structure, and Function. Neurath H (ed) 2d ed, Vol 1. New York, Academic Press, 1963

13. Cantor H, Asofsky R: Synergy among lymphoid cells mediating the graft-versus-host syndrome. II. Synergy in G. v H. reactions produced by Balb/c lymphoid cells of differing anatomic origin. J Exp Med 131:235, 1970

14. Chin AH, Saiki HJ, Trujillo JM, Williams RC Jr: Peripheral blood T- and B-lymphocytes in patients with lymphoma and acute leukemia. Clin Immunol Immunopathol 1:499–510, 1973

15. Cohen EP: On the mechanism of immunity: In defense of evolution. Ann Rev Microbiol 22:283, 1968

16. Cooper HL: Studies on RNA metabolism during lymphocyte activation. Transplant Rev 11:3–38, 1972

17. Claman HN, Chaperon EA, Triplett RF: Thymus-marrow cell combinations: Synergism in antibody production. Proc Soc Exp Biol Med 122:1167, 1966

18. Claman HN, Mosier DE: Cell-cell interactions in antibody production. Prog Allergy 16:40–80, 1972

18a. Cooper MD, Lawton AR III: The development of the immune system. Sci Am 231:58, 1974

19. Coutinho A, Gronowicz E, Bullock W, Möller G: Mechanism of thymus independent immunocyte triggering mitogenic activation of B cells results in specific immune responses. J Exp Med 139:74, 1974

20. David CS, Shreffler DC, Frelinger JA: New lymphocyte antigen system (Lna) controlled by the Ir region of the mouse H-2 complex. Proc Natl Acad Sci (USA) 70:2509–2514, 1973

21. Dutton RW, Eady JD: An in vitro system for the study of the mechanism of antigen stimulation in the secondary response. Immunology 7:40, 1964

22. Dutton RW, Campbell P, Chan E, Hirst J et al: Cell cooperation during immunologic responses of isolated lymphoid cells. In Cellular Interactions In The Immune Response. Basel Karger, 1971

23. Dutton RW, Falkoff R, Hirst JA, Hoffmann M, et al: It there evidence for a non-antigen specific diffusable chemical mediator from the thymus-derived cell in the initiation of the immune response? In Progress in Immunology, Amos B (ed). New York, Academic Press, 1971, pp 355–368

24. Ehrlich P: On immunity, with special reference to cell life. Proc R Soc Lond [Biol] 66:424, 1900

25. Ehrlich P: Studies In Immunity. New York, Wiley, 1910

26. Elfenbein GJ, Shevach EM, Green I: Proliferation by bone-marrow derived lymphocytes in response to antigenic stimulation in vitro. J Immunol 109:820, 1972

27. Epstein CH, Goldberger RF, Anfinsen CG: The genetic control of teriary protein structure: Studies with model systems. Cold Spring Harbor Symp Quant Biol 28:439, 1963

28. Everett NB, Tyler RW: Lymphopoiesis in the thymus and other tissues: Functional implications. Int Rev Cytol 22:205–237, 1967

29. Feldmann M: Cell interactions in the immune response in vitro. V. Specific collaboration via complexes of antigen and thymus-derived cell immunoglobulin. J Exp Med 136:737, 1972
30. Feldmann M, Basten A: The relationship between antigenic structure and the requirement for thymus derived cells in the immune response. J Exp Med 134:103, 1971
31. Feldmann M, Nossal GJV: Tolerance, enhancement and the regulation of interactions between T cells, B cells and macrophages. Transplant Rev 13:3, 1972
32. Fishman M: Antibody formation in vitro. J Exp Med 114:837, 1961
33. Gajl-Peczalska KJ, Lim SD, Jacobson RR, Good RA: B lymphocytes in lepromatous leprosy. N Engl J Med 288:1033–1035, 1973
34. Gasser DL, Silbers WK: Genetic determinants of immunologic responsiveness. Adv Immunol 18:1–66, 1974
35. Gell PGH, Benacerraf B: Delayed hypersensitivity to simple protein antigens. Adv Immunol 1:319–343, 1961
36. Goldschneider I, McGregor DD: Migration of lymphocytes and thymocytes in the rat. J Exp Med 127:155, 1968
37. Goldschneider I, McGregor DD: Anatomical distribution of T and B lymphocytes in the rat. Development of lymphocyte specific antisera. J Exp Med 138:1443–1465, 1973
38. Goldstein AL, White A: Thymosin and other thymic hormones: Their nature and roles in the thymic dependency of immunological phenomena. In Davis AJS, Carter RL (eds). Contemporary Topic In Immunology. Vol 2. New York, Plenum Publishing Co, 1973, p 339.
39. Gloub ES: Brain-associated θ antigen: Reactivity of rabbit anti-mouse brain with mouse lymphoid cells. Cell Immunol 2:353–361, 1971
40. Gottlieb AA, Schwartz RH: Review: Antigen-RNA interactions. Cell Immunol 5:341, 1972
41. Götze D, Reisfeld RA, Klein J: Serologic evidence for antigens controlled by the Ir region in mice. J Exp Med 138:1003–1008, 1973
42. Gowans JL: Lifespan, recirculation and transformation of lymphocytes. Int Rev Exp Pathol 5:1, 1966
43. Greaves MF: Biological effects of anti-immunoglobulins: Evidence for immunoglobulin receptors on "T" and "B" lymphocytes. Transplant Rev 5:45–75, 1970
44. Greaves MF, Hogg NM: Immunoglobulin determinants on the surface of antigen binding T and B lymphocytes in mice. In Progress in Immunology. Amos B (ed). 1:111–126, 1971
45. Green I, Paul WE, Benacerraf B: A study of the passive transfer of delayed hypersensitivity to DNP-poly-L-lysine and DNP-GL in responder and nonresponder guinea pigs. J Exp Med 126:959, 1967
46. Grey HM: Phylogeny of immunoglobulins. Adv Immunol 10:51, 1969
47. Grey HM, Rabellino E, Pirofsky B: Immunoglobulins on the surface of lymphocytes. IV. Distinction in hypogammaglobulinemia, cellular immune deficiency and chronic lymphatic leukemia. J Clin Invest 50:2368, 1971
48. Gutman GA, Weissman IL: Lymphoid tissue architecture: Experimental analysis of the origin and distribution of T-cells and B-cells. Immunology 23:465–480, 1972
49. Habe, E: Recovery of antigenic specificity of denaturation and complete reduction of disulphides in a papain fragment of antibody. Proc Natl Acad Sci USA 52:1099, 1964
50. Hadden JW, Hadden EM, Haddox MK, Goldberg ND: Guanosine 3′,3′ — cyclic monophosphate: A possible intracellular mediator of mitogenic influences in lymphocytes. Proc Nat Acad Sci USA 69:3024, 1972
51. Hämmerling GJ, Deak BD, Mauve G, Hämmerling U, McDevitt HO: B lymphocyte alloantigens controlled by the Ir region of the major histocompatibility complex in mice. Immunogenetics 1:68–81, 1974
52. Haurowitz F: Antibody formation and the coding problem. Nature 205:847, 1965
53. Hood L, Talmadge DW: Mechanism of antibody diversity: Germ line basis for variability. Science 168:325, 1970
54. Jerne NK: The natural selection theory of antibody formation. Proc Natl Acad Sci USA 41:849, 1955
55. Jondal M, Holm G, Wigzell H: Surface markers on human T and B lymphocytes.

I. A large population of lymphocytes forming non-immune rosettes with sheep red blood cells. J Exp Med 136:207–215, 1972

56. Jost JP, Rikenberg HV: Cyclic AMP, Annu Rev Biochem 40:741, 1971

57. Kantor FS, Ojeda A, Benacerraf B: Studies on artificial antigens. I. Antigenicity of DNP-poly-lysine and DNP-copolymer of lysine and glutamic acid in guinea pigs. J Exp Med 117:55, 1963

58. Katz DH: The allogeneic effect on immune responses: Model for regulatory influences of T lymphocytes on the immune system. Transplant Rev 12:141–179, 1972

59. Katz DH, Benacerraf B: The regulatory influence of activated T cells on B cell response to antigen. Adv Immunol 15:1–94, 1972

60. Katz DH, Hamaoka T, Dorf ME, Benacerraf B: Cell interactions between histoincompatible T and B lymphocytes. The H-2 gene complex determines successful physiologic lymphocytes interactions. Proc Nat Acad Sci USA 70:2624–2628, 1973

61. Katz DH, Hamaoka T, Dorf ME, Maurer PH, Benacerraf B: Cell interactions between histoincompatible T and B lymphocytes. IV. Involvement of the immune response (IR) gene in the control of lymphocyte interactions in responses controlled by the gene. J Exp Med 138:734–739, 1973

62. Kettman J, Dutton RW: Radioresistance of the enhancing effect of cells from carrier-immunized mice in an in vitro primary immune response. Proc Nat Acad Sci USA 68:699, 1971

63. Kirchner H, Oppenheim JJ, Blaese MR, Hofstrand HJ: Defective in vitro spleen cell proliferation response to antigens in agammaglobulinemic chickens. J Immunol 109:348, 1972.

64. Klein J, Park JM: Graft versus host reaction across different regions of the H-2 complex of the mouse. J Exp Med 137:1213–1225, 1973

65. Komuro K, Boyse EA: Induction of T lymphocytes from precursor cells in vitro by a product of the thymus. J Exp Med 138:479–482, 1973

66. Landsteiner K: The specificity of serological reactions, 2d ed. Cambridge, Harvard University Press, 1945

67. Lay WH, Mendex NF, Bianco C, Nussenzweig V: Binding of sheep red blood cells to a large population of human lymphocytes. Nature 230:531, 1971

68. Lederberg J: Genes and antibodies. Science 129:1649, 1959

69. Ling NR: Lymphocyte stimulation. Amsterdam, North Holland Publishing Co, 1968

70. Levine BB, Benacerraf B: Genetic control in guinea pigs of immune response to conjugates of haptens and poly-L-lysine. Science 147:517, 1965

71. Lieberman R, Humphrey W: Association of H-2 types with genetic control of immune responsiveness to IgA allotypes in the mouse. Proc Natl Acad Sci (USA) 68:2510, 1971

72. Lieberman R, Paul WE, Humphrey W, Stimpfling JH: H-2-linked immune response (Ir) genes. Independent loci for Ir-IgG and Ir-IgA genes. J Exp Med 136:1231–1240, 1972

73. Linthicum DS, Sell S: Surface immunoglobulin on rabbit lymphoid cells. I. Ultrastructural distribution and endocytosis of b4 allotypic determinants on peripheral blood lymphocytes. Cell Immunol 12:443, 1974

74. Livnat S, Klein J, Bach FH: Graft versus host reaction in strains of mice identical for H-2K and H-2D antigens. Nature [New Biol] 243:42, 1973

75. Lucas DO, Shohet SB, Merler E: Changes in phospholipid metabolism which occur as a consequence of mitogenic stimulation of lymphocytes. J Immunol 106:768, 1971

76. Mäkelä O, Cross A, Kosunen TV (eds): Cell Interactions and Receptor Antibodies in Immune Responses. New York, Academic Press, 1971

77. Makinodan T, Albright JF: Proliferative and differentiative manifestations of cellular immune potential. Prog Allergy 10:1, 1967

78. Marshall WH, Valentine FT, Lawrence HS: Cellular immunity in vitro: Clonal proliferation of antigen-stimulated lymphocytes. J Exp Med 130:327, 1969

79. McDevitt HP, Bechtol KB, Hämmerling GJ: Histocompatibility-linked genetic control of specific immune responses. In Cellular Selection and Regulation in the Immune Response. Edelman GM (ed). New York, Raven Press, 1974, pp 101–120

80. McDevitt HO, Benacerraf B: Genetic control of specific immune responses. Adv Immunol 11:31, 1969

81. Mendelsohn J, Multer MM, Boone RF: Enhanced effects of prostaglandin E_1 and

dibutyryl cyclic-AMP upon human lymphocytes in the presence of cortisol. J Clin Invest 52:2129, 1973

82. Mendelsohn J, Skinner SA, Kornfeld S: The rapid induction by phytohemogglutinin of increased α-aminoisobuteic acid uptake by lymphocytes. J Clin Invest 50:818, 1971

83. Mercier P: The rosettes and the immuno-cyto-adherence: Analytic essay. Biomedicine (Paris) 20:17, 1974

84. Miller JFAP, Basten A, Sprent J, Cheers C: Interaction between lymphocytes in immune response. Cell Immunol 2:469–495, 1971

85. Miller JFAP, Mitchell FG: Cell to cell interaction in the immune response. I. Hemolysin forming cells in neonatally thymectomized mice reconstituted with thymus or thoracic duct lymphocytes. J Exp Med 128:801, 1968

86. Miller JRAP, Osoba D: Current concepts of the immunological function of the thymus. Physiol Rev 47:437, 1967

87. Mills JA: The immunologic significance of antigen induced lymphocyte transformation in vitro. J Immunol 97:239, 1966

88. Mitchell J: Lymphocyte circulation in the spleen. Marginal zone bridging channels and their possible role in cell traffic. Immunology 24:93–107, 1973

89. Mitchison NA: In Immunologic Tolerance, Landy M, Braun W (eds). New York, Academic Press, 1969, pp 149–151

90. Mitchison NA: The carrier effect in the secondary response to hapten-protein conjugates. II. Cellular cooperation. Eur J Immunol 1:18, 1971

91. Möller G (ed): Lymphocyte activation by mitogens. Transplant Rev 11:1972

92. Möller G (ed): Lymphocyte immunoglobulin. Transplant. Revs. Vol 14. Copenhagen, Munksgaard, 1973

93. Möller G (ed): T and B lymphocytes in humans. Transplant Rev 16:1973

93a. Möller G (ed): B₂-microglobulin and HL-antigen. Transplant Rev 21:1974

94. Mosier DE, Coppleson LW: A three-cell interaction required for the induction of the primary response in vitro. Proc Natl Acad Sci (USA) 61:542, 1968

95. Mosier DE, Johnson BM, Paul WE, McMaster PRB: Cellular requirements for the primary in vitro antibody response to DNP-ficoll. J Exp Med 139:1354, 1974

96. Movat HZ, Fernando MVP: The fine structure of lymphoid tissue during antibody formation. Exp Mol Pathol 4:155, 1965

97. Nilsson B, Sultzer BM, Bullock WW: Purified protein derivative of tuberculin indices immunoglobulin production in normal mouse spleen cells. J Exp Med 137:126, 1973

98. Nossal GJV, Ada GL: Antigens, lymphoid cells and the immune response. New York, Academic Press, 1971

99. Nossal GJV, Ada GL, Austin CM: Antigens in immunity. IV. Cellular localization of ¹²⁵I-labeled flagella in lymph nodes. Aust J Exp Biol Med Sci 42:311, 1964

100. Oppenheim JJ, Wostencroft RA, Gell PGH: Delayed hypersensitivity in the guinea pig to a protein-hapten conjugate and its relationship to in vitro transformation of lymph node, spleen, thymus and peripheral blood lymphocytes. Immunology 12:89, 1967

101. Ovary Z, Benacerraf B: Immunological specificity of the secondary response with dinitrophenylated proteins. Proc Soc Exp Biol Med 114:72–76, 1963

102. Parrott DM, DeSousa MA: Thymus dependent and thymus independent populations, origin, migratory patterns and lifespan. Clin Exp Immunol 8:663, 1971

103. Paul WE: Function specificity of antigen-binding receptors of lymphocytes. Transplant Rev 5:130–166, 1970

104. Pauling LA: A theory of the structure and process of formation of antibodies. J Am Chem Soc 62:2643, 1940

105. Pearmain G, Lycette RR, Fitzgerald PH: Tuberculin-induced mitosis in peripheral blood leukocytes. Lancet 1:637, 1963

106. Perkins WD, Karnovsky MJ, Unanue ER: An ultrastructural study of lymphocytes with surface-bound immunoglobulin. J Exp Med 135:267, 1972

107. Perlmann GE, Diringer R: The structure of proteins. Ann Rev Biochem (Stanford) 29:151, 1960

108. Raff MC: Two distinct populations of peripheral lymphocytes in mice distinguishable by immunofluorescence. Immunology 19:637–650, 1970

109. Raff MC: Surface antigenic markers for distinguishing T and B lymphocytes in mice. Transplant Rev 6:52, 1971
110. Raff MC, Cantor H: Subpopulations of thymus cells and thymus derived cells. In Progress in Immunology. Amos B (ed). New York, Academic Press, 1971, p 83
111. Raff MC, Wortis HH: Thymus dependence of θ-bearing cells in peripheral lymphoid tissue of mice. Immunology 18:931–942, 1970
112. Resch K, Ferber E: Phospholipid metabolism of stimulated lymphocytes. Effects of phytohemogglutinin, concanavalin A and an anti-immunoglobulin serum. Eur J Biochem 27:153, 1972
113. Robinson GA, Butcher RW, Sutherland EW: Cyclic AMP. Academic Press, New York, 1971
113a. Rosenthal AS, Shevach EM: Function of macrophages in antigen recognition by guinea pig T lymphocytes. I. Requirement for histocompatible macrophages and lymphocytes. J Exp Med 138:1194, 1974
114. Ross GD, Rabellino EM, Polley MJ, Grey HM: Combined studies of complement receptor and surface immunoglobulin-bearing cells and sheep erythrocyte rosette-forming cells in normal and leukemic lymphocytes. J Natl Cancer Inst 52:377–385, 1973
115. Rowley DA, Fitch FW, Stuart FP, Köhler H, Cosenza H: Specific suppression of immune responses. Science 181:1133–1141, 1973
116. Rowe DS, Hug K, Forni L, Pernis B: Immunoglobulin D as a lymphocyte receptor. J Exp Med 139:965–972, 1973
117. Santos GW: Adoptive transfer of immunologically competent cells. III. Comparative ability of allogenic and syngeneic spleen cells to produce a primary antibody response in the cyclophosphamide treated mouse. J Immunol 97:587–593, 1966
118. Schrader SW: Mechanism of activation of the bone marrow-derived lymphocyte. III. A distinction between a macrophage-produced triggering signal and the amplifying effect on triggered B lymphocytes of allogeneic interaction. J Exp Med 138:1466, 1973
119. Schwartz RS, Ryder RJW, Gottlieb BAA: Macrophages and antibody synthesis. Prog Allergy 14:81, 1970
120. Schweet R, Owen RD: Concepts of protein synthesis in relation to antibody formation. J Cell Physiol (Suppl. 1) 50:199, 1957
121. Sell, S: Development of restrictions in the expression of immunoglobulin specificities by lymphoid cells. Transplant. Rev. 5:19, 1970
122. Sell S: Studies on rabbit lymphocytes in vitro. XIX. Kinetics of reversible antiallotypic stimulation and restimulation of blast transformation. Cell Immunol 12:119–126, 1974
123. Sell S, Asofsky R: Lymphocytes and immunoglobulins. Prog Allergy 12:86, 1968
124. Sell S, Gell PGH: Studies on rabbit lymphocytes in vitro. I. Stimulation of blast transformation with an antiallotype serum. J Exp Med 122:423, 1965
125. Sell S, Rowe DS, Gell PGH: Studies on rabbit lymphocytes in vitro. III. Protein, RNA and DNA synthesis by lymphocyte cultures after stimulation with phytohemagglutinin, staphylococcal filtrate, anti-allotype serum, and heterologous antiserum to rabbit whole serum. J Exp Med 122:823–839, 1965
126. Sell S, Sheppard HW: Rabbit blood lymphocytes may be T cells with surface immunoglobulin. Science 182:586, 1973
127. Shevach EM, Paul WE, Green I: Histocompatibility-linked immune response gene function in guinea pigs. Specific inhibition of antigen-induced lymphocyte proliferation by alloantisera. J Exp Med 136:1207, 1972
127a. Shevach EM, Rosenthal AS: Function of macrophages in antigen recognition by guinea pig T lymphocytes. II. Role of the macrophage in the regulation of genetic control of the immune response. J Exp Med 138:1213, 1974
128. Shreffler DC: Genetic fine structure of the H-2 gene complex. In Cellular Selection and Regulation in the Immune Response. Edelman GM (ed). New York, Raven Press, 1974, pp 83–100
129. Silveira NPA, Mendes NF, Tolnai MEA: Tissue localization of two populations of human lymphocytes distinguished by membrane receptors. J Immunol 108:1456–1460, 1972

130. Smith JW, Steiner AL, Parker CW: Human lymphocyte metabolism. Effects of cyclic and noncyclic nucleotides on stimulation by phytohemagglutin. J Clin Invest 50:442, 1971
131. Smith T: Active immunity produced by so-called balanced or neutral mixtures of diphtheria toxin and anti-toxin. J Exp Med 11:241, 1909
132. Smithies O, Poulik MD: Initiation of protein synthesis at an unusual position in an immunoglobulin gene. Science 175:187, 1972
133. Snell GD: Histocompatibility genes of the mouse. II. Production and analysis of isogenic resistant lines. J Natl Cancer Inst 21:843, 877, 1958
134. Snell GD, Stimpfling JH: Genetics of tissue transplantation. In Biology of the Laboratory Mouse (2d ed). Green EL (ed). New York, McGraw-Hill, 1966, pp 457–491
135. Solheim BG, Thorsby E: β-2-microglobulin. Part of the HL-A molecule in the cell membrane. Tissue Antigens (Munksgaard) 4:83, 1974
136. Stobo JD: Phytohemagglutinin and concanavalin A probes for murine "T" cell activation and differentiation. Transplant Rev 11:60–86, 1972
137. Stutman O, Good RA: Thymus hormones. In Contemporary Topics in Immunology: Thymus Dependency. Vol 2. Davis AJS, Carter RL (eds). New York, Plenum Publishing Co, 1973, p 299
138. Szilard L: The molecular basis of antibody formation. Proc Natl Acad Sci USA 46:293, 1960
139. Taylor RB, Duffus PH, Raff MC, dePetris S: Redistribution and pinocytosis of lymphocyte surface immunoglobulin molecules induced by anti-immunoglobulin antibody. Nature [New Biol] 233:225–229, 1971
140. Taylor RB, Iverson GM: Hapten competition and the nature of cell cooperation in the antibody response. Proc R Soc Lond [Biol] 176:393–418, 1971
141. Tigelaar RE, Asofsky R: Synergy among lymphoid cells mediating the graft-versus-host response. V. Derivation by migration in lethally irradiated recipients of two interacting subpopulations of thymus derived cells from normal spleen. J Exp Med 137:239, 1973
142. Tranin N, Small M: Thymic humoral factors. In Contemporary Topics in Immunology. Vol. 2. Davis AJS, Carter RL (eds). New York, Plenum Publishing Co, 1973, p 321
143. Uhr JW, Moller G: Regulatory effect of antibody on the immune response. Adv Immunol 8:81, 1968
144. Unanue ER: The regulatory role of macrophages in antigenic stimulation. Adv Immunol 15:95, 1972
145. Valentine FT: The transformation and proliferation of lymphocytes in vitro. In Cell-Mediated Immunity: In vitro correlates. Revillard JP (ed). Baltimore, University Park Press, 1971
146. White RG: Functional recognition of immunologically competent cells by means of fluorescent antibody technique. In The immunologically competent cell. Wolstenholme GEW, Knight J (eds). London, Churchill, 1963
147. White RG, French VI, Stark JM: Germinal center formation and antigen localization in Malpighian bodies of the chicken spleen. In Germinal Centers in Immune Responses. Cottier H (ed). Berlin, Springer, 1966, pp 131–142
148. Whitney RB, Sutherland RM: Enhanced uptake of calcium by transforming cells. Cell Immunol 5:137, 1972
148a. Winkelmann RK (ed): Symposium on the Sézary Cell. May Clinic Proceedings 49:513, 1974
149. Wortis HH: Immunological responses of "nude" mice. Clin Exp Immunol 8:305, 1971
150. Wybran J, Carr MC, Fudenberg HH: The human rosette-forming cell as a marker of thymus-derived cells. J Clin Invest 51:2537–2543, 1972
151. Wybran S, Fudenberg HH: Thymus-derived rosette-forming cells in various human disease states: Cancer, lymphoma, bacterial and viral infections, and other diseases. J Clin Invest 52:1026–1032, 1973

5

Antibodies and Immunoglobulins

Antibodies belong to a group of structurally related protein molecules known collectively as immunoglobulins (6). Most, if not all, immunoglobulins are the products of plasma cells, which secrete these proteins into serum and tissue fluids. While some immunoglobulins are produced at all times in most normal animals, specific antibodies are a unique group of proteins produced in response to antigenic stimulation. Given the great number of antigenic specificities identifiable, an individual must have the ability to produce a large variety of antibody molecules. Immunoglobulins possess a degree of structural heterogeneity not found in other proteins, but at the same time immunoglobulins also have structural similarities.

IMMUNOGLOBULIN CLASSES

Five major immunoglobulin classes have been identified in man (6,10). Some of the characteristics of each of these immunoglobulins are given in Table 5–1, and their structural relations are summarized in Fig. 5–1. The five classes now identified include immunoglobulins G (IgG), A (IgA), M (IgM), D (IgD), and E (IgE). The designation of γ for Ig (e.g., γG instead of IgG) has been discontinued because many European typewriters do not have a key for γ. These five classes have antigenic determinants in common, so that an antiserum produced by immunizing an animal with one class cross reacts with the other classes. This cross reaction is the result of shared structural components. On the other hand, each immunoglobulin class also contains antigenic determinants unique to that class which elicit the production of specific antibodies that react only with that immunoglobulin class,

STRUCTURE OF IMMUNOGLOBULINS

The basic structural unit of each immunoglobulin class consists of two pairs of polypeptide chains joined by disulfide bonds (Fig. 5–1)

TABLE 5-1
Some Properties of Human Immunoglobulins

Property	Immunoglobulin class				
	IgG	**IgA**	**IgM**	**IgD**	**IgE**
Serum concentration (gm/100 ml)	1.2	0.4	0.12	0.003	< .0005
Sedimentation coefficient (S)	7	7 (9, 11, 13)*	19 (24, 32)	7	8
Molecular weight	140,000	160,000†	900,000	180,000	200,000
Electrophoretic mobility	γ	Slow β	Between γ and β	Between γ and β	Slow β
H-chains	γ	α	μ	δ	ϵ
L-chains	λ or κ	λ or κ	λ or κ	λ or κ	λ or κ
Complement fixation	Yes	No	Yes	No	No
Placental transfer	Yes	No	No	No	No
Per cent intravascular	40	40	70	70	?
Half-life (days)	23	6	5	3	2.5
Percent carbohydrate	3	10	10	13	10
Antibody activity	Most Ab to infections; major part of secondary response; Rh isoaggluti-nins; LE factor	Present in external secretions	First Ab formed; ABO iso-agglutinins; rheumatoid factor	Antibody activity rarely demonstrated, found on lymphocyte surface	Reagin

* Figures in parentheses indicate the existence of other molecular forms, i.e., polymers.
† Serum IgA 160,000 MW; secretory IgA 350,000 MW.
Modified from Fahey JL. JAMA 194:183, 1966

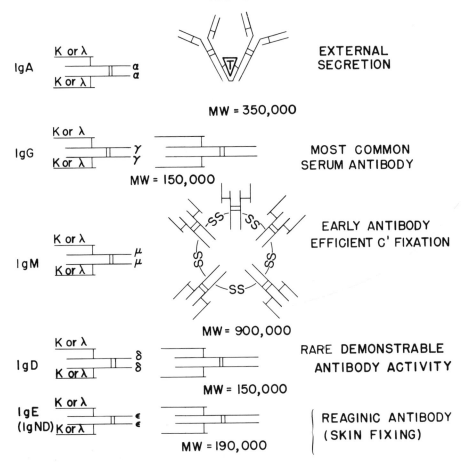

Fig. 5–1. **Human immunoglobulin classes.** Human humoral or circulating antibodies belong to five classes: IgA, IgG, IgM, IgD and IgE. Basic units of all immunoglobulin molecules are two pairs of polypeptide chains joined by disulfide bonds. All immunoglobulins have the same L- (light) chain components, identifiable antigenically as kappa (κ) or lambda (λ), with any given immunoglobulin molecule having two κ-chains or two λ-chains. No naturally occurring immunoglobulin molecule has one κ-chain and one λ-chain. H- (heavy) chains of each immunoglobulin class are unique for that class and determine its biologic properties. H-chains of each immunoglobulin class are designated by Greek letter corresponding to capital letter identifying the class.

(5,11,20,24,25). The disulfide bonds may be reduced by mercaptoethanol, resulting in the liberation of four polypeptide chains: two L- (light) and two H- (heavy) chains. The intact molecule may be digested by enzymes to give other fragments (Fc and Fab fragments; Fig. 5–2). The L-chains are shared by immunoglobulins of the different classes and can be antigenically divided into two subclasses—kappa (κ) and lambda (λ). A given immunoglobulin molecule is either type κ or type λ. Approximately 60%

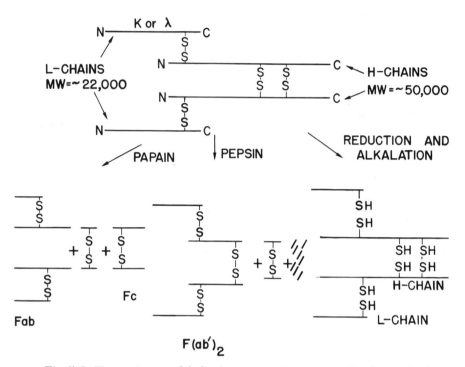

Fig. 5–2. Human immunoglobulin fragments. Intact IgG molecule may be fragmented by different reagents into subunits. Digestion with papain results in two major fragments, Fab and Fc, and a minor fragment. Fab fragment consists of L-chain and half of H-chain joined by a disulfide bond. Fc fragment is carboxy terminal segment of H-chains joined by a disulfide bond. An additional small peptide containing a disulfide bond has been recognized. Fab fragment contains antigen-binding site and reacts with, but does not precipitate, antigen because it is monovalent. Fc portion is responsible for biologic properties such as complement fixation, placental transfer, catabolic rate and skin fixation. Digestion with pepsin results in two Fab fragments joined by a disulfide bond due to preservation of one of the disulfide bonds joining H-chains. This fragment, F(ab')₂, reacts with and precipitates antigen since it is divalent (contains two antigen-binding sites). Additional peptide fragments, some containing disulfide bonds, are produced by action of pepsin, presumably due to further digestion of Fc fragment. Reduction and alkalation results in liberation of polypeptide chains—two L-chains (MW 22,000) and two H-chains (MW 50,000). Contribution of each polypeptide chain to antigen-binding site is unclear, although separated chains have only small fraction of antigen-binding capacity of intact Fab fragment. That portion of H-chain present in Fab fragment is called Fd piece. (Modified from Metzger H: JAMA 202:129, 1967)

of the immunoglobulin molecules of a given individual contain κ-type L-chains and 40% λ-type L-chains. The H-chains are unique for each immunoglobulin class and are designated by the Greek letter corresponding to the capital letter designation of the immunoglobulin class (α-chains for the H-chains of IgA, γ-chains for the H-chains of IgG). IgM and IgA have a third chain component, the J-chain (18,34), which is believed to join the monomeric 7s units. The J-chain may play a role in holding together the 7s units of these immunoglobulins.

BIOLOGIC PROPERTIES OF IMMUNOGLOBULINS

The five classes of immunoglobulins have different biologic properties and are distributed differently in the intact animal (5,10,11). The structure responsible for the biologic properties of each immunoglobulin class is located on that part of the immunoglobulin molecule that is unique for each class (the Fc portion of the H-chain).

Antibody activity is most frequently detected in the IgG class. Each IgG molecule consists of one four-chain unit with a molecular weight of about 150,000. Molecules of the IgG class have the ability to cross the placenta and to provide passive immunity to the newborn infant at a time when the infant's immune mechanisms are not developed. IgG is widely distributed in the tissue fluids and is equally distributed in the intravascular and extravascular spaces.

IgM is the first immunoglobulin class produced by the maturing fetus and may be the first immunoglobulin class representing a given antibody specificity following immunization (primary response) (40). IgM occurs as five four-chain units joined by disulfide bonds located on the Fc part of the molecule; its molecular weight is 900,000. IgM is found mainly in the intravascular fluids (80%). It is also the most efficient class of immunoglobulin in fixing complement and therefore is highly active in cytotoxic and cytolytic reactions (see Chapter 11). IgM does not normally cross the placenta from mother to fetus, but may be produced actively by the fetus prior to birth, especially if the fetus has been exposed to antigens by infection.

IgA is found in relatively low concentration in serum and tissue fluids, but is present in high concentration in external secretions such as colostrum, saliva, tears, and intestinal and bronchial secretions (39). The IgA molecules in these fluids exist as dimers (two four-chain units) joined by an extra fragment ("transport" piece) which appears to facilitate the secretion of the IgA into the external fluids. Because IgA antibodies are prominent in external secretions, such antibodies are part of the first line of defense against infectious agents.

IgE is present in very low concentrations in serum and tissue fluids, but has a particular affinity to fix to tissues (see Chapter 12). The significance of this biologic property of IgE antibodies is the ability to sensitize certain cells (mast cells) so that upon contact with antigen, biologically active materials present in mast cells are released. Antibody with this biologic property is termed reaginic antibody, or reagin.

IgD is present in very low concentrations in the serum and is distributed mainly in the intravascular space. Antibody activity in the IgD class of immunoglobulins has rarely been demonstrated, the biologic function of IgD remains unknown, but IgD has been found on the surface of a high proportion of human lymphocytes, suggesting that IgD may serve as a cellular receptor for antigen (31).

All antibodies are immunoglobulins; it is not clear that all immunoglobulins are antibodies. At the present time most immunoglobulins of a given individual cannot be demonstrated to have antibody activity. However, this may be the result of inability to identify the antigens with which they might react.

IMMUNOGLOBULIN SUBCLASSES

In addition to the five major classes of immunoglobulins in man, subclasses of IgG, IgA, and IgM have been recognized (5,10,11). For example, four subclasses of IgG may be identified. These subclasses are designated IgG_1, IgG_2, IgG_3 and IgG_4 (10,25). The subclasses differ in their antigenic specificities, amino acid sequence, genetic control, and biologic properties (Table 5–2). IgG_1 molecules predominate in normal serum (9 mg/ml; the serum content of IgG_2 is 2.5 mg/ml; and the serum content of IgG_3 and IgG_4 is 0.5 to 1.0 mg/ml) (10). The biologic significance of these immunoglobulin subclasses is not well understood. However, IgG_1 and IgG_3 are more active in fixing complement, while IgG_4 does not fix complement. IgG_2 does not cross the placenta with the same efficiency as the other IgG subclasses. Therefore, the different IgG subclasses do have different properties.

ANTIGEN-BINDING SITE

The antigen-binding site of immunoglobulins is located on the Fab portion of the antibody molecule (5,10,11,24,25). The ability to combine specifically with a given antigenic determinant may be shared by immunoglobulins belonging to different classes. The actual site of antigen binding is small, but the complete site involves both the L- and the H-chains of a given antibody molecule (see Fig. 5–3).

PRIMARY STRUCTURE OF ANTIBODIES

The primary structure of a protein molecule is the sequence of amino acids that make up the polypeptide chain(s) (23). Considerable insight

TABLE 5–2
Biologic Properties of IgG Subclasses

Property	IgG_1	IgG_2	IgG_3	IgG_4
Complement fixation	++	+	+++	0
Placental transfer	+++	+++	+++	+++
Passive cutaneous anaphylaxis*	+++	0	+++	+++
Receptor for macrophage	+++	0	+++	0
Reaction with staph A protein	+++	+++	0	+++
Prominant antibody activity	Anti-Rh	Anti-Levan Anti-Dextran	Anti-Rh	Anti-Factor VIII

* Heterocytophilic antibody (see Chapter 12)

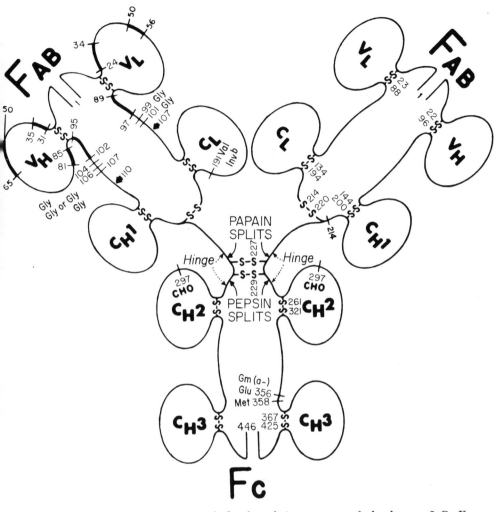

Fig. 5–3. Schematic view of the four-chain structure of the human IgG₁ K-molecule. The numbers on the right side are the actual residue numbers in protein EU (8); those on the Fab fragment (left side) are aligned for maximum homology; the light chains are numbered according to Kabat (20). Eu hypervariable regions are accentuated by heavier lines. V_L and V_H are the light and heavy chain variable region, C_H1, C_H2 and C_H3 are the domains of the constant region of the heavy chain and C_L is the constant region of the light chain. The hinge region in which the two heavy chains are linked by disulfide bonds is indicated approximately. Attachment of carbohydrate is at residue 297. Arrows at residues 107 and 110 denote the transition from variable to constant regions. The sites of action of papain and pepsin and the locations of a number of genetic factors are given (see Human Immunoglobulin Allotypes, p. 76).

into the structure and function of antibodies has been obtained by analysis of amino acid sequence and peptide maps of purified antibodies with different specificities and of isolated homogeneous myeloma immunoglobulins (1,19) (see below). Antibodies of different specificities have different primary structures. The amino acid sequences of the immunoglobulins studied to date have two regions in the L-chains. Of the total of 212 amino acids, those located at the carboxy terminal are virtually identical for each L-chain of a given type (κ or λ); the primary structure of the amino terminal (that portion presumably containing the antigen-binding site) varies for each of the proteins studied. The H-chain consists of four regions, each containing about 106 amino acids. The amino terminal segment of the H-chain is variable; the other three segments are constant. Therefore, a variable region exists at the amino terminal of the L-chain and the H-chain of each immunoglobulin molecule (4,16,19,25). The primary structure responsible for antigen binding is located in this variable portion. A schematic view of an IgG molecule is presented in Fig. 5–3. The antigen-binding site most likely corresponds to the heavier lines indicated in the figure. These segments of the variable region are folded to juxtapose in three dimensions in a manner that forms an appropriate pocket for antigen to be bound (see Antibody–Antigen Reactions, Chapter 6). In addition, immunoglobulin molecules have a high degree of segmented flexibility because of a "hinge" region between the first and second constant regions (between Fab and Fc) of the heavy chain. This permits the individual combining sites to move over great distances and assume different angles on reaction with antigenic sites.

Within the variable portion are constant segments containing up to 30 amino acids and "hot spots" of 4–7 amino acids where variability is marked. Constant portions exist over the carboxy terminal segments of the L-chain and the H-chain. This situation provides a structural basis for antibodies of different antigen-binding specificity (variable portion) in immunoglobulin molecules with similar or different biologic properties (constant portion). A variable region is needed to form antigen-binding sites of great diversity, while a constant region preserves the biologic properties of each immunoglobulin class.

HIGHER ORDER STRUCTURE OF IMMUNOGLOBULINS

In addition to primary structure (amino acid sequence), immunoglobulins, like other protein molecules, have higher orders of structure: 1) secondary, the coiling of the individual polypeptide chains; 2) tertiary, the folding of the polypeptide coils; and 3) quarternary, the arrangement and association of the folded chains (23,38). The results of chemical analysis and enzymatic cleavage studies have provided considerable insight into the secondary and tertiary structure of immunoglobulins. The chain relations of the immunoglobulins have been presented above and in Figs. 5–1 and 5–2. Sedimentation, diffusion, and viscosity measurements indicate a tightly ordered structure for the polypeptide chains, with a considerable amount of helical coiling. In addition to disulfide bonds, the coiled chains of the immunoglobulin unit are folded together. Reduction of the disulfide bonds does not separate the component chains until ionic bonds (van der Waals) are also broken. Details of the secondary and tertiary structure of immunoglobulins are not precisely known because of technical difficulties in the methods used and the complex nature of the structure.

The quarternary structure of the different immunoglobulins has been studied by hydrodynamic measurements, x-ray diffraction, and electron microscopy, and the results compared with those obtained by chemical analysis. The electron density map of an Fab fragment of a mouse myeloma protein with binding activity for the hapten phosphorylcholine gives a structure which can be divided into four distinct globular regions. The regions correspond to the four domains of the molecule as defined by amino acid sequence analysis (30). The hapten binding site lies between two domains near one end of the molecule interpreted to represent the variable domains of the light and heavy chain. Electron microscopic studies provide additional observations on the shape and form of immunoglobulin molecule (1,15). Immunoglobulin molecules cannot be examined directly, but produce areas of low density in films of a suitable salt (phosphotungsate) and carbon. In this way a replica of the molecule in a uniform layer of a stain of high density can be obtained (negative staining).

IgG unbound to antigen is an irregular globular particle lacking a characteristic structure, with a maximum dimension of 120 Å. IgG antibody bound to antigen (virus particle, ferritin) appears as a Y-shaped molecule. Removal of the Fc piece of IgG causes loss of the stem of the Y. The structure identified has a thickness of 40 Å. Each arm of the Y measures 65 Å in length; the stem measures 50Å. The arms and stem are inflexible, but the junction of the arms with the stem is flexible. The angle between the arms may vary from 10° to 180°. The arms are most likely the Fab pieces and contain the antibody combining site. Thus, the flexibility of the junction angle permits bridging of antigen particles by binding sites that stretch between two antigen particles as well as looping and joining of two antigen sites on the same molecule (15).

In fine structure, IgM consists of a central thin disk about 180 Å in diameter with five projecting arms measuring 35 by 125 Å; the entire molecule has a diameter of 270 Å. The structure is consistent with that postulated from chemical studies, i.e., five basic 150,000-MW units jointed together. If each arm represents a Fab piece, the molecule would be expected to have 10 arm-like extensions. Therefore, either each arm consists of two Fab pieces, or one of each pair of Fab pieces is incorporated into the central disk (15).

IgA also has a Y-shaped appearance in which two basic units are superimposed on each other in a close-packed state (37). The additional fragment found in secretory IgA is located at the stem area of two Y-shaped units. This fine structure is consistent with that proposed from chemical studies.

IMMUNOGLOBULIN ANTIGENIC SPECIFICITIES

The great variety of antigenic specificities that may be recognized on a given molecule is exemplified by antibodies to immunoglobulins (14,17,21,27).

Interspecies Specificity

Antisera produced in distantly related species such as rabbit anti-human immunoglobulin, may not only recognize specificities in human immunoglobulin but also react with immunoglobulin from other primate species.

Species Specificity

The above antisera may also recognize specificities present on essentially all human immunoglobulins but not in any other species. The term *isotypy* is given to species-specific antigenic systems.

Class Specificity

Antisera may also recognize specificities limited to a given immunoglobulin class, such as anti-immunoglobulin G that does not react with IgA, IgM, IgD, or IgE.

Subclass Specificity

Antisera may specifically identify the IgG subclasses (IgG_1, IgG_2, IgG_3, IgG_4). Such antisera usually require absorption to remove IgG common specificities.

Fragment Specificity

Antisera may also be specific for the Fab, Fc, or Fd fragment of an immunoglobulin. This specificity may be so exact as to require the fragment as antigen; reaction with native IgG does not occur.

Chain Specificity

Similar specificities may also be produced for L-chains or H-chains.

Allotype Specificity

Immunoglobulins also carry genetically controlled antigenic specificities termed allotypes (21). Allotypes are antigenic specificities which differ among individuals of the same species. In experimental animals antisera to allotypes are produced by immunizing an animal that does not carry the given specificity with immunoglobulin from an individual that does carry the specificity. As many as 30 different allotype specificities have been identified in humans. Human immunoglobulin allotypes are discussed below.

Denatured Immunoglobulin Specificity

Antisera produced to heat denatured or chemically denatured immunoglobulin may react only with denatured immunoglobulins and not with native immunoglobulins. Denaturation, if not extensive, causes the unfolding or refolding of the molecule so that determinants not present on the native molecule are revealed (9).

Anti-Antibody Specificity

An antibody that reacts with another antibody is termed anti-antibody (14). Anti-antibody reacts with an immunoglobulin molecule because that molecule is an antibody, not just because it is an immunoglobulin. Anti-antibody is best produced by immunizing an animal with an antibody–antigen complex. An animal so immunized may produce 1) antibody that reacts with the antigen; 2) antibody that reacts with the antibody, but also reacts with normal immunoglobulin; 3) antibody that reacts with the complex of antibody and antigen, but not with either uncomplexed antibody or antigen (anti-complex); and 4) antibody that reacts with the antibody itself in native form, but does not react with other normal immunoglobulin. In this last example, individual determinants wholly specific to particular antibodies in a mixture of immunoglobulins are recognized. Such characteristic specificity limited to a single group of proteins (antibody) within a larger population of molecules (immunoglobulins) common to all individuals of a species is termed an *idiotype* (14). The simplest explanation is that such anti-antibodies are directed toward the antigen-binding site of the reactant antibody molecules and that this site is not present in detectable amounts in the normal immunoglobulin population. If this were so then antiidiotypic antibodies should be limited in their specificity of reactivity. Indeed, some different individuals in a given strain of mouse produce antibody with the same idiotypic specificity when immunized with the same antigen (22). However, antibodies to the same antigen may also elicit anti-antibodies that are specific for each antibody and do not cross-react, and anti-antibodies of this type may not interfere with the antigen binding activity of the first antibody. In addition, reaction of the antibody with the specific antigen may not block reaction with the antiidiotypic antibody (2). Therefore sites on the antibody not responsible for antigen-binding, but genetically codetermined with the antigen-binding site, must be responsible. The original antigen must elicit the production of antibody in a restricted population of immunoglobulins that are not present, or are present in undetectable amount, in normal sera of other animals or in the preimmunization serum of the same animal. On the other hand, antiidiotypic antibodies have been produced which do react with the antigen-binding sites of some antibodies (2,35).

Antireceptor Antibodies

Antireceptor antibodies (antibodies that react with the recognition site of antibody molecules) may be produced by 1) immunization with myeloma proteins with antigen binding activity (3), 2) immunization with antibody (Rajewsky, unpublished data), or 3) reaction of the host to receptor sites on cells producing a graft-vs-host reaction (30a). In this latter situation, the antireceptor antibody also reacts with immunoglobulin antibody that reacts with the antigen responsible for graft rejection. This, plus the findings that

T cell activity of mice can be blocked by antireceptor antibody (1a) and antibody production can be inhibited by antireceptor, strongly suggests that the antigen receptor of T and B cells is the same (see also page 40).

Complex Specificity

Anti-complex anti-antibody is formed to new determinants revealed by alteration of the quarternary structure of the antibody, the antigen, or both as a result of formation of the antibody–antigen complex (14). This is similar to the determinants revealed by partial denaturation of immunoglobulins. Anti-complex antibody reacts with the antibody only when it is complexed with antigen. Anti-complex antibodies have been recognized that require the whole antibody molecule in complex form for reaction, while other anti-complex antibodies react with the Fab or Fc fragment of the complexed molecule.

HUMAN IMMUNOGLOBULIN ALLOTYPES

Human immunoglobulins carry genetically controlled antigenic speci-ficities termed allotypes (17,27). Human immunoglobulin allotypes are detected by hemagglutination inhibition (see Chapter 6). This detection system depends upon the ability of antigenic immunoglobulin to inhibit the agglutination of erythrocytes coated with antigen when the coated cells are treated with antibody. The detection system is as follows: O RH + human red cells are coated with subhemagglutinating doses of im-munoglobulin by the addition of anti-Rh, or by cells coated with myeloma proteins of a given allotype using chromic chloride as the coupling agent. These coated cells are then used as the indicator particles. The coated cells are agglutinated by antibody that reacts with the immunoglobulin coating the red cell (direct Coombs' test). Antibodies to human immuno-globulin allotypes may be found in the sera of normal individuals (serum normal agglutinators, SNagg) or in the sera of patients with rheumatoid arthritis (rheumatoid agglutinators, Ragg) that agglutinate cells coated with immunoglobulins of some individuals but do not agglutinate cells coated with immunoglobulins of other individuals. For the detection of human immunoglobulin allotype Gm 1, a serum containing Gm 1 is mixed with a SNagg that reacts with Gm 1 so that the anti-Gm 1 is neutralized. The mixture is then added to cells coated with immunoglobulin containing the Gm 1 specificity. Since the anti-Gm 1 has been neutralized, it is unable to agglutinate the Gm 1-coated cells. If the serum tested did not contain Gm 1, it would be unable to inhibit the reaction of anti-Gm 1 with the Gm 1-coated cells. Careful testing of the system must be done to rule out the other immunoglobulin specificities described above.

Allotypic Specificities

Using such techniques, up to 30 different allotypic specificities have been identified in humans (17,27,28). These are divided into two groups–the Gm, with up to 25 specificities, the Inv, with 3 specificities, in addition, allotypes restricted to IgA and IgM classes have been reported (12). The properties of these specificities are tabulated in Table 5–3. The allotypes are given numerical designation herein, although many workers still use the earlier alphabetical notation (28). The Gm specificities are found only in IgG and are located on the γ-chain. Different specificities are found in the IgG subclasses and are inherited in fixed combinations. In order to simplify the data, the alleles for each subclass are termed a and b.

TABLE 5–3
Allotypic Markers of Human Immunoglobulins Gm and Inv

Spe-cificity	Ig class	Allelic cistron	Molec-ular localiza-tion	Frequency (%)		Comment
				white	negro	
Gm 1*	IgG_1	a	Fc	60	100	Inherited en bloc with Gm 17
2	IgG_1	a	Fc	25	0	Rarely found in Gm (−1) individuals
3	IgG_1	b	Fd	90	0	Expression requires association with L-chain
4*	IgG_1	b	Fd	90	0	Expression requires association with L-chain
5*	IgG_3	b	Fc	90	100	Almost always found with Gm 3
6	IgG_3	b	Fc	<1	40	Always associated with Gm 5
7	IgG_1	a		50	100	Associated with Gm 1 and Gm 20
8	IgG_1	b		95	50	Associated with Gm 4
9	IgG_1	b	Fc	85	40	Associated with Gm 4
10	IgG_3	b		95		Probably same as Gm 13
11	IgG_3	b		90	90	Associated with Gm 5
12	IgG_3	b		90	100	Probably same as Gm 5
13	IgG_3	b		90	90	Associated with Gm 5
14	IgG_3	b		90	90	Almost always found with Gm 5
15	IgG_3	b		<1	20	Always associated with Gm 13
16	IgG_3	b		<1	0	Frequency of 30% in Mongoloids
17	IgG_1	a	Fd	60	100	High association with Gm 1
18	IgG_1	a	Fc	20	50	High association with Gm 1 and Gm 2
19				12		Data insufficient
20	IgG_1	a	Fc	45	90	High association with Gm 1, 7
21	IgG_3	a		50	<10	Found only in Gm (−11) individuals
22	IgG_1	b	Fc	90	0	Inherited en bloc with Gm 4
23	IgG_2	a†	Fc	90	0	Only Gm specificity detected by precipitation; rarely occurs in Gm (−4) individuals
Am 1	IgA_2	?	Fc	90	0	
Inv 1	All	a	κ	20	30	Rarely found in Inv (−2) individuals
2	All	a	κ	20	30	Found only with Inv 1
3	All	b	κ	80	70	Inv (−1, −2, −3) individuals rare

* Gm 1 and Gm 4, as well as Gm 1 and Gm 5, are inherited as alleles in Caucasians, but are found associated in some Mongoloids.
† Gm specificity for the allele of Gm 23 has not been identified.

TABLE 5–4
Allelic Distribution of Gm Specificities

IgG class	Percent of IgG	Alleles	Gm specificities
IgG₁	70	a	1, 17 (2, 7, 18, 20)
		b	22, 4 (3, 8, 9)
IgG₂	18	a	23
		b	—23
IgG₃	8	a	21
		b	5, 11, 13, 14 (10, 12, 14, 15, 16)
IgG₄	3		None identified

* Inconsistently found Gm specificities are given in parentheses. No Gm specificity has been identified as the allele for Gm 23 and no Gm specificities have been identified for the IgG₄ subclass.

For the IgG₁ subclass the two alleles are IgG₁ₐ and IgG₁ᵦ. The Gm specificities controlled by each allele for each subclass are given in Table 5–4. This type of designation is really oversimplified as the genetic analysis of the actual serologically defined specificities is much more complicated (28). Most of the specificities are located on the Fc fragment of the appropriate IgG subclass, but IgG₁ molecules also have specificities on the Fd piece. No Gm specificities have been identified by the IgG₄ subclass. The Inv specificities are located on the κ light chains of each immunoglobulin class and are determined by a single amino substitution of position 191 of the κ-chain.

As indicated in Table 5–3, data on many of the Gm specificities are incomplete. Some specificities, such as Gm 5, 10, 11, 12, 13, 14, and 15, may be identical or part of a common larger specificity. Gm 2 is never found in the absence of Gm 1, but only about one-quarter of Gm 1 Caucasions are Gm 2, and essentially all Negroes are Gm 1, 2. Gm 2 may represent a part of a Gm 1 specificity not expressed in all Gm 1 individuals.

Nonmarkers

Through the study of unique Ig molecules represented by myeloma proteins, genetically controlled antigenic determinants present in only one subclass but allelic with determinants shared by two or more subclasses have been identified (28). Since one allelic specificity is unique for a subclass while the other specificity is shared by subclasses, the shared specificity is termed a "nonmarker." An example of such a nonmarker is non-Gm 1. This specificity is found in all Gm 1 negative IgG₁ proteins as well as in all IgG₂ and IgG₃ proteins regardless of genetic type. Therefore, Gm 1 may represent a genetic event occuring in the cistron for IgG₁ only and producing the allelic specificities Gm 1 and non-Gm 1 for the IgG₁ subclass but not for IgG₂ or IgG₃ subclasses which contain non-Gm 1 only.

The IgG$_4$ subclass illustrates a unique relationship between two antigens shared by the other subclasses. Two specificities 4a and 4b are present on different IgG$_4$ protein molecules; IgG$_4$ molecules either contain 4a or 4b but not both. Among the other subclasses 4a is found in all IgG$_1$ and IgG$_3$ proteins, but IgG$_2$ proteins have 4b. Since all human sera contain both 4a and 4b determinants, these specificities can only serve as markers for IgG$_4$ when detected on isolated IgG$_4$ molecules. When the IgG$_1$, IgG$_2$ and IgG$_3$ subclasses are removed, the 4a and 4b determinants can be used as markers for the IgG$_4$ subclass, and behave as if controlled by alleles. These nonmarkers have valuable uses in characterizing some of the rare IgG gene complexes. Even though our understanding of human Ig allotypes is incomplete, considerable analysis of the genetics of human immunoglobulin allotypes is possible.

GENETIC ANALYSIS OF HUMAN GM ALLOTYPES

Human immunoglobulin allotypic markers are highly specific, inbuilt, genetically dependent labels which may be used to analyze the genetic control of immunoglobulin structure. Allotypic determinants show strict adherence to Mendelian law and are inherited as codominant alleles. Studies of amino acid sequence of the polypeptide chains of immunoglobulins reveal that the allotypic specificities are associated with amino acid sequence. The number of amino acid substitutions between two allelic allotypes is one, or at the most two. The known genetic markers are located on "constant" portions of the immunoglobulin chain. No human genetic marker has been found on the amino terminal quarter of the H-chain or the amino terminal half of the L-chain. Therefore, allotypic determinants are not believed to be involved in the antibody-combining site. The simultaneous variability and stability within regions of the immunoglobulin polypeptide chains and the sharing of multiple antibody-combining activity in different classes of immunoglobulins indicate that an array of structural information in the genome is active in the production of a given immunoglobulin chain.

To clarify the following discussion of the genetics of the human allotype system, certain genetic terms must be defined. A *codon* is a trinucleotide sequence of chromosomal DNA that codes for one amino acid. A *cistron* is a linear array of codons, the total number of which is required for the synthesis of a given polypeptide chain. (The term gene, because of its historical connotation, is not used here, but may be considered as synonymous with cistron). A *locus* is the location of a cistron on a chromosome as determined by genetic mapping. *Alleles* are alternative cistrons. Any given diploid individual normally carries a pair of allelic cistrons. A *mutation* is a change in one or more nucleotides of a codon which causes the codon to code for a different amino acid. A *crossover* is a partial exchange of codons between allelic cistrons or an exchange of cistrons between paired chromosomes. A *chromosome* is a sequence of linked cistrons usually inherited as a unit.

The number of cistrons coding for the Gm allotypes of IgG must be no less than eight. This does not include cistrons coding for other immunoglobulins or other allotypes. The variability controlled by the Gm cistrons is in the germ line of the individual and is represented by eight different IgG γ-chains that can be recognized. These eight cistrons also include the genetic information coding for antibody-binding sites of the IgG molecules. The wide variety of antigen-binding specificities of antibodies within the IgG class suggests an almost infinite number of cistrons coding for antigen binding. The most intriguing problem in immunology today involves an explanation of antibody variability on the basis of present genetic theory.

The cistrons controlling Gm specificities are closely linked. Crossing-over between IgG cistrons has been directly observed in some family studies (27). The recombination frequencies have been estimated as follows: IgG_1 and IgG_3, 1:1,000 to 1:10,000; IgG_1 and IgG_2, 1:100 to 1:1000. The recombination data indicate the order of H-chain cistrons as IgG_2, IgG_3, IgG_1. The IgG_4 cistron may be next to that of IgG_2. This order is in agreement with linkage analysis and gene complexes in various population groups (see Table 5–5) (27). The existence of a hybrid IgG_1–IgG_3 molecule in rare individuals is direct evidence for the existence of cistron crossover.

The association of IgG_1 Gm markers in different populations indicates that crossing-over within IgG_1 cistrons may occur. Gm 1 is located on the Fc piece of IgG_1, and Gm 17 is located on the Fd piece of IgG_1. These markers are invariably found together, as are Gm 4 and Gm 22 which represent the allelic cistron. This evidence indicates that the Fc and Fd markers are not coded for by separate cistrons. Gm 1 is the Fc marker associated with the Fd marker Gm 17, and Gm 4 is the Fd marker associated with the Fc marker Gm 22 in Caucasians. However, Gm 1 and Gm 4 are controlled by the same cistron in some Chinese, and analysis of myeloma proteins containing Gm 1 and Gm 4 from Chinese patients demonstrates that Gm 1 and Gm 4 specificities appear on the same immunoglobulin molecule.

There appears to be a series of codon sequences within a given cistron coding for variable and constant segments of the immunoglobulin polypeptide chain. Considerable segments of the chains of IgG_1, IgG_2, and IgG_3 have the same amino acid sequences. This observation is also true among

TABLE 5–5
Frequency of Gm Allelic Combinations in Different Populations

Allelic combinations			Frequency among			
IgG_2	IgG_3	IgG_1	Caucasian	Negro	Japanese	Chinese
a	b	b	0.52	0	0	0
a	a	a	0.005	0	0	0
b	b	b	0.17	0	0	0
b	a	a	0.30	0	0.65	0.05
b	b	a	0.008	1	0.25	0.2
a	a	b	0.005	0	0	0
b	a	b	0.005	0	0	0
a	b	a	0	0	0	0
a	b	a/b*	0	0	0.1	0.75

* Gm (1, 4)

the immunoglobulin classes IgG, IgA, IgM, etc. Approximately 30 out of every 100 amino acids are the same. Even within the variable sequence areas, the amino terminal half of L-chains and the amino terminal quarter of H-chains, there are many amino acid homologs among immunoglobulin classes (4,16,19). The variable sequences contain "hot spots" of 4–7 amino acids that have great variability. Therefore γ chain-cistrons must contain arrays of identical codons mixed with arrays of different codons. This interpretation has been used to support the concept of cistron duplication in the evolution of immunoglobulins (see Phylogeny of Immunoglobulins, later in this chapter).

Further evidence for cistron duplication is the presence of a single amino acid substitution at position 190 of human light chains producing two different chains OZ (+) and OZ (−). The OZ (+) determinant is recognized by a rabbit antiserum and is present in λ chains of all individuals; neither the OZ (+) nor OZ (−) chains are produced by allelic cistrons; rather they are products of recently duplicated λ chain constant region genes.

Population Studies of IgG Allotypes

Since IgG allotypic determinants are inherited in classic Mendelian codominant fashion, the distribution of these markers can be used by anthropologists to study population mixing. Thirty percent Caucasian admixture in American Negroes has been estimated using Gm factors, a figure that is essentially identical with that proposed from studies using the hemoglobulin S marker (12). Analysis of Gm factor distribution in Europe indicates that the highest frequency of Gm 1 occurs at the northeast corner with a steady decline toward the south and west (12,36).

MYELOMA PROTEINS

The study of the structure and function of human immunoglobulins has been made possible by the production of homogeneous immunoglobulins by plasma cell neoplasms (multiple myeloma, macroglobulinemia) (1,29). From the sera of individuals with such tumors relatively homogeneous proteins can be isolated. These homogeneous immunoglobulins can then be studied and structural analyses made that are not possible using normal immunoglobulins because of the great heterogeneity of normal immunoglobulins. Myelomas producing proteins representing each of the major immunoglobulin classes and each of the four subclasses of IgG have been found.

Waldenström's macroglobulinemia is caused by a tumor of IgM-producing cells, which may be considered a variant of multiple myeloma. In addition, myelomas may produce only part of an immunoglobulin molecule (1,29,33). Those found include synthesis of L-chain, H-chain (H-chain disease), and Fc fragment of γ-chain. Patients with myelomas that produce an excess of L-chain will excrete free L-chain in their urine (Bence Jones protein). The presence of Bence Jones proteins has been used as a diagnostic test for myeloma for over 100 years, but the identification of this

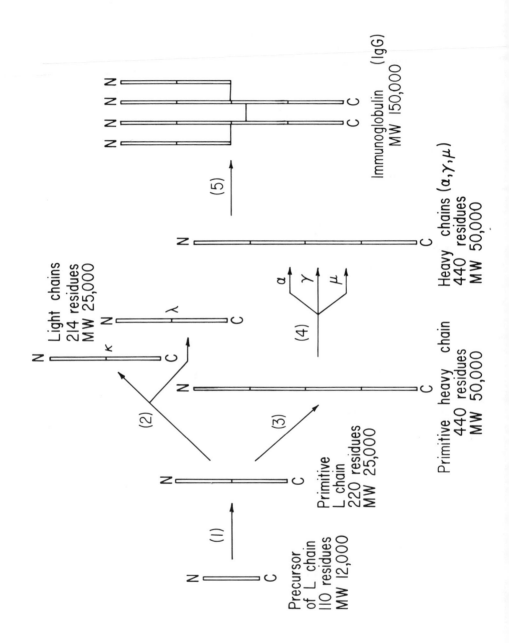

Precursor
of L chain
110 residues
MW 12,000

(1)

Primitive
L chain
220 residues
MW 25,000

(2)

Light chains
214 residues
MW 25,000

κ

λ

(3)

Primitive heavy chain
440 residues
MW 50,000

(4)

α
γ
μ

Heavy chains (α,γ,μ)
440 residues
MW 50,000

(5)

Immunoglobulin (IgG)
MW 150,000

protein as L-chains of immunoglobulins has only recently been made. When urine containing Bence Jones protein is heated to 50–60°C, a white cloudy precipitate appears; but when the temperature is raised to near the boiling point, the precipitate redissolves. Bence Jones protein is observed in about 50% of myeloma patients. Recent developments in immunoglobulin quantitation permit identification of other myeloma proteins in sera and have aided in the diagnosis of myeloma and macroglobulinemia.

SYNTHESIS AND ASSEMBLY OF IMMUNOGLOBULINS

Immunoglobulin molecules are synthesized, assembled, and secreted by plasma cells (33). This process is generally the same as protein synthesis in other mammalian cells, knowledge of which has largely been extrapolated from studies of bacterial systems (7). Genetic information is encoded in DNA (deoxyribonucleic acid) of the nucleus and is transcribed in messenger RNA (ribonucleic acid). The messenger RNA molecules are released into the cytoplasm where they become associated with a number of ribosomes to form a polyribosome. The polyribosome is the basic unit of protein synthesis. The messenger RNA is aligned on the ribosome in such a way that transfer RNA molecules charged with the proper amino acids become arranged so that, with the help of specific enzymes, the amino acids are incorporated into a polypeptide chain. When translation of the message is completed, the newly synthesized polypeptide is released with the cytoplasm.

The production of immunoglobulins by myelomas is the model system used to study immunoglobulin synthesis (33). L-chains and H-chains are produced on different sized ribosomes. H-chain polyribosomes contain 12–18 ribosomes and L-chain polyribosomes 7 or 8. Newly synthesized L-chains enter a rapidly turning-over pool and then become associated with H-chains. Disulfide bonds usually form between free L-chains and H-chains still on the H-chain ribosome. However, assembly differs among different myelomas. In some cases one L- and one H-chain are formed prior to formation of the inter-H-chain bond, while in others the inter-H-chain bond forms first, followed by bonding of the L-chains. Partially assembled molecules, such as half molecules of one L- and one H-chain joined together, may be formed, as well as L-chains alone (Bence Jones proteins) or H-chains alone (H-chain disease). However, normal lymphoid cells pro-

---

Fig. 5–4. **Development of immunoglobulin diversity—germ line theory.** According to a germ line theory, germ cells contain all the DNA required for the structural genes of immunoglobulins and these genes have developed from duplication of a single ancestral precursor during evolution (see text). These genes are not modified during somatic development. Stimulation of antibody formation is accomplished by selection by the antigen of cells that have the capacity to produce the specific antibody, clonal selection. (Reproduced, with permission, from "On the Mechanism of Immunity—In Defense of Evolution," by EP Cohen, Ann Rev Microbiol. Vol. 22. © 1968 by Annual Reviews, Inc. All rights reserved.)

duce essentially equal numbers of L- and H-chains. The mechanisms of initiation of polypeptide synthesis by ribosomes, of release of formed chains from ribosomes, and of secretion of immunoglobulins from plasma cells are poorly understood but are under study.

THEORIES OF ORIGIN OF IMMUNOGLOBULIN DIVERSITY

GERM LINE THEORY

Immunoglobulin molecules have been identified and studied in a variety of fish, amphibian, reptile, bird, and mammalian species (4,16,19). A phylogenetic tree based on the homology in primary structure (amino acid sequence) and intrachain linkages has been assumed (16,19). It is postulated that a primitive immunoglobulin gene coding for a peptide chain equal in length to one-half an L-chain developed in the prevertebrate era. The most primitive immunoglobulins yet found in vertebrates consist of fully developed L- and H-chains. The genes responsible for fully developed chains are believed to have developed through gene duplication (germ line theory) (4,16,19) (Fig. 5–4). One duplication would result in a gene for a complete L-chain (constant and variable half). Additional duplications would be required for production of a polypeptide chain the length of the H-chain (four primitive units). A subsequent duplication of the L-chain gene produced genes for the two L-chains, κ and λ. The most primitive H-chain identified (cyclostomes) is homologous to the μ-chain of IgM. Further gene duplication and divergence in teleosts and amphibians resulted in a gene coding for a chain homologous to the γ-chain of IgG. The α-chain may have resulted from a further duplication of the μ-chain gene, and the δ- and ϵ-chains from duplication of the γ-chain gene. Later duplication of the γ-chain gene resulted in evolution of the IgG subclasses. This scheme is highly speculative and is mainly dependent on the observation that L-chain consists of two ~12,000-MW units (the variable and constant regions) and the H-chain consists of four ~12,000-MW units (one variable region similar to that of the L-chain and three constant regions). Thus duplication of a gene coding for ~12,000-MW polypeptide chain could account for the evolution of human immunoglobulins (2,16,19).

SOMATIC MUTATION THEORY

According to the somatic mutation theories, a small number of germ line genes become highly diversified during development of the individual resulting in the formation of a large number of differentiated immunocompetent cells capable of recognizing individually a variety of antigens. This may be accomplished by point mutations occurring successively, perhaps through the influence of antigenic contact (26) or by recombination of inherited germ line V genes during somatic cell division (13) (Fig. 5–5).

At the present time it is impossible to choose between the gene line and somatic mutation theories for the generation of immunoglobulin diversity. The basic genetic information is probably derived from germ line diversity developed during evolution, and additional diversity arises during somatic development.

POINT MUTATION   RECOMBINATION

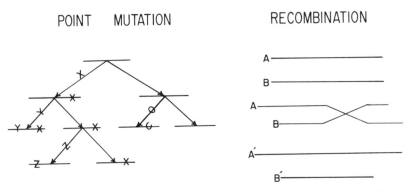

Fig. 5–5. Development of immunoglobulin diversity—somatic theories. Somatic generation of immunoglobulin diversity may occur as the result of point mutations or because of recombination (crossing over) of DNA strands. During the process of point mutation, some of the bases on a DNA strand are disrupted. The disruption is repaired, but during repair a base substitution is made. Replication of this substitution gives rise to cells that produce new types of Ig molecules. Recombination occurs during cell division, producing misalignment of the two strands. This crossing over leads to creation of new cistron alignments, new Ig classes and different specific antibodies.

REFERENCES

1. Bernier GM: Structure of human immunoglobulins: Myeloma proteins as analogues of antibody. Prog Allergy 14:1, 1970
1a. Binz H, Lindeman J, Wigzell H: Cell-bound receptors for alloantigens on normal lymphocytes. II. Antialloantibody serum contains specific factors reacting with relevant immunocompetent T lymphocytes. J Exp Med 140:731, 1974
2. Brient BW, Nisonoff A: Quantitative investigations of idiotypic antibodies. IV. Inhibition of specific haptens of the reaction of anti-hapten antibody with its anti-idiotypic antibody. J Exp Med 132:951, 1970
3. Cosenza H, Kohler H: Specific suppression of the antibody response by antibodies to receptors. Proc Natl Acad Sci USA 69:2710, 1972
4. Cohen EP: On the mechanism of immunity: In defense of evolution. Ann Rev Microbiol (Stanford) 22:283, 1968
5. Cohen S, Milstein C: Structure and biologic properties of immunoglobulins. Adv Immunol 7:1, 1967
6. Committee on Nomenclature of Human Immunoglobulins. Notation for genetic factors of human immunoglobulins. Bull WHO 30:447, 1964
7. Crick FHC: On protein synthesis. Symp Soc Exp Biol 12:138, 1958
8. Edelman GM, Cunningham BA, Gall WE, Gottlieb PD, Rutishauser U, Waxdal MJ: The covalent structure of an entire γG-immunoglobulin molecule. Biochemistry 63:78, 1969
9. Epstein CH, Goldberger RF, Anfinsen CB: The genetic control of tertiary protein structure: Studies with model systems. Symp Quant Biol 28:439, 1963
10. Fahey JL: Antibodies and immunoglobulins. JAMA 194:141, 183, 1966
11. Franklin EC: Immune globulins: Their structure and function and some techniques for their isolation. Prog Allergy 8:58, 1964
12. Fudenberg HH, Pink JRL, Stites DP, Wang A-C: Basic Immunogenetics. New York, Oxford University Press, 1972
13. Gally JA, Edelman GM: Genetic control of immunoglobulin synthesis. Ann Rev Genet 6:1, 1972
14. Gell PGH, Kelus AS: Anti-antibodies. Adv Immunol 6:461, 1967
15. Green NM: Electron microscopy of the immunoglobulins. Adv Immunol 11:1, 1969

16. Grey HM: Phylogeny of immunoglobulins. Adv Immunol 10:51, 1969
17. Grubb R: The Genetic Markers of Human Immunoglobulins. In Molecular Biology, Biochemistry, and Biophysics. Vol 9. Kleinzeller A, Springer GF, Wittmann HG (eds). Berlin, Springer, 1970
18. Halpern MS, Koshland ME: The stoichiometry of J chain in human secretory IgA. J Immunol 111:1563–1660, 1973
19. Hood L, Talmadge DW: Mechanism of antibody diversity: Germ line basis for variability. Science 168:325, 1970
20. Kabat EA: General features of antibody molecules. In Specific Receptors of Antibodies, Antigens and Cells. Pressman D, Tomasi, Jr TB, Grossberg AL, Rose NR (eds) Basel, Karger, 1973
21. Kelus AS, Gell PGH: Immunoglobulin allotypes of experimental animals. Prog Allogy 11:141, 1967
22. Kuettner MG, Wang AL, Nisonoff A: Quantitative investigations of idiotypic antibodies. VI. Idiotypic specificity as a potential genetic marker for the variable regions of mouse immunoglobulin polypeptide chains. J Exp Med 135:579, 1972
23. Linderstrøm-Lang K: Proteins and Enzymes. Lane Medical Lectures, Stanford University Medical Series 6. Palo Alto, Calif., Stanford University Press, 1952
24. Merler E, Rosen FS: The gamma globulins. I. The Structure and synthesis of the immunoglobulins. N Engl J Med 275:480, 536, 1964
25. Metzger H: The chemistry of the immunoglobulins. JAMA 202:129, 1967
26. Milstein C, Pink JRL: Structure and evolution of immunoglobulins. Prog Biophys Mol Biol 21:211, 1970
27. Natvig JB, Kunkel HG: Genetic markers of human immunoglobulins: The Gm and InV systems. Ser Haematol 1:66, 1968
28. Natvig JB, Kunkel HG: Human immunoglobulins: classes, subclasses, genetic varients and idiotypes. Adv Immunol 16:1, 1973
29. Osserman EF, Takatsuki K: Plasma cell myeloma: Gamma globulin synthesis and structure. Medicine 42:357, 1963
30. Padlan EA, Segal DM, Spande TF, Davis DR, Rudikoff S, Potter M: Structure at 4.5 Å resolution of a phosphorylcholine-binding Fab. Nature [New Biol] 245:165, 1973
30a. Ramseier H, Lindenmann J: Aliotypic antibodies. Transplant Rev 10:57–96, 1972
31. Rowe DS, Hug K, Forni L, Pernis B: Immunoglobulin D as a lymphocyte receptor. J Exp Med 138:965, 1973
32. Rowley DA, Fitch FW, Stuart FP, Köhler H, Cosenza H: Specific suppression of immune responses. Science 181:1133, 1973
33. Scharff MD, Laskov R: Synthesis and assembly of immunoglobulin polypeptide chains. Prog Allergy 14:37, 1970
34. Speigelberg H: D Immunoglobulin. In Contemporary Topics in Immunochemistry. Inman FP (ed). Plenum Publishing Co, New York, 1:165–180, 1972
35. Spring-Stewart S, Nisonoff A: Effect of blocking the active site of an antibody on the expression of its idiotypic determinants during immunization. J Immunol 110:679, 1973
36. Steinberg AC: Globulin polymorphisms in man. Ann Rev Genetics 3:25, 1969
37. Svehag SE, Bloth B: Ultrastructure of secretory and high-polymer serum immunoglobulin A of human and rabbit origin. Science 168:847, 1970
38. Talmadge DW, Cann JR: The Chemistry of Immunity in Health and Disease. Springfield Ill, Thomas, 1961
39. Tomasi TB, Bienenstock J: Secretory immunoglobulins. Adv Immunol 9:1, 1968
40. Uhr JW: The heterogeneity of the immune response. Science 145:457, 1964

6

Antibody–Antigen Reactions

The ultimate result of immunization with an antigen is the production of specifically modified immunoglobulin molecules (antibodies) or specifically sensitized cells that react with the immunizing antigen. The joining of antibody to antigen to form an antibody–antigen complex depends upon the close physical approximation of oppositely charged ionic groups (31).

ANTIGENIC DETERMINANTS

The unit or part of an antigen molecule with which an antibody reacts is an antigenic determinant. Although the concept of an antigenic determinant or antigenic site is a convenient one for understanding antigen–antibody reactions, the actual identification of a specific antigenic determinant is difficult (18).

ANTIBODY SPECIFICITY AND ANTIGENIC DETERMINANTS

In order to investigate the antigenic determinant, use has been made of low molecular weight incomplete antigens (haptens). Chemically defined haptens, such as p-azobenzoate, are combined with a protein carrier for immunization (induction of antibody to p-azobenzoate). The specificity of reaction of the antibodies formed is tested by reacting the antibodies with chemically related haptens attached to the same or to different carrier proteins. Using such a technique, Kitagawa et al. (22) determined that there was a great heterogeneity in the specificity of antibodies to even a simple hapten (Fig. 6–1). An ideal binding of an antibody to an antigenic site is shown at the left of the figure, where the antibody-combining site fits snugly over the entire surface of the hapten. For a high-affinity bond, there would be a close apposition of oppositely charged ionic groups between the surfaces of the antibody-combining site and the antigen site. When the antibodies to such a hapten were actually tested, a range of combining specificities was found, as illustrated in the right-hand drawing

87

ANTIBODY   ANTIBODIES

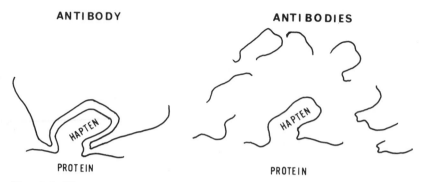

PROTEIN   PROTEIN

Fig. 6–1. **Heterogeneity of antibody specificity.** Outline of hapten represents
van der Waals' outline of *p*-azobenzoate group coupled to protein carrier. Drawing
(**left**) represents idealized antibody that might be formed to such an antigenic
structure. Since strength and specificity of antibody–antigen binding depend upon
close approximation of oppositely charged ionic groups between antibody and antigen, binding site of ideal antibody would present configuration that would fold
closely over antigenic determinant (in this case, hapten) and provide close apposition of ionic groups oppositely charged to those of antigenic determinant. Antibodies actually produced to such a hapten (**right**) consist of a mixed group of
specificities and avidities. Some antibodies appear to bind to some parts of antigenic determinant and others to other parts of determinant, with varying degrees
of overlapping specificity. (Modified from Kitagawa M, Yagi Y, Pressman D: J
Immunol 95:455, 1965. © Copyright 1965, The Williams & Wilkins Co.)

of Figure 6–1. Thus, even to a relatively simple chemical configuration
a wide variety of antibody-combining sites on different antibody molecules
is produced upon immunization. If such heterogeneity of specificity is found
in antibodies to a simple hapten, it is not difficult to imagine the wide
range of specificities that might be found in antibodies produced in response
to immunization by more complex protein molecules containing many antigenic sites or by contact with infectious agents containing multiple antigenic
specificities of different molecules.

ANTIBODY–ANTIGEN BINDING SITES

The strength of binding of antibody and antigen depends upon the
closeness of geometric apposition and the number of ionic groups of opposite charge that occur in the binding site (31). The specificity of the reaction is thus determined by the complementarity of antigen and antibody
(21). A tight fit is important because the combining forces involved act
only at short range and are weak, so that fairly large areas of the reacting
molecules must come into close contact.

PRIMARY ANTIBODY–ANTIGEN REACTIONS

The combination of antigen with antibody to form an antigen–antibody
complex is termed the primary reaction. This primary reaction may be

considered as an establishment of equilibrium between free antigen and free antibody on one side, and bound antigen and antibody (complex) on the other side of the equilibrium equation.

Attempts have been made to measure directly the primary reaction of antigen and antibody without relying on secondary effects such as precipitation and lysis (see below). Perhaps the most satisfactory attempt at such measurements has been made by Farr (13) in his studies of the equilibrium between bovine serum albumin (BSA) and rabbit antibody to bovine serum albumin (anti-BSA). This method depends on the fact that radiolabeled BSA (BSA*) is soluble in 50% saturated ammonium sulfate, whereas the anti-BSA (γ-globulin) and BSA*—anti-BSA complexes are not.

Antigen-Binding Capacity

The antigen-binding capacity (ABC) of a given antiserum is determined by diluting the antiserum in normal serum until 33% of a constant concentration of BSA* is precipitated as BSA*—anti-BSA complexes by 50% saturated ammonium sulfate. The ABC-33 value is calculated from the dilution of antiserum that gives 33% precipitation and is expressed as micrograms of BSA* bound per milliliter of antiserum.

Affinity

The strength of attractiveness between antibody and antigen is termed affinity. The effect of dilution of antiserum may be used as a measure of qualitative differences in the ability of antibody to bind antigen. Antisera collected during the first 2 weeks of a primary response are more affected by dilution than antisera collected later in the primary response or after a booster immunization (secondary response). If the antibodies present in a dilute solution are able to bind to antigen as well as antibodies in a more concentrated solution, the antibodies have a strong affinity for the antigen. This dilution effect measures the antigen–antibody reaction represented by the reaction to the right of the equilibrium equation:

$$Ab + Ag \rightarrow AgAb$$

Avidity

Avidity is the strength of the antibody–antigen bond after formation of antibody–antigen complexes. This property is a measure of the reaction to the left of the equilibrium equation:

$$Ab + Ag \leftarrow AgAb$$

The avidity of an antibody–antigen reaction can be measured by the degree of dissociation of antigen–antibody complex to free antibody and free antigen after formation of the complex. The time required for dissociation of antigen–antibody complexes should be independent of the concentration of free antigen present, since the concentration of free antigen affects only the association time. Farr studied the rate of exchange between antibody-bound BSA* and unlabeled, unbound BSA. To a series of tubes containing a fixed amount of BSA* bound to anti-BSA was added an excess of un-labeled BSA. When BSA*—anti-BSA dissociated, unlabeled antigen would replace the labeled antigen in the association reaction because of its presence in excess. At intervals after addition of the excess of unlabeled BSA, the percent of the labeled BSA still bound to antibody was determined. The avidity of an antiserum can be estimated by the time required for the dissociation of a given amount of labeled antigen. From such determinations the relative binding strength of different antisera can be compared.

Antigen-Precipitating Capacity

The antigen-precipitating capacity of an antiserum may also be measured with Farr's method. The end point is that dilution of antiserum at which 80% of 0.1 mg BSA* nitrogen is precipitated (see Precipitin Reaction, below) and is designated the P80. The P80 for an antiserum is expressed as γBSA N precipitable per milliliter of undiluted serum.

The relation between the antigen-binding capacity (ABC-33) and the antigen-precipitating capacity (P80) of a given antiserum is revealing. The P80 is usually 15–30% of the ABC-33. However, occasional antisera have a P80 of less than 5% of the ABC-33. This indicates that such antisera contain antibody that binds with antigen but does not precipitate (nonprecipitating antibody). The explanation for this heterogeneity in the properties of different antisera to the same antigen lies in the diversity of immunoglobulin molecules. Antibody molecules directed toward the same antigen may belong to different immunoglobulin classes or subclasses and therefore behave differently when complexed with antigen.

SECONDARY ANTIBODY–ANTIGEN REACTIONS

Following the combination of antibody and antigen, a number of different phenomena may be observed, depending upon the conditions under which the primary reaction takes place (45). These phenomena are termed secondary reactions:

$$\text{Ag} + \text{Ab} \underset{\substack{\text{Primary} \\ \text{reaction}}}{\rightleftharpoons} \underset{\text{complex}}{\text{AgAb}} \rightarrow \text{Secondary reactions}$$

Secondary reactions due to the formation of antigen–antibody complexes depend upon the nature of the antigen, the nature of the antibody, and the presence of a wide variety of other factors such as complement. A partial list of secondary reactions includes precipitation of the antigen–antibody complex, agglutination of antigen-containing particles by antibody, lysis of antigen-containing cells or organisms, complement fixation, immobilization of motile organisms or cells, destruction of organisms or biologically active molecules, and various effects upon tissues if antigen–antibody complexes are formed in vivo (1,45). A designation of the secondary effect elicited by a given antiserum has been used to name that antiserum. Thus, the antibody in a serum that elicits precipitation when combined with antigen is called precipitin. Other such terms include hemolysin (lysis of red blood cells), agglutinin (agglutination of antigen particles), and opsonin (enhancement of phagocytosis). These terms may be used functionally, but they are not mutually exclusive. Thus, a precipitin may also be an hemolysin, an agglutinin, or an opsonin, depending upon the secondary reaction used to measure it. The antigen used to elicit antibody with a given secondary effect is named by the suffix "-ogen." For example, antigen used to produce and elicit precipitin is called precipitinogen; that used to produce agglutinin is agglutinogen; that used to produce opsonin is opsinogen (19).

PRECIPITIN REACTION

Insoluble Antibody–Antigen Complexes

Most naturally occurring circulating antibody molecules (except for IgM antibodies) contain two antigen-binding sites of identical specificity (are divalent), and most antigens contain more than two antigenic determinant sites (are multivalent). Because of this, when multivalent antigen is mixed in the proper portions with divalent antibodies, each antibody molecule usually combines with two antigen molecules. As antibody molecules connect molecules of soluble antigen, a lattice-like conglomeration of antigen molecules connected by antibody molecules may occur (17). This results in the formation of large conglomerates which become insoluble, presumably owing to a decrease in affinity for water as a result of an interaction of the solubilizing polar groups of the antigen and antibody. If the antigen is soluble, this reaction with antibody results in precipitation of the complex, and visible precipitates may be observed when the appropriate amounts of antibody and antigen are mixed.

Agglutination

If the antigen is particulate (large enough to be visible by itself), agglutination of the particulate antigen occurs as the individual particles of antigen are joined together by the antibody. This agglutination can be seen with the naked eye.

Soluble Antibody–Antigen Complexes

If the antigen is soluble and contains one or two determinant sites (is monovalent or divalent as opposed to multivalent), precipitation does not occur and soluble complexes are formed. Similar soluble antibody–antigen complexes are formed if the antibody is monovalent and the antigen multivalent. In these last two situations the number of combining sites of antigen or antibody is insufficient for a lattice-like structure to be built up.

Nonprecipitating (soluble) antibody–antigen complexes are also formed if the proportions of soluble antigen to specific antibody are such that a lattice-like conglomeration of antibody and antigen is not formed (Fig. 6-2). Such a situation exists in reactions where antigen or antibody is in excess. In the zone of antigen excess each divalent antibody reacts with two separate multivalent antigen molecules, and there are not enough anti-

I ANTIBODY EXCESS

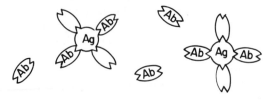

II EQUIVALENCE

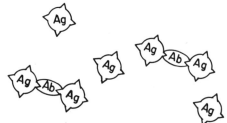

III ANTIGEN EXCESS

Fig. 6–2. **Lattice theory of precipitation reactions of antibody and antigen.** Formation of insoluble precipitate due to reaction of divalent antibody molecules with multivalent soluble antigen molecules depends upon relative concentration of antibody and antigen. I) **Antibody excess.** With excess antibody, all antigenic sites are covered with antibody and no sites are available for given antibody to join two molecules of antigen. Here, largest antibody–antigen complex formed is Ab4Ag. II) **Equivalence.** If concentrations of antibody and antigen are approximately balanced, each divalent antibody molecule can bind with two antigenic sites on different antigen molecules. Shown is a large lattice-like complex of antibody and antigen. With large complexes, affinity for water decreases due to interaction of solubilizing polar groups and loss of solubility (precipitation). III) **Antigen excess.** With excess antigen, each site of divalent antibody molecule may be occupied by antigen molecule, but not enough antibody molecules are available to join two antigen molecules together. Maximum complex size formed is AbAg2.

body molecules to form larger complexes by binding such antigen–antibody complexes together. The complexes formed consist of only two antigen molecules and one antibody molecule. A complex of this size may not be large enough to be insoluble. Similarly, in the zone of antibody excess each binding site of a multivalent antigen molecule is occupied by an antibody molecule, and not enough antigen sites are available so that a divalent antibody molecule can join or bridge two antigen molecules. The resulting complex consists of one antigen molecule and the number of antibody molecules sufficient to cover its antigenic sites. Such a complex may not be of a form or size to be insoluble, and a soluble antigen–antibody complex is the result.

Effect of Antigen Concentration on Precipitin Reaction

A precipitin reaction may be divided into three zones in relation to increasing amounts of antigen (17) (Fig. 6–3): 1) the zone of antibody excess, in which soluble complexes are the result of inadequate antigen and free antibody remains after all the antigen sites are covered by antibody; 2) the zone of equivalence, in which the amount of antigen is sufficient to bind all or most of the antibody in an insoluble form, and in which most or all of the antigen and antibody is insoluble and neither unbound antibody nor antigen remains in a soluble form; 3) the zone of antigen excess, in which the amount of antigen is sufficient to bind all the antibody to the extent that few antibody molecules can bind two antigen molecules together and free antigen remains after all the antibody molecules are bound to antigen.

QUANTITATIVE PRECIPITIN TEST

Expression of Antibody Activity in Titers

Earlier tests for antibody depended upon effects such as neutralization (destruction) or agglutination of bacteria which gave end points in the dilution of the antiserum that was still effective. The results of such tests were expressed as a titer (dilution). As stressed by Heidelberger (17), the expression of the activity of an antiserum as a titer or highest dilution effective for a certain secondary reaction does not actually indicate how much antibody there is. For example, comparisons of titers of antipneumococcal sera and antityphoid sera cannot be made directly. Although the titer (effective dilution) of one antiserum may be higher than that of another antiserum, much more antibody may be required to agglutinate or neutralize one kind of microorganism than another. Therefore, a direct comparison of titers in different systems is misleading.

Determination of Antibody by Weight

The quantitative precipitin reaction (17) permits measurement of antibody on a weight basis (Fig. 6–3). A series of test tubes each containing the same amount of antiserum is prepared. To this series of test tubes are added increasing amounts of antigen of known quantity. At the equiv-

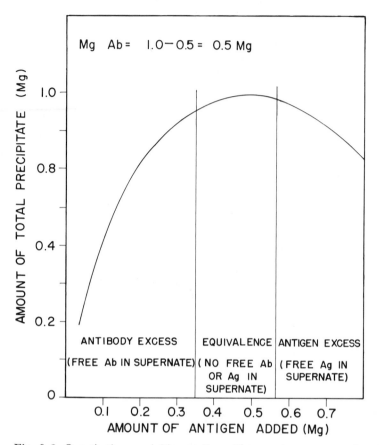

Fig. 6–3. **Quantitative precipitin reaction.** If increasing amounts of antigen are separately added to constant amounts of antiserum, increase in amount of precipitate occurs to maximum point, and further addition of antigen results in decrease in amount of total precipitate. This phenomenon is due to formation of antibody–antigen complexes of different composition (Fig. 6–2). At point of maximum precipitate, all antibody and antigen should be in precipitate (equivalence zone). If amount of antigen added at equivalence is known, amount of antibody can be determined by subtracting amount of antigen added at equivalence from amount of total precipitate formed. For example, if total precipitate is 1.0 mg and antigen added at equivalence is 0.5 mg, antibody present is 1.0 minus 0.5, or 0.5 mg.

alence zone all the antibody and all the antigen-added precipitate. The quantity of protein in the precipitate is determined by chemical or spectrophotometric measurement. Since the amount of antigen added is known, this quantity can then be subtracted from the value of total precipitate to determine the amount of specific antibody present. The validity of this technique depends upon at least three factors: 1) The antibody-antigen reaction must be specific. If a reaction of mixed specificity (more than one antigen and more than one antibody) occurs, it is virtually impossible to reach an equivalence zone since two or more separate antigen–antibody reactions are occurring at the same time. 2) The antiserum being measured must not contain monovalent (nonprecipitating) antibody, as these may not be carried down with the precipitate. 3) Other proteins which may affix to antigen–antibody complexes (such as complement, see below) must be eliminated or an erroneously high value for specific antibody will be obtained because of nonspecific binding of the other proteins.

PRECIPITATION-IN-AGAR TECHNIQUES

Precipitation reactions as a result of antibody–antibody combinations also occur in agar media (9,17). Precipitation-in-agar reaction is most valuable for analysis of multiple antigenic components.

Simple Gel Diffusion Technique

The simple gel diffusion technique evolved directly from the precipitin reaction in solution. If a solution of soluble antigen is layered over antiserum in a small caliber tube, a line appears at the interface of these solutions as a precipitation reaction occurs. If the antiserum is placed in agar in the tube and a solution of antigen layered over the antiserum–agar base, a precipitation line appears at the interface. This is known as an Oudin tube (29). Since the antigen is in solution and the antiserum is distributed evenly in the agar, the location the precipitation line assumes depends upon six factors: 1) concentration of the antigen, 2) diffusion coefficient of the antigen, 3) concentration of the antibody, 4) time, 5) temperature, and 6) concentration or density of the agar (9). If the last four variables are held constant, then for a given antigen the distance the precipitation line moves into the antiserum–agar layer depends upon the concentration of the antigen. If the concentration of the antigen is not sufficient to overcome the concentration of the antibody in the agar layer, the line remains at the interface. If the concentration of the antigen is sufficient to overcome the adjacent antibody concentration in the antiserum–agar layer, the precipitation line moves into the agar layer. This occurs as antigen diffuses into the precipitate, converting precipitates formed at antibody–antigen equivalence into soluble complexes due to antigen excess and creating a new zone of equivalence below this zone. The distance a precipitation line migrates into the antibody–agar layer may be used to quantitate the concentration of antigen if the distance of migration caused by the unknown antigen solution is compared with that caused by known concentrations of the same antigen. This distance can be calibrated on a standard log graph since, given constant temperature, antiserum–agar concentrations, and time, the log of the concentration of the antigen plotted against the distance of migration gives a straight line.

Two or more antigens in solution placed over an antiserum–agar layer containing antibody to the two or more antigens may result in separate precipitation bands for each specific antigen–antibody system. Since the location of the precipitation band formed by each system depends upon an independent set of variables, the number of precipitation lines formed in a tube containing an antiserum–agar base by layering over this base a mixture of antigens gives the minimum number of separate antibody–antigen systems present. Simple gel diffusion may also be carried out on a flat surface (24). Antiserum is incorporated into agar which is allowed to gel as a layer on a glass slide. A hole is cut into the agar, and antigen solution is placed into the hole. The antigen will diffuse out into the antibody-containing agar, producing a ring of precipitation, the area of which depends upon the relative concentration of antigen and antibody. Using a constant dilution of antiserum, quantitation of antigen may be accomplished by comparing the diameter of the ring of precipitation produced by a solution of known antigen concentration to that of an unknown (24).

Double Diffusion-in-Agar Technique

A better technique for analysis of mixtures of antibody–antigen systems is provided by the double diffusion-in-agar (Ouchterlony) technique (28). When this technique is used, antigen and antisera are separately placed in small holes cut out of a layer of agar on a plate. The antibody and antigen are permitted to diffuse toward each other. A precipitation band forms where the antibody and antigen meet in the concentrations necessary to meet the requirements of the equivalence zone of the precipitin reaction. If the concentration of the antigen is relatively greater than the concentration of the antibody, the precipitation line appears nearer the antibody hole; if the concentrations are equal, the line appears midway between the antibody and the antigen holes; and if the antibody concentration is greater than the antigen concentration, the precipitation line appears closer to the antigen hole. If multiple antibody–antigen systems are present, a separate line may be observed for each system. The patterns precipitation lines form when two or more antigens are compared with one antiserum, or vice versa, may be used to characterize an antigen or antibody preparation (Fig. 6–4).

Immunoelectrophoresis

If multiple antigen–antibody systems react in agar, it may be difficult to identify and differentiate the number of precipitation bands present. An example is an antiserum prepared in one species (rabbit) by immunizing with the whole serum proteins of another species (rat). The rabbit antiserum to whole rat serum may produce up to 30 separate precipitation bands when reacted in agar with rat serum. In order to identify the components of such a complicated system, a combination of electrophoresis of rat serum in agar and the double diffusion-in-agar technique is employed (Fig. 6–5). This method is called immunoelectrophoresis (9). A variation of single radial immunodiffusion employing electrophoresis—electroimmunodiffusion—may be used to quantitate antigens in dilute fluids (25). Antiserum is incorporated into the agar layer and an electric current applied across the agar after placing an antigen solution into a well cut into the agar. The electric field pulls the antigen into the antibody–agar layer. The distance that the antigen–antibody precipitate migrates into the agar layer is proportional to the amount of antigen in the solution.

I IDENTITY (FUSION)

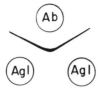

II NONIDENTITY (CROSS)

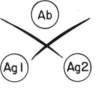

III PARTIAL IDENTITY (SPUR)

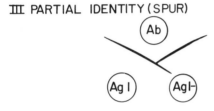

Fig. 6–4. Double diffusion-in-agar precipitation patterns. If solution of antigen is placed in one hole on flat layer of agar and appropriate antiserum placed in adjacent hole, antigen and antibody migrate toward each other and precipitation line forms when concentrations of antibody and antigen are in equivalence. If two identical antigen solutions (Ag1) are placed in holes in agar at base of triangle, and appropriate antiserum (Ab) placed in hole at apex of triangle, precipitation line forms between each antigen-containing hole and antiserum hole. Since both antigen solutions are the same, separate lines fuse where they meet in center of triangle (reaction of identity). If different antigen (Ag1 and Ag2) solutions are placed in base holes, and antiserum-containing antibodies (Ab) directed against both antigens is placed in apex hole, precipitation lines do not fuse, but cross, because independent systems are involved (reaction of nonidentity). If one antigen solution containing molecules with several antigenic specificities present on same molecule (Ag1) and a second antigen solution containing molecules with only some of the antigenic specificities of first antigen (Ag1—) are placed in adjacent holes against antiserum (Ab) which contains antibodies directed toward all specificities present in first antigen solution, line of partial identity, or spur formation, is observed. Precipitation line formed between antiserum and antigen with limited antigenic specificities fuses with line formed by antiserum and antigen containing additional specificities, but this second line extends past first line, resulting in spur effect.

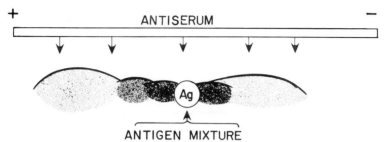

Fig. 6–5. Immunoelectrophoresis. Reaction of antiserum (rabbit anti-whole-rat-serum) with mixture of antigens (whole rat serum) separated by electrophoresis in agar. Mixture of antigens is placed in small hole in layer of agar on glass plate or slide. Electric current is applied to agar. Current acts upon protein components and results in migration into agar of proteins in whole serum. Distance each serum protein migrates is proportional to electrostatic charge of that protein. Since proteins in whole serum differ in charge, separation of proteins due to different migration distance occurs. Location of proteins as they diffuse in agar is represented by shaded areas. Following electrophoretic separation, a trough is cut in agar a short distance from hole in which whole serum was originally placed. Trough is cut so that its long axis is parallel to electrophoretic separation. Antiserum to whole serum (rabbit anti-whole-rat-serum) is then placed in trough and allowed to diffuse into agar. Antibody to each rat serum protein then separately reacts with rat proteins in agar, forming precipitation lines where antibody and antigen are in equivalence (solid curved lines). Because rat serum proteins have been separated by electrophoresis, individual antibody–antigen reactions are easier to identify and differentiate. Many variations in this basic procedure have been utilized to provide more exact immunochemical analysis of complex antibody–antigen systems.

AUTORADIOGRAPHY OF IMMUNOELECTROPHORESIS

Autoradiography of immunoelectrophoresis is a qualitative technique for the identification of proteins synthesized by a given organ in vitro or by a living animal. Newly synthesized proteins contain incorporated radiocarbon-labeled amino acids (1). Tissue extracts, serum, or culture fluids containing the labeled proteins are fractionated by electrophoresis in agar, and the proteins present are precipitated in the agar by specific antisera. The labeled proteins are then identified by autoradiography of the washed, dried immunoelectrophoresis slide. Labeled precipitation bands are revealed by exposure of a film or a photographic emulsion overlying the labeled band in the immunoelectrophoretic pattern. Newly synthesized proteins may also be identified by coprecipitation of labeled proteins with specific antisera, using the tube-precipitation method, but such techniques require rigid controls to rule out nonspecific precipitations.

IMMUNOFLUORESCENCE

The binding of a dye-labeled antibody to antigens in tissue sections permits the specific identification and localization of antigens in tissue (1). The most commonly employed dyes are fluorescein and rhodamine. These compounds may be attached to antibody molecules and emit light (fluoresce) when exposed to ultraviolet light of the appropriate wave length. Fluorescein- or rhodamine-labeled antibody preparations are applied to frozen sections of the tissue to be examined. The antibody adheres to the antigen if the latter is present in sufficient amounts in the tissue section, forming microprecipitates. If the treated tissue section is then washed to remove excess unbound labeled antibody and observed under ultraviolet light, the areas of the tissue section containing the antigen fluoresce. Variations of this technique are illustrated in Fig. 6–6.

Immunofluorescence studies must be carefully controlled to prevent mis-

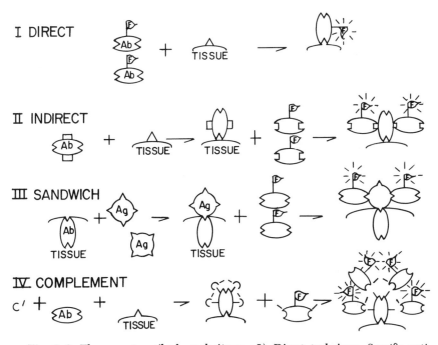

Fig. 6–6. Fluorescent antibody techniques. I) Direct technique. Specific antibody is labeled with fluorescent compound (F) and added to tissue sections. Reaction of specific antibody to antigenic sites in tissue section can then be detected by exposing section to ultraviolet light and visualizing areas of fluorescence. II) Indirect technique. Unlabeled antibody is reacted with tissue antigen. Fluorescein-labeled antibody to first antibody is then added. Second antibody reacts with first, which in turn has reacted with tissue antigen. First antibody added provides more binding sites for second antibody than was provided by tissue antigen, thus increasing sensitivity of technique. III) Sandwich technique. This is used to identify antibody in tissue sections rather than antigen. Antigen is added to tissue and is bound by specific antibody present in tissue. Specific fluorescein-labeled antibody to antigen is then added which reacts with antigen now fixed to tissue. IV) Complement technique. Reaction of specific antibody with tissue antigen usually results in fixation of complement if complement is present while antibody–antigen reaction takes place. Presence of complement can then be detected by addition of a fluorescein-labeled antibody to complement. Since many molecules of complement may be fixed by antibody–antigen reaction, sensitivity of detection may be greatly increased by this technique.

interpretation of the staining patterns. 1) The specificity of the labeled antibody must be carefully checked by immunochemical techniques. This is absolutely necessary, as minute amounts of contaminating antibody to an antigen other than the one of interest may give erroneous results. 2) The fluorescence produced by the labeled antibody must be differentiated from nonspecific tissue fluorescence. This can usually be done because natural tissue fluorescence gives a different color from fluorescein or rhodamine fluorescence at the wave length of ultraviolet light employed. 3) The staining pattern produced by the labeled specific antibody must be clearly different from that which may occur if an adjacent tissue section is treated with labeled nonantibody (normal) immunoglobulins, since the labeled antibody may be nonimmunologically (nonspecifically) bound to the tissue section. 4) The staining pattern should not occur if the tissue section is treated with nonlabeled antibody prior to the addition of the labeled antibody. This specific blocking should also occur if the labeled antiserum is treated with nonlabeled antigen prior to the addition of the antiserum to the tissue section. Even if these controls are carefully done, the investigator must not overinterpret the results of immunofluorescence. Used appropriately, immunofluorescence is a valuable, highly specific technique for tissue antigen identification.

IMMUNOELECTRONMICROSCOPY

The ultrastructural location and distribution of antigens on tissues or cells can be accomplished using a variety of techniques employing markers which are localized by antigen–antibody reactions. Such markers include ferritin (37), peroxidase (23,27,41), hemocyanin (20), viral particles (16) and radiolabeled antibody (36). These may be coupled directly to the antibody used by chemical means (37). In addition, markers coated with antigen may be bound to antigenic determinants by bivalent antibody which serves as a bridge; one binding site of the antibody joins to the antigen on a given cell while the other binding site joins to and holds the marker coated with the antigen (2,3,43). It is also possible to use artificially produced hybrid antibody molecules which contain one binding site for the antigen on the tissue and another site for an antigen on the marker (3,15). Using larger marker particles, such as latex, these methods may be adapted to localization of antigenic markers by scanning electron microscopy (26).

AGGLUTINATION

Agglutination of visible antigen particles by antibody occurs by the same mechanism as precipitation of soluble antigen (1,45). Simple agglutination results when the antigen is an integral part of the particle, as when antibody to erythrocytes or to bacteria causes the agglutination of these particles. Passive agglutination results when a soluble antigen is placed on an insoluble particle and antibody to the soluble antigen is used to agglutinate the coated particle. Materials that have been used for this purpose include latex and bentonite particles and erythrocytes (passive hemagglutination). Addition of the soluble antigen in sufficient amounts to react with the antibody to passively coated particles inhibits the agglutination reaction. Inhibition of passive hemagglutination reactions is an extremely sensitive method for detecting antigen. The reaction of specific antibody with erythrocytes or other walled structures (bacteria, other cells) in the presence of a series of normal serum proteins—collectively termed complement—results in the eventual destruction of the red cell (hemolysis). The complement system and the role of complement proteins in tissue reactions is described in Chapter 11.

LYSIS (COMPLEMENT FIXATION)

The effect of antibody and antigen upon the complement system may be used to measure an antibody–antigen reaction (1,19). The reaction of antibody and antigen in the presence of complement consumes components of the complement system (complement fixation). Normal serum-containing complement causes the lysis of erythrocytes coated with complement-fixing antibody (sensitized erythrocyte). If a separate antibody–antigen reaction is allowed to take place in a given volume of normal complement-containing serum, the complement activity is removed by adsorption of active complement components to the antibody–antigen complexes formed. If this mixture is then added to sensitized erythrocytes, lysis does not occur, as the necessary complement components have been exhausted. This complement-fixation reaction provides a sensitive and accurate measurement of antibody or antigen if the fixation reaction is properly controlled. For complement fixation to occur, a type of antibody that can react with complement must be active (complement-fixing antibody); all immunoglobulins do not have the capacity to fix complement. For more details about the complement system, see page 153.

IMMUNOABSORBENTS

Specific antibody or antigen may be coupled to insoluble carriers such as cellulose (6,46), bentonite (32), sephorose (47) or glass beads (44) or made insoluble by cross linking (4,5,7). These solid antibody or antigen reagents provide valuable methods for isolation of antigen (by insoluble antibody) or antibody by insoluble antigen. For instance, a specific antiserum to a given antigen may be utilized to purify that antigen. The antiserum is coupled to an insoluble carrier, and a solution of a mixture of proteins is added. The specific antigen attaches to the insoluble antibody. The contaminating proteins are washed off and the bound specific antigen eluted from the insoluble antibody by lowering the pH of the buffer sufficiently to disrupt the antibody–antigen electrostatic bond, but not the covalent bond leaking the antiserum to the insoluble carrier.

RADIOIMMUNOASSAY

The practical importance of the use of antigen–antibody reactions for the quantitation of antigenic materials is exemplified by the use of radioimmunoassay· for quantitation of hormones and other biologically active molecules (1). Hormones, being macromolecules with species-specific antigenic determinants, elicit antibody when injected into other species. If care is taken to produce a specific antiserum to a given hormone, this antiserum may be used to identify and quantitate the hormone, even if it represents only a small fraction in a mixture of a number of other proteins. The basic principle is the inhibition of the reaction of a specific antibody and a known amount of antigen by the addition of antigen in unknown amounts. This principle may be used in many antigen–antibody secondary reactions, such as hemagglutination inhibition and precipitation inhibition. However, the use of radiolabeled antigen greatly increases the sensitivity of the test. Radioimmunoassay has been used to measure a large variety of antigenic molecules including hormones, enzymes and serum proteins (42).

The principle of a radioimmunoassay is given in the following reactions:

$$Ab + Ag^* \quad \rightarrow AbAg^*$$
$$Ab + Ag + Ag^* \rightarrow AbAg \quad + Ag^*$$

In the first reaction, antibody (Ab) is reacted with a radiolabeled antigen (Ag*) under conditions that result in essentially complete precipitation of the antigen. In the second reaction, excess unlabeled antigen (Ag) is included in the reaction mixtures. Since the unlabeled antigen is in excess, little or no labeled antigen is obtained in the precipitate. By varying the amount of unlabeled antigen present, a quantitative relation can be obtained between the amount of antigen present and the amount of radioactivity in the precipitate or supernate. Once such a relation has been determined, a standard graph may be constructed plotting the percent of label in the precipitate (or, inversely, the percent in the supernate) against the amount of unlabeled antigen added. The amount of antigen in an unknown may then be found by determining the effect of the addition of dilutions of the unknown upon the antibody-labeled antigen system. The amounts of antibody and labeled antigen are kept constant in each determination.

Other properties of an antibody–antigen system may be used to quantitate a given antigen. Most involve the reaction of varying amounts of the antigen or unknown with constant amounts of specific antiserum. As increasing amounts of antigen are added 1) the amount of unbound antibody decreases, 2) the amount of complex increases, and 3) after exceeding equivalence, increasing amounts of free antigen are present. The extent of any of these changes, in the presence of a fixed amount of antibody, depends upon the amount of antigen added. This permits variations in the final measurement used to quantitate an antigen by immunoassay (33).

IMMUNORADIOMETRIC ASSAY

A variation of radioimmunoassay, immunoradiometric assays, use purified radiolabeled antibody instead of labeled antigen (34). Radiolabeled antibody is added to a solution of antigen. A solid immunoabsorbent is then used to separate unbound antibody leaving the labeled antibody bound to the soluble antigen in the supernate. The sensitivity of immunoradiometric assays is comparable to that of radioimmunoassays. The choice of which assay to use depends on the feasibility and applicability of a given antibody–antigen system to the method (34).

IDENTIFICATION OF INDIVIDUAL ANTIBODY-CONTAINING CELLS

The secondary effects of antibody–antigen reactions may be used to identify individual antibody-containing cells. The methods include immunoadherence, the use of microdrops, localized hemolysis in agar and immunofluorescence.

Immunoadherence

The adherence of antigen particles to lymphoid cells containing antibody results in the formation of rosettes or clusters of the antigen particles around the lymphoid cells. The antigen particles may be erythrocytes, bacteria, or soluble antigen-coated particles (bentonite).

Use of Microdrops

Single lymphoid cells may be isolated in small drops of medium and the capacity of such isolated cells to exhibit reaction with antigen determined. Reactions used have included immunoadherence and neutralization of bacteriophage.

Localized Hemolysis in Agar

Cells containing antibody to erythrocytes may be identified by the specific formation of hemolytic areas in agar or other media containing a suspension of erythrocytes. When hemolysin-containing cells are mixed with a suspension of erythrocytes in agar and plated, a lymphoid cell in the center of the lytic plaques can be identified.

Immunofluorescence

Antibody-containing cells in suspension or in tissue sections can be identified by a two-step immunofluorescence procedure. First the antigen is added to the suspension or tissue sections. Cells containing the specific antibody bind the antigen. Second, the suspension or section is washed and fluorescein-labeled specific antibody is added. The labeled antibody binds with the antigen on the cells. The antibody-containing cells fluoresce when exposed to ultraviolet light. Other labels that may be used for tracing antibody molecules are enzymes (peroxidase), which may be identified by their reaction with substrate, and ferritin, which because of its density and configuration may be identified with the electron microscope.

MICROBIOLOGIC TESTS IN VITRO

The effect of bactericidal antibody and complement on certain organisms provides the basis for the laboratory tests described below.

Treponema Pallidum Immobilization (TPI)

A specific serologic test for syphilis depends upon the presence in an affected individual's serum of antibodies to the causative agent; *T. pallidum.* Mobile organisms are mixed with the test serum and normal guinea pig serum (complement source); the mixture is incubated for 16–18 hours at 35°C under anaerobic conditions and then examined microscopically. Normally, the *T. pallidum* organisms are motile and are observed to move actively. The action of specific antibody and complement results in loss of this motility. The TPI test is difficult to perform routinely because the fastidiousness of the organisms makes it necessary to maintain a source of test organisms.

Opsonic Index

Opsonization is the reaction of specific antibody and complement with a particle or organism to facilitate or augment phagocytosis of the organism (1). An opsonic index can be obtained by determining the ratio of activity of a patient's serum to that of normal serum. The activity is determined by the degree of phagocytosis of the test material by microscopic examination of mixtures of serum, complement, and organisms cultured in the presence of macrophages.

Neutralization Tests

The activity of antisera to bacteria, viruses or phage may be tested by the ability of such sera to reduce the viability of suspensions of these organisms when cultured in vitro. The effect is usually measured by the activity of dilutions of the antisera or by the rate of neutralization of the target organism by a dilution of the antiserum.

MICROBIOLOGIC TESTS IN VIVO

Neutralization of the activity of a biologically active molecule or infective organism may also be tested in vivo (19). The two classic examples described here are the mouse protection test for the activity of antipneumococcal sera and the toxin neutralization test for antidiphtheria toxin sera.

Mouse Pneumococcus Protection Test

In the mouse protection test for standardization of antipneumococcal sera, 1 mouse protective unit is that fraction of a milliliter of antiserum which will protect a proportion of mice against 1 million fatal doses of an 18-hour serum–broth culture of such virulence that 3–10 organisms will produce death of mice in 36–48 hours when injected intraperitoneally. Mice are injected with 0.5 ml of a 1:200 dilution of an 18-hour broth culture (500,000 lethal doses) mixed with an equal volume of the dilution of the antiserum to be tested. Dilutions of antiserum ranging from 1:20 to 1:2,000 are used, and three mice are injected with each dilution. The highest dilution protecting two of three mice for 96 hours is taken as the number of protective units.

Diphtheria Toxin Neutralization

The neutralization potency of an antisera to diphtheria toxin (antitoxin) is measured by comparison with a standard sample of antitoxin. To test a toxin preparation, increasing amounts of toxin are added to a series of tubes containing 1 unit of a standard antitoxin, and each of the mixtures is injected into a 250-gm guinea pig. The amount of toxin which must be mixed with 1 unit of antitoxin to cause death in 4 days is taken as the end point and is called the L_+ dose. The amount of toxin which can just be neutralized by 1 unit of antitoxin is called the L_0 dose. To determine the potency of the unknown antiserum, increasing dilutions of the antitoxin are each mixed with one L_+ dose of the toxin and the mixtures injected into guinea pigs. The volume of serum which when mixed with one L_+ dose of toxin results in death in 4 days contains 1 unit of antitoxin.

SECONDARY REACTIONS IN VIVO

The activity of antibodies in an actively immunized animal or an animal that has received antibody by passive transfer of an antiserum prepared in another animal may be tested by a number of methods. Intravenous injection of antigen into an actively or passively sensitized animal may result in an acute systemic reaction (see Chapter 12). If the antigen is injected into the skin, a particular type of inflammatory skin reaction may be observed (see Chapters 12 through 14). These reactions depend upon tissue inflammatory responses initiated by reactions of antibody or sensitized cells with antigen. The induction of antibody production also leads to the rapid elimination of antigen from the circulation (immune elimination; Fig. 6–7).

Schick Test

In vivo neutralization of diphtheria toxin by antibody may be determined by skin testing. A small amount of diphtheria toxin injected intradermally produces a local inflammatory reaction which is maximal at 4–5 hours and then fades. In an immunized individual who has antibody to diphtheria toxin, no reaction occurs; the antibody neutralizes the effects of the toxin. This test was pioneered by Bela Schick between 1910 and 1930 and is known as the Schick test (38), although intradermal tests for small amounts of toxin and antitoxin were first described by Römer (35). A delayed hypersensitivity reaction to diphtheria toxin may also occur. This is known as a pseudoreaction and can usually be differentiated from the effects of the toxin as the delayed reaction reaches a maximum at 2–3 days and fades by 4–5 days.

Schultz-Charlton Phenomenon

In 1918 Schultz and Charlton (39) described the observation that human serum injected into a patient with a characteristic scarlet fever

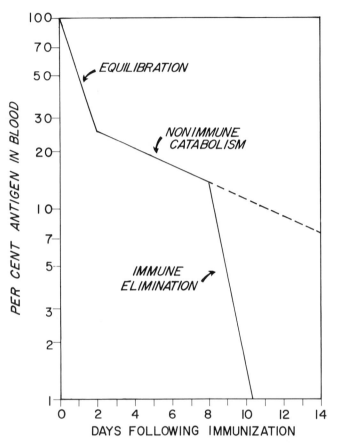

Fig. 6–7. Immune elimination. If antibody is present in vivo, antigen is rapidly cleared from blood stream. A three-stage elimination of diffusible antigen from bloodstream of previously nonimmunized animal has been recognized. Upon intravascular injection, blood level of antigen rapidly drops until only about 40% of injected antigen remains in blood. This is due to equilibrium of diffusible antigen between intravascular and extravascular fluids. Following this rapid equilibration, antigen is slowly removed by normal metabolic processes (nonimmune catabolism) until onset of antibody production between 7–10 days after antigen injection. Appearance of antibody results in rapid elimination of antigen (immune elimination) due to formation of antibody–antigen complexes and their removal by reticuloendothelial system. During phase of immune elimination, soluble antibody–antigen complexes (formed in antigen excess) may be demonstrated in blood. After antigen is completely removed, free antibody appears. If antigen is injected into an animal that already has circulating antibody, antigen is removed in one rapid immune elimination phase.

rash (scarlatina) could produce a blanching of the rash at the site of injection. It was later demonstrated that not all human sera could induce this blanching (12) and that the effect was due to the presence of specific antibody to the erythrogenic toxin. These observations led to the development of the Dick test for scarlet fever.

Dick Test

An intradermal test for antibody to hemolytic streptococcal antigens is known as the Dick test (10,11). Filtrates of cultures of the scarlatenal strains (strains responsible for scarlet fever) of streptococci contain a toxic substance that produces a typical skin reaction in immunized individuals. Individuals with neutralizing antibody do not react to this erythrogenic toxin. The reaction induced by erythrogenic toxin appears as a bright red flush within 6–12 hours, is maximum at 24 hours and fades rapidly. This test only measures resistance to strains of streptococci causing scarlet fever and does not measure protection or susceptibility to streptococcal throat infection (40).

SENSITIVITY OF SECONDARY ANTIBODY–ANTIGEN REACTIONS

The sensitivity of some methods for detection of antibody–antigen reactions is given in Table 6–1. For further information on how to detect and measure both primary and secondary antibody–antigen reactions, the text Experimental Immunochemistry by Kabat and Mayer is recommended (19).

TABLE 6–1
Sensitivity of Some Methods of Measuring Antibody–Antigen Reactions

Method	Sensitivity (μg antibody N/ml)
Quantitative precipitin	4–10
Simple agar diffusion	5–10
Bacterial agglutination	0.01
Bactericidal	0.0001–0.001
Hemagglutination	0.003–0.006
Hemolysis	0.001–0.03
Complement fixation	0.1
Toxin neutralization	0.01
Passive systemic anaphylaxis (guinea pig)	30
Uterine muscle in vitro*	0.01
Passive cutaneous anaphylaxis	0.003
Radioimmunoassay	<0.001

* Schultz-Dale test, see under Reaginic Antibody in Chapter 12.
Modified from Humphrey JH, White RG: Immunology for Students of Medicine. 2d ed. Oxford, Blackwell, 1963, p 201; (see also reference 14)

REFERENCES

1. Ackroyd JF: Immunological Methods. Oxford, Blackwell, 1964
2. An T, Miyai K, Sell S: Electron microscopic localization of rabbit immunoglobulin allotype b4 on blood lymphocytes by an indirect ferritin immune complex labelling technique. J Immunol 108:1271, 1972
3. Avrameas S: Indirect microenzyme techniques for intracellular detection of antigens. Immunochemistry 6:825, 1969
4. Avrameas S, Ternynck T: Biologically active water-insoluble protein polymers. I. Their use for isolation of antigens and antibodies. J Biol Chem 7:1651–1659, 1967
5. Avrameas S, Ternynck T: The cross-linking of proteins with glutaraldehyde and its use for the preparation of immunoadsorbents. Immunochemistry 6:53–66, 1969
6. Campbell DH, Luescher E, Lerman LS: Immunologic absorbents. I. Isolation of antibody by means of cellulose protein antigen. Proc Natl Acad Sci USA 37:575, 1951
7. Centeno ER, Sehon AH: The use of ethylene maleic anhydride for the preparation of versatile immunosorbents. Immunochemistry 8:887–900, 1971
8. Coons AH: Histochemistry with labelled antibody. Int Rev Cytol 5:1, 1956
9. Crowle AJ: Immunodiffusion. New York, Academic Press, 1961
10. Dick GF, Dick GH: A skin test for susceptibility to scarlet fever. JAMA 82:265, 1924
11. Dick GF, Dick GH: Results with the skin test for susceptibility to scarlet fever. Preventive immunization with scarlet fever toxin. JAMA 84:1477, 1925
12. Dochez AR: Etiology of Scarlet Fever. Medicine 4:251, 1925
13. Farr RS: A quantitative immunochemical measure of the primary interaction between I*BSA and antibody. J Infect Dis 103:239, 1958
14. Gill TJ III: Methods for detecting antibody. Immunochemistry 7:997–1000, 1970
15. Hämmerling U, Aoki T, de Harven E, Boyse EA, Old LJ: Use of hybrid antibody with anti-G and anti-ferritin specificities in locating cell surface antigens by electron microscopy. J Exp Med 128:1461, 1968
16. Hämmerling U, Aoki T, Wood HA, Old LJ, Boyse EA, deHarven E: New visual markers of antibody for electron microscopy. Nature (Lond) 223:1968
17. Heidelberger M: Lectures in Immunochemistry. New York, Academic Press, 1956
18. Kabat EA: The nature of an antigenic determinant. J Immunol 97:1, 1966
19. Kabat EA, Mayer MM: Experimental Immunochemistry, 2d ed. Springfield, Ill, Thomas, 1961
20. Karnovsky MJ, Unanue ER, Leventhal M: Ligand-induced movement of lymphocyte membrane macromolecules. II. Mapping of surface markers. J Exp Med 136:907, 1972
21. Karush F: Immunological specificity and molecular structure. Adv Immunol 2:1, 1962
22. Kitagawa M, Yagi Y, Pressman D: The heterogeneity of combining sites of antibodies as determined by specific immunoabsorbents. J Immunol 95:446, 991, 1965
23. Kraenenbuhl JP, Galardy RE, Jamieson JD: Preparation and characterization of an immunoglobulin microscope tracer consisting of a heme-octopeptide coupled to Fab. J Exp Med 139:208, 1974
24. Mancini G, Carbonara AO, Heremans JF: Immunochemical quantitation of antigens by single radial immunodiffusion. Immunochemistry 2:235, 1965
25. Merrill D, Hartley TF, Claman HN: Electroimmunodiffusion (EID): A simple, rapid method for quantitation by immunoglobulins in dilute biological fluids. J Lab Clin Med 69:151, 1967
26. Linthicum DS, Sell S: Topography of lymphocyte surface immunoglobulin using scanning immunoelectron microscopy. J Ultrastruct Res (In press)
27. Nakane PK, Pierce GB Jr: Enzyme labelled antibodies for the light and electron microscopic localization of tissue antigens. J Cell Biol 33:307, 1967
28. Ouchterlony O: Diffusion-in-gel methods for immunological analysis. Prog Allergy 6:30, 1962
29. Oudin J: Method of immunochemical analysis by specific precipitation in gel medium. C R Acad Sci [D] (Paris), 222:115, 1946

30. Perkins WD, Karnovsky MJ, Unanue ER: An ultrastructural study of lymphocytes with surface-bound immunoglobulin. J Exp Med 135:267, 1972
31. Pressman D, Grossburg AL: The Structural Basis of Antibody Specificity. New York, Benjamin, 1968
32. Reisberg MA, Rossen RD, Butler WT: A method for preparing specific fluorescein-conjugated antibody reagents using bentonite immunoadsorbents. J Immunol 105:1151–1161, 1970
33. Rodbard D, Catt KJ: Mathematical theory of radioligand assays: The kinetics of separation of bound from free. J Steroid Biochem 3:255–273, 1972
34. Rodbard D, Weiss GH: Mathematical theory of immunoradiometric (labeled antibody) assays. Anal Biochem 52:10–44, 1973
35. Römer PH: Veber Den Nachweis Sehr Kleiner Mengen Des Diphtheriegiftes. Z Immunitaetsforsch 3:208, 1909
36. Santer V, Bankhurst AD, Nossal GJV: Ultrastructural distribution of surface immunoglobulin determinants on mouse lymphoid cells. Exp Cell Res 72:377, 1972
37. Schick AF, Singer SJ: On the formation of covalent linkages between two protein molecules. J Biol Chem 236:2477, 1961
38. Schick B: Die Diphtherietoxin-Hautreaktion Des Menschen Als Vorprobe Der Prophylaktischen Diphtherieheilserum Injection. Munch Med Wochenschr 60:2608, 1913
39. Schultz W, Charlton W: Serologische Beobachtungen Am Scharlachexanthum. Z Kinderheilkd 17:328, 1917
40. Schwentker FF, Hodes HL, Kingsland LC, Chenoweth BM, Peck JL: Streptococcal infections in a naval training station. Am J Public Health 33:1455, 1943
41. Shnitka TK, Seligman AM: Ultrastructural localization of enzymes. Ann Rev Biochem 40:375, 1971
42. Skelley DS, Brown LP, Besch PK: Radioimmunoassay. Clin Chem 19:146–186, 1973
43. Steinberger LA, Hardy PH Jr, Cuculis JJ, Meyer HG: The unlabeled antibody enzyme method of immunochemistry. Preparation and properties of soluble antigen–antibody complex (Horseradish peroxidase antihorseradish peroxidase) and its use in identification of spirochetes. J Histochem Cytochem 18:315, 1970
44. Weetall HH: Preparation and characterization of antigen and antibody adsorbents covalently coupled to an inorganic carrier. J Biochem 117:257–261, 1970
45. Weir DM: Antigen–Antibody Reactions. In Modern Trends in Immunology. Cruickshank R (ed). London, Whitefriar, 1963
46. Weliky N, Weetall HH: Studies of antigen–antibody interaction on some specific solid adsorbents derived from cellulose. Immunochemistry 9:967–978, 1972
47. Wilchek M, Bocchini V, Becker M, Givol D: A general method for the specific isolation of peptides containing modified residues, using insoluble antibody columns. Biochemistry 10:2828–2834, 1971

7

Immune Tolerance

Immune tolerance may be defined as the specific failure of a normally responsive individual to make an immune response to a known antigen. It is specific for a given antigen; immune responses to other antigens are not affected. Burnett (7,8) first postulated immune tolerance to explain why an individual does not normally make an immune response to his own antigenic material, although his macromolecules may be immunogenic when they are given to a different individual. He further explained immune tolerance as a means of recognition of "self" and "non-self," and the mechanism of immune self-recognition as not innate, but a process of maturation.

NATURAL TOLERANCE

Natural tolerance was postulated to develop during fetal life when the individual does not yet have the capacity to produce an immune response. Contact with antigens at this time would affect the maturation of the immune system so that recognition and reaction of immune mechanisms to the antigen would not develop. Under usual conditions the fetus only contacts its own antigens and therefore develops immune tolerance to them. However, Burnet predicted that if a foreign antigen were presented to the fetus before or during maturation of its immune system, specific immune tolerance could be produced to this antigen (7,8).

Burnet's theories were largely stimulated by Owen's demonstration of acquired tolerance to foreign antigens in dizygotic twins of cattle (29). Such twins are genetically different but have a common circulation during fetal life so that there is a continuous exchange of proteins and blood cells. When mature, such twins tolerate and do not manifest an immune response to each other's antigens. Since Owen's observation, many other instances of immune tolerance to foreign antigens have been produced in experimental animals (13,23,25). If a potential immunogen is introduced to an animal early in its life, the animal may develop specific immune tolerance to it. Upon second contact with the same antigen at an age when an immune response would be expected, the tolerant animal does not respond. Immune tolerance to non-self antigens is called *acquired tolerance* to contrast this phenomenon with the spontaneous tolerance to self antigens, i.e., *natural tolerance.*

TABLE 7-1
Relation of Degree of Immunogenicity to Source and Complexity of Antigen

Complexity of antigen	Autogeneic (same individual)	Syngeneic (genetically identical individual)	Allogeneic (different individual, same species)	Xenogeneic (different species)
Serum proteins	0	0	± †	++
Altered serum proteins*	+	+	+	++
Erythrocytes	0	0	++	++++
Tissue grafts	0	0	+++	+++++

* Denatured or conjugated with haptens.

† An immune response may occur to some serum proteins (see Allotypes, Chapter 4).

0, no response; ±, inconsistent response; + weak response; ++ through +++++, rough indication of degree of immunogenicity.

ACQUIRED TOLERANCE

Acquired tolerance may not only be produced by contact of the individual with non-self antigens early in development, but it may also be instituted by contact with antigen after exposure of the adult individual to systemic events such as the administration of irradiation or large doses of antimetabolic agents. An antigen which induces tolerance is called a tolerogen; the same antigen presented under different circumstances may stimulate an immune response (immunogen). Some of the characteristics of the acquired tolerant state that have been discovered from experimental work are discussed below.

1. Tolerance is most easily induced by antigens that are closely related to those of the host; induction of the tolerant state becomes more difficult as the complexity of the antigen increases. In other words, the ability to induce acquired tolerance to a given antigen is inversely related to the degree of immunogenicity of the antigen (Table 7–1).
2. Tolerance is of finite duration, and the duration of the tolerant state depends upon the presence of antigen. Newborn rabbits made tolerant to an antigen so that no immune response can be elicited at 4 months of age may give an immune response at 12 months of age. If such animals are given repeated doses of the antigen, they remain tolerant at 12 months of age (13,23,25).
3. Either high or low doses of an antigen may induce tolerance to an antigen that will elicit an antibody response when an intermediate dose is used (high and low dose tolerance) (27).
4. The state of tolerance may be terminated by injection of antigens that contain antigenic determinants (specificities) in common with the antigen to which the individual is tolerant but also contain antigenic determinants to which the same individual is not tolerant (32).

5. Tolerance is not terminated by the transfer of cells from a normal (nontolerant) animal to a tolerant animal.
6. The transfer of cells from an immunized animal to a tolerant animal results in a temporary loss of tolerance due to the activity of the transferred cells. However, when the host animal reacts against the transferred cells (allograft rejection) and destroys them, its tolerance is reestablished.
7. Cells transferred from a tolerant animal to an irradiated animal (i.e., an animal whose own immune system has been destroyed) restore the general immune responsive state of the irradiated animal. However, tolerance to the specific antigen to which the original donor of the cells was tolerant is also transferred (adoptive tolerance) (2,3).
8. Transfer of cells from a tolerant donor to a normal syngeneic host may institute specific tolerance in the recipient. This effect is not produced if the T cells of the donor are killed prior to transfer (6,31).
9. Both T cells and B cells may be made tolerant (10). T cells are made tolerant for long periods of time by low doses of antigen while B cells require high doses of antigen and the tolerant state induced is temporary (11). Tolerance of either T or B cells leads to tolerance in the animal. However, the B cells recover after a relatively short time while T cells remain tolerant.

The breaking of tolerance by related antigens can be explained by a two-cell system (Fig. 7-1). Antigens that cross react (i.e., contain some determinants in common) with the antigen used to induce tolerance are processed by recognition cells that are specific for the immunogenic antigen. These recognition cells are able to present the cross-reacting specificities to responsive precursor lines that have recovered from the tolerant state. The recovery of recognition or production cells from a tolerant state may be due to 1) the reformation from uncommitted stem cells of cells with the ability to react with the specific antigen, 2) the resynthesis of sites by cells whose sites have been blocked or destroyed, or 3) the removal of some block to a potentially reactive cell. T cells and B cells may become tolerant as the result of different mechanisms.

MECHANISMS OF TOLERANCE

For many years the explanation of tolerance was based on the clonal selection theory of Burnet (7,8). While his theory may still explain some types of tolerance, more recent studies have identified tolerant situations that require a different explanation—Four theories which deserve comment are: 1) *Clonal Elimination*—cells responsible for recognizing and responding to the given antigen are eliminated from the tolerant animal (Clonal Selection Theory). 2) *Suppressor Cells*—specific cells actively inhibit reactive cells, preventing the tolerant animal from making an immune response. 3) *Blocking Antibody*—specific antibody or antibody–antigen complexes block reaction of potentially responding cells. 4) *Immunogen Processing*—immunogen catabolism in the tolerant animal bypasses reactive cells, preventing release of immunogen to potential responding cells.

ANTIGEN   THYMUS   BONE   MARROW

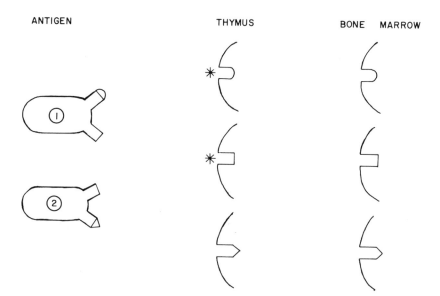

Fig. 7–1. Interplay of cells derived from thymus and bone marrow in "breaking" of tolerance by related antigens. Antigen 1 contains two types of determinants—one different from antigen 2 and one shared by antigen 2. Antigen 2 also contains two types of determinants—one shared by antigen 1 and one different from antigen 1. Thymus-derived and bone marrow-derived cells, both required for maximum primary antibody responses, contain individual cells or populations of cells that separately recognize the three types of determinants. Both T and B cells can become tolerant to these antigens, but experimental data show that thymus-derived cells are made tolerant for long periods by low doses of antigen while bone marrow-derived cells require large doses of antigen to become tolerant for even a short period. Thus, recovery of responsiveness of bone marrow cells occurs rapidly. However, thymus-derived cells are needed to present antigen to bone marrow cells for antibody production to occur. If an animal is made tolerant to antigen 1, thymus-derived cells recognizing antigenic determinants of antigen 1 are functionally absent (indicated by asterisk) while bone marrow cells recognizing determinants of antigen 1 recover in a short time and are available to respond. If antigen 2 is presented as an immunogen, thymus-derived cells for unique determinant are available, and present antigen to bone marrow cells recognizing not only unique determinant but also shared determinant. Thus antibody to antigen 1 is produced, but only to those determinants shared by antigen 2. It is also possible that each thymus-derived cell is able to recognize a range of antigenic determinants and that tolerance of such cells is achieved by "blocking" of specific receptor sites of tolerogen, leaving other receptor sites free to function. Bone marrow precursors, however, appear to be restricted to recognition of only one determinant. (Explanation supplied by WO Weigle, Scripps Clinic and Research Foundation, La Jolla, Calif. See Proc Natl Acad Sci USA 65:551, 1970)

CLONAL ELIMINATION

The clonal selection theory of Burnet (7,8) designates that the ability of an individual to recognize an immunogen lies in individual reactive cells or cell lines (clones). Upon contact with the antigen, the cells with the capacity to recognize the antigen are stimulated to multiply and differentiate. The property of antigen recognition is restricted in the sense that each reactive cell recognizes only one or a very few antigens. In fetal life, or under special situations in adults, contact of the reacting cell with antigen causes the death of this cell and therefore a loss of the ability of the individual to make an immune response to that antigen (tolerance). The death or loss of immunologically reactive precursor cells in fetal life, upon contact of these cells with the individual's own tissues, usually results in the establishment of natural tolerance. In adult animals the establishment of acquired tolerance may be preceded by a brief period of antibody production. This is explained by antigen-driven differentiation leading to depletion of antigen recognition cells (exhaustive differentiation) (11).

The clonal selection theory of tolerance is weakened by the results of many experiments in which tolerance is easily broken. Such experiments indicate that tolerance depends not upon the loss of immunologically reactive precursor cells, but upon an altered reactivity of cells that can be redirected to immune responsiveness by certain procedures. Thus in most instances tolerance is most likely due not to the elimination or failure of development of specifically reactive cells, but to blocking of expression or temporary inactivation of cells required for a specific response. The breaking of tolerance by cross-reacting antigens can be explained by a different range of tolerogenic recognition by T and B cells (Fig. 7–1).

SUPPRESSOR T CELLS

The ability of populations of lymphocytes to inhibit certain immunologic reactions has been ascribed to a subpopulation of T cells with a suppressor activity (6,18,19). Perhaps the first clues to the presence of suppressor T cells came with the observations concerning the effects of transfer of normal or immune cells to tolerant hosts and of tolerant cells to normal irradiated or syngeneic recipients. Antilymphocytic serum (ALS) treatment (see p. 320) of syngeneic lymphoid cells could in turn increase or reduce a subsequent antibody response in irradiated recipients (4) and inactivated a cell type that normally suppresses the antibody response (5). Further studies demonstrated that thymectomized, lethally irradiated, bone marrow-grafted mice reconstituted with thymocytes and pretreated with antigen did not respond with antibody production after a second challenge while mice not receiving thymocytes were able to respond (18). This phenomena as been termed *infectious tolerance* (19) and strongly implies a role for suppressor T cells in the induction and maintenance of tolerance.

A number of additional findings support a role for suppressor T cells in controlling the response of B cells. 1) An increase in antibody production to thymus-independent antigens may be obtained after thymectomy (26). 2) Thymocytes from rats treated with antigen 48 hours previously, when transferred to syngeneic recipients, may specifically suppress the response of the recipients to the same antigen (21). 3) An increase in homocyto-trophic antibody occurs in sublethally irradiated rats, but this increased production is markedly reduced 2 days after transfer of thymocytes or T cells containing spleen cell populations from hyperimmunized rats (28). 4) ATS treatment of young New Zealand Black (NZB) mice increases antibody response to certain antigens, but this effect is not seen in older NZB mice who may have lost their suppressor T cell population (12), thus rendering them prone to development of certain "autoallergic" diseases (see p. 244). 5) Lymphocytes from mice with chronic suppression of a given immunoglobulin allotype produce suppression of expression of that allotype by normal cells in vitro or upon passive transfer (24). 6) Lymphocytes stimulated by certain mitogens such as Concanavalin A, will inhibit the immune response of normal cells (14). 7) Treatment of tolerant cells with anti-thy serum plus complement abolishes the ability of these cells to transfer tolerance (adoptive tolerance) to irradiated recipient mice (6).

Each of these observations supports the concept that a certain population of T cells controls the response of B cells, although the mechanism through which they do is unclear. Suppressor T cells may prevent recognition of antigen, inhibit antigen-induced metabolic changes in B cells, limit the extent of B cell proliferation, block differentiation of B cells to antibody secreting cells or interfere with helper T cell–B cell interaction.

Suppressor T cells may also limit the activity of other T cells. The percentage of the T cell population that exerts a suppressor effect is probably about 10–20%. Certain T cells inhibit the blastogenic response to phytohemagglutinin (16), and to specific antigens (17), which are believed to be T cell functions. In addition, treatment of recipient rats with antithymocyte serum may increase the severity of a graft-vs-host reaction (see p. 236) produced upon transfer of thymus cells. Since that reaction is T cell mediated, the ATS may depress suppressor T cells that control the GvH T cells (9).

Suppressor T cells may be the primary mechanism for preventing antibody production by B cells or for cellular immunologic reaction by other T cells in the tolerant animal. Suppressor T cells may be specific for a given antigen, thus explaining the fact that immune reactions to other antigens are not suppressed in animals rendered tolerant to a given antigen.

BLOCKING ANTIBODY

Earlier it was pointed out that specific antibody acted as a feedback to limit the production of more specific antibody and control the extent of an immune response (p. 58). During the induction of tolerance a phase of antibody production sometimes occurs prior to the establishment of the tolerant state (27). It is tenuous to postulate that such an antibody can induce tolerance since it is impossible to induce adoptive tolerance with antiserum. It has been suggested that the immunologic activities of T cells can be blocked by antigen–antibody complexes (20). Although there is little concrete data to support this role in induction of antibody formation it is possible that antigen–antibody complexes could react with the surface receptors of helper T cells in such a way as to block reaction with free antigen and prevent carrier cell function. Such blocking effects have been described as preventing tumor and tissue graft rejection (see p. 336).

ANTIGEN CATABOLISM

The establishment of the tolerant state may be caused by an inability of the affected animal to metabolize the antigen properly whereby the information necessary for a specific immune response is not made available (1). An immunogen may be processed by an immature or suppressed immune system so that it is not recognized as foreign by specifically reactive cells and becomes sequestered in immune recognition cells with the result that future contacts with the antigen do not evoke a response. This explanation is inconsistent with the fact that tolerance lasts considerably longer than the calculated duration of antigen present in the tolerant animal. However, sensitive assays indicate that in fact antigens may be sequestered in tolerant animals longer than was previously recognized (1).

Studies with cell transfer systems using populations enriched with lymphocytes or macrophages, or combinations thereof, suggest that tolerance may be a function of the cell type that first contacts the antigen (13,23,25,30). According to this concept the induction of an immune response requires the processing of antigen by macrophages (see Chapter 3), which prepares the antigen for recognition by specific immunologically reactive cells (lymphocytes). If the antigen is not processed by macrophages, the direct interaction of the antigen with the specific reactive cells results in a loss of the ability of these cells to be stimulated immunologically (tolerance). The processing of immunogen by macrophages is an immunologically nonspecific event, the specificity of tolerance being determined by the loss of recognition by specifically reactive lymphocytes.

In summary, no single theory can explain all of the natural and experimental phenomena that are grouped under the umbrella of tolerance. Different mechanisms may explain different phenomena or more than one mechanism may be operative in a given situation. Cells with the capacity of responding to a specific antigen (immunologically competent cells) may undergo induction in four directions upon contact with the antigen. They may become immune (antibody-producing plasma cells or sensitized lymphocytes), or tolerant; they may become memory cells, or suppressor cells (Fig. 7-2). The final direction depends upon the dose and type of antigen and the state of the potentially responding individual. It is also possible that some reactive cells are killed by reaction with the tolerogen or that an immunogen may be presented in a nonimmunogenic manner in a tolerant animal. However, tolerance is best considered as an active process involving either the production of tolerant cells that cannot respond to an immunogen or suppressor cells that inhibit potentially responding cells.

TOLERANCE AND IMMUNITY

Immune tolerance may be a more common or more natural state than immune reactivity. An individual is more likely to be presented with small amounts of antigen (everyday contact with nonpathogenic organisms) or

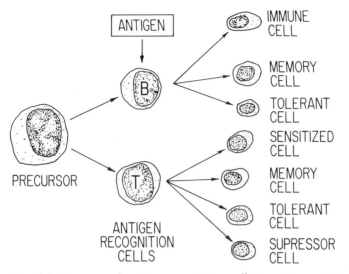

Fig. 7–2. Response of antigen recognition cells to antigen. Both T cells and B cells are capable of recognizing, reacting with and being changed by specific antigen. B cells that react with antigen may be converted to antibody-producing plasma cells, B memory cells or tolerant B cells. T cells that react with antigen may become sensitized, memory, tolerant or suppressor cells. The final effect in a given animal depends upon the balance of effect of the different populations produced. This balance may be determined by factors such as dose, route and form of the antigen and age and condition of the responding animal. There is also some evidence for the development of suppressor B cells.

very high and continued doses of antigen (an individual's own serum proteins), in a manner more conducive to the production of tolerance (nonaggregated) than to the production of active immunity. The immunologist has worked most often in dose ranges likely to result in active immunity and commonly uses nonspecific adjuvants to enhance immune responses. These adjuvants generally have the effect of mobilizing lymphoid cells and concentrating reactive cells at the site of antigen deposition; a similar effect would occur in the case of an infection with an organism capable of producing a nonimmune inflammatory response. The role of tolerance or lack of tolerance is important for the understanding of autoallergic diseases and the principles of transplantation, which will be covered in later chapters.

IMMUNE PARALYSIS

An effect similar to tolerance [Felton's immune paralysis (15)] may be induced by injection of moderate amounts of nondegradable antigen. In such cases, antibody-producing cells may be identified if they are removed from the animal, but secreted antibody is rapidly bound to the circulating antigen. Usually antigens bound to antibody (complexes) are taken up by macrophages (phagocytosis), and both antigen and antibody are degraded. When an antigen is undegradable, only the antibody is destroyed; the antigen is released so that it may again combine with antibody. Thus, any antibody formed is removed rapidly by antigen so that circulating antibody is not detectable (22). Under these circumstances, transient states of antibody formation may be detected, but the continued presence of the undegradable antigen continues to stimulate differentiation of plasma cells, resulting in a situation similar to high-dose tolerance (exhaustive differentiation).

REFERENCES

1. Ada GL, Nossal GJV, Pye J: Antigens in immunity. XI. The uptake of antigen in animals previously rendered immunologically tolerant. Aust J Exp Biol Med Sci 43:337, 1965
2. Argyris BF: Adoptive tolerance; transfer of the tolerant state. J Immunol 90:29–34, 1963
3. Argyris BF: Adoptive tolerance transferred by bone marrow, spleen, lymph node or thymus cells. J Immunol 96:273–278, 1966
4. Baker PJ, Stashak PW, Amsbaugh DF, Prescott B: Regulation of the antibody response to type III pneumococcal polysaccharide. II. Mode of action of thymic-derived suppressor cells. J Immunol 112:404–409, 1974
5. Baker PJ, Stashak PW, Amsbaugh DR, Prescott B, Barth RF: Evidence for the existence of two functionally distinct types of cells which regulate the antibody response to type III pneumococcal polysaccharide. J Immunol 105:1581–1583, 1970
6. Basten A, Miller JFAP, Sprent J, Cheers C: Cell-to-cell interaction in the immune response X T cell-dependent suppression in tolerant mice. J Exp Med 140:199, 1974
7. Burnet FM: The Clonal Selection Theory of Acquired Immunity. London, Cambridge University Press, 1959
8. Burnet FM: The Integrity of the Body: A Discussion of Modern Immunological Ideas. Cambridge, Mass, Harvard University Press, 1962
9. Cantor H, Asofsky R: Paradoxical effect of anti-thymocyte serum on the thymus. Nature 243:39–41, 1973
10. Chiller JM, Habicht GS, Weigle WO: Cellular sites of immunologic unresponsiveness. Proc Natl Acad Sci USA 65:551, 1970
11. Chiller JM, Rombard CG, Weigle WO: Induction of immunological tolerance in neonatal and adult rabbits. Cell Immunol 8:28, 1973
12. Chused TM, Steinberg AD, Parker LM: Enhanced antibody response of mice to polyinosinic polycytidylic acid by antithymocyte serum and its age-dependent loss in NZB/W mice. J Immunol 111:52–57, 1973
13. Dresser DW, Mitchison NA: The mechanism of immunological paralysis. Adv Immunol 8:129, 1968
14. Dutton RW: Inhibitory and stimulatory effects of Concanavalin A on the response of mouse spleen cell suspensions to antigen. II. Evidence for separate stimulatory and inhibitory cells. J Exp Med 138:1496–1505, 1973
15. Felton LD: The significance of antigen in animal tissue. J Immunol 61:107, 1949
16. Folch H, Yoshinaga M, Waksman BH: Regulation of lymphocyte responses in vitro. III. Inhibition by adherent cells of the T-lymphocyte response to phytohemagglutinin. J Immunol 110:835–839, 1973
17. Gershon RK, Cohen P, Hencin R, Liebhaber SA: Suppressor T cells. J Immunol 108:586–590, 1972
18. Gershon RC, Kondo K: Cell interactions in the induction of tolerance: The role of thymic lymphocytes. Immunology 18:723, 1970
19. Gershon RK, Kondo K: Infectious immunological tolerance. Immunology 21:903–914, 1971
20. Gorczynski R, Kontiainen S, Mitchison NA, Tigelar RE: Antigen–antibody complexes as blocking factors on the T lymphocyte surface. In Cellular Selection and Regula-

tion in the Immune Response. Edelman GM (ed). New York, Raven Press, 1974, p 143.
21. Ha T-Y, Waksman BH, Treffers HP: The thymic suppressor cell. I. Separation of subpopulations with suppressor activity. J Exp Med 139:13–23, 1974
22. Halliday WJ: Immunological paralysis of mice with pneumococcal polysaccharide antigens. Bacteriol Rev 35:267, 1971
23. Hašek M, Langerová A, Hraba T: Transplantation immunity and tolerance. Adv Immunol 1:1, 1961
24. Herzenberg LA, Chan EL, Ravitch MM, Riblet RJ, Herzenberg LA: Active suppression of immunoglobulin allotype synthesis. III. Identification of T cells as responsible for suppression by cells from spleen, thymus, lymph node, and bone marrow. J Exp Med 137:1311–1324, 1973
25. Hraba T: Mechanisms and Role of Immunological Tolerance. Monographs in Allergy. In Kallós P, Goodman HC, Hašek M, Inderbitzen T (eds). Basel, Karger, 1968
26. Kerbel RS, Eidinger D: Enhanced immune responsiveness to a thymus-independent antigen early after adult thymectomy: Evidence for short-lived inhibitory thymus-derived cells. Eur J Immunol 2:114–118, 1972
27. Mitchison NA: Induction of immunological paralysis with two zones of dosage. Proc R Soc Lond (Biol) 161:275, 1966
28. Okumura K, Tada T: Regulation of homocytotropic antibody formation in the rat. VI. Inhibitory effect of thymocytes on the homocytotropic antibody response. J Immunol 107:1682–1689, 1971
29. Owen RD: Immunogenetic consequence of vascular anastomoses between bovine twins. Science 102:400, 1945
30. Schwartz RS, Ryder RJW, Gottlieb BAA: Macrophages and antibody synthesis. Prog Allergy 14:81, 1970
31. Weber G, Kölsch E: Transfer of low zone tolerance to normal syngeneic mice by θ-positive cells. Eur J Immunol 3:767, 1973
32. Weigle WO: Termination of acquired immunological tolerance to protein antigens following immunization with altered protein antigens. J Exp Med 116:913, 1962

8

Phagocytosis and the Reticuloendothelial System

PHAGOCYTOSIS

Phagocytosis is the engulfing of microrganisms, other cells or foreign particles by living cells (1,2) known as phagocytes or macrophages, the most active of which make up the reticuloendothelial system. Monocytes and histiocytes are the blood and tissue phagocytes respectively. Phagocytes possess cellular structures which contain enzymes that are usually able to digest ingested particles (Fig. 8–1). The structures, called primary lysosomes, are membrane-limited cytoplasmic vacuoles containing high concentrations of acid hydrolases (1), and are believed to be formed from the endoplasmic reticulum of the phagocyte and released into the cytoplasm of the cell by a tubular array of membranes known as the Golgi apparatus. Phagocytized particles enter the cell via invagination of the cytoplasmic membrane. This invagination forms around the particles so that they enter the cytoplasm surrounded by a layer of cytoplasmic membrane. Thus, another membrane-limited body, termed a phagosome, is formed. As the phagosome enters into the cytoplasm, fusion occurs between the enzyme-containing primary lysosome and the particle-containing phagosome, with mixing of the contents of the vacuoles. The enzymes of the lysosome, which include acid phosphatase, β-glucuronidase, cathepsin and other acid hydrolases, then digest the particles in a membrane-limited body formed by the fusion of the primary lysosome and the phagosome. This fusion vacuole is called a secondary lysosome. The particles are then destroyed. Undigested debris may remain in the secondary lysosome or may be extruded from the cell (cell defecation).

In some cases, either because of the nature or the amount of the phagocytized material or because of an insufficiency in lysosomal hydrolases, ingested particles or organisms are not digested. Some organisms (*Histoplasma capsulatum*) have the ability to survive phagocytosis and reproduce

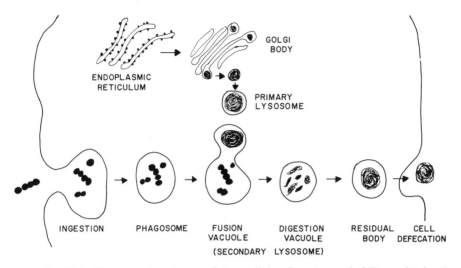

ENDOPLASMIC RETICULUM

GOLGI BODY

PRIMARY LYSOSOME

INGESTION   PHAGOSOME   FUSION VACUOLE   DIGESTION VACUOLE   RESIDUAL BODY   CELL DEFECATION

(SECONDARY LYSOSOME)

Fig. 8–1. Phagocytosis. Stages of intracellular digestion and different kinds of lysosomes. Foreign material is ingested into a phagosome. Phagosome fuses with primary lysosome (formed by Golgi body) which contains enzymes to digest ingested material. Resulting fusion vacuole is secondary lysosome. When digestion is ended, some material may remain in residual body which is then eliminated from cell by cell defecation. (Modified from de Duve C: Sci Am 208:64, 1963. © Copyright 1963 by Scientific American, Inc. All rights reserved)

within phagocytes. Infection with such an agent may result in the presence of large numbers of viable organisms in the cytoplasm of phagocytic cells. Some particles (silica) cannot be digested, remain in phagocytic cells, and eventually cause destruction of the phagocyte (phagocytic suicide) and the formation of collections of dead phagocytes (see Chapter 15). A congenital deficiency in acid hydrolases in phagocytes and an increased susceptibility to infection (chronic granulomatous disease).

THE RETICULOENDOTHELIAL SYSTEM

The reticuloendothelial system is a multiorgan collection of cells whose primary property is phagocytosis (2). Two general types of phagocytes are recognized—wandering and fixed. The wandering cells are the monocytes of the peripheral blood. These cells may be found in other organs, such as the sinusoids of lymphoid organs or the connective tissue stroma of many organs where they may be only temporary residents. The fixed cells (histiocytes) are more permanent residents in these tissue locations. Histiocytes may be found in liver (Kupffer cells or sinusoid-lining cells), spleen (sinusoid-lining cells, reticular cells, dendritic macrophages), lymph nodes, connective tissue, brain (microglia), bone marrow, adrenals, thymus and lungs. If particles such as carbon or vital dyes are injected into the blood, the Kupffer cells of the liver and the phagocytic cells of the spleen ingest most of them; if the particles are inhaled, the pulmonary alveolar macrophages ingest them; if they are injected into connective tissue, the local node phagocytes ingest them; if the particles are injected into the brain, the microglia destroy them. All these cells have in common the ability to ingest foreign materials.

PHAGOCYTIC INDEX

Measurement of the phagocytic capacity of an animal may be accomplished by determining the rate of disappearance of stable, inert, uniform particles such as gelatin-stabilized carbon particles (2). Upon intravenous injection of such particles, about 90% are taken up by the liver and most of the remainder by the spleen. Carbon clearance is measured after saturation of the clearing mechanism, since a dose of particles lower than the saturation dose is cleared during the first few passages of the blood through the liver. Determination of carbon clearance under these conditions primarily measures liver blood flow. If a dose large enough to saturate the reticuloendothelial system is given, a two-stage elimination occurs: 1) a rapid clearance as the particle-laden blood first passes through the liver and spleen, and 2) a slower clearance which occurs upon recirculation through the previously saturated reticuloendothelial system. The slope of this second curve is the phagocytic index. It measures regeneration of phagocytic capacity after saturation.

Determination of Phagocytic Index

The clearance of particles from the blood by the reticuloendothelial system follows first-order reaction kinetics:

$$Reactant \rightarrow product$$
$$or$$
$$particles\ in\ blood \rightarrow ingestion\ by\ RES$$

The change in concentration of the particles in the blood over a given time is related to the concentration at the start of the experiment, as follows:

$$dC/dt + KC_o$$

This becomes:

$$Ct = C_o 10^{-Kt}$$

where Ct = concentration at time t
C_o = initial concentration
t = time
K = constant (phagocytic index)

solving for K:

$$K = \frac{\log C_1 - \log C_2}{t_2 - t_1}$$

After injection of a dose of carbon particles sufficient to saturate the reticuloendothelial system, the concentration of carbon in the blood at a given time is determined (C_1, t_1). After a period of several hours, the animal is bled and the concentration of carbon again determined (C_2, t_2). K, the phagocytic index, can then be determined from the formula given above.

STIMULATION OF THE RETICULOENDOTHELIAL SYSTEM

The effect of a number of treatments on the phagocytic index has been determined (2). Products of microorganisms such as the cell wall of yeast (zymosan), bacterial endotoxins, extracts of *Mycobacterium tuberculosis*, living and killed organisms; simple lipids such as triglycerides; and hormones such as estrogen, have all been shown to increase carbon clearance. The ability of some organisms, such as *Salmonella typhimurium* to increase phagocytic activity results in increased resistance of the host to other infecting microorganisms (Nonspecific Macrophage Activation, see Chapter 15). Immunoglobulin antibody to a given organism or particle may increase the capacity of the host to phagocytize antibody-coated particles. Antibody with such properties is called opsonin. The mechanisms of action of agents that stimulate phagocytic clearance is not clear. Such stimulation may occur by increasing the number of lysosomes per cell, by increasing the amount of hydrolytic enzymes in each lysosome, or by changing the surface properties of the particle being ingested so that it is more easily recognized or more easily catabolized by phagocytes.

BLOCKADE OF THE RETICULOENDOTHELIAL SYSTEM

Phagocytic clearance may be depressed by overloading the reticuloendothelial system (2). Thus, a saturating dose of carbon may decrease the clearance of a second dose of carbon. Blockade of the reticuloendothelial system with fibrin results in a decreased clearance of fibrin formed after blockade (see Chapter 22). Agents that blockade the system have similar properties. Colloidal carbon blockades the system for a second dose of carbon or for similar agents but does not affect the clearance of chromic phosphate. This suggests different phagocytic receptors for different particles.

Phagocytic Dysfunction

Certain human diseases are characterized by abnormalities in phagocytosis. Such phagocytic deficiencies are usually associated with susceptibility to infections. These diseases are presented in more detail in Chapter 19.

REFERENCES

1. Cohn ZA: The structure and functions of monocytes and macrophages. Adv Immunol 9:163, 1968
2. Stuart AE: The Reticuloendothelial System. Edinburgh, Livingstone, 1970

II

Immunopathology

Immune reactions of both humoral and cellular types play important roles in the defense of the host against infectious agents. Antibody is generally operative against bacteria or bacterial products, whereas cellular reactivity is prominent in the defense against viral and mycotic organisms. The protective effect of immune reactions is called immunity and is the subject of the third part of this text. However, we increasingly recognize instances in which the immune reaction of the host produces tissue damage (disease). The destructive effect of immune reactions is termed *allergy* or *hypersensitivity*. Immunopathology is the study of tissue alterations made manifest by various types of hypersensitivity or allergic reactions, the subject of the following section (Part II).

The terms *immunity* and *allergy* should be reserved for effects mediated through immune mechanisms. In a strict sense, some instances of altered reactivity due to a previous exposure are not reactions of allergy or immunity. These phenomena include the Shwartzman reaction (alteration in the state of blood coagulation), adaptive enzyme synthesis (substrate selection of enzyme production), anaphylactoid reactions (pseudoallergic reactions resulting from liberation of pharmacologically active agents that may also be liberated by allergic reactions), reactions to drugs caused by nonallergic physiologic hyperreactivity (idiosyncrasy), and other types of environmental adaptations (heat, cold, altitude, emotion) produced by nonimmune physiologic or psychologic mechanisms.

9

Classification of Immunopathologic Disorders

The tissue alterations caused by various allergic reactions may be considered variations of the inflammatory reaction. Because more than one organ system may be involved with the same allergic process and because the alterations in different organ systems caused by the same process have pathologic similarities, the lesions produced by allergic reactions are best classified according to the particular type of allergic mechanisms involved (1). In the systematic study of pathology, disease conditions are usually classified according to the anatomic location of the pathologic process. From a strictly pathologic standpoint, the organ system classification has definite advantages. From an immunopathologic standpoint, however, it leaves much to be desired.

CLASSIFICATION BY IMMUNE MECHANISM

Immunopathologic processes may be divided into six major classes: 1) neutralization or inactivation, 2) cytotoxic or cytolytic, 3) atopic or anaphylactic, 4) Arthus (toxic complex), 5) delayed hypersensitivity (cellular), and 6) granulomatous.

The first four types of reactions are mediated by humoral antibodies; the fifth and sixth by specifically sensitized cells (Fig. 9–1). The features of each type of reaction are summarized in Table 9–1. This classification is an extension of the original classification of Gell and Coombs (1) which has contributed greatly to the understanding of immunopathologic mechanisms.

CLASSIFICATION BY ORIGIN OF RESPONSE AND SOURCE OF ANTIGEN

A second method of classification, which provides considerable insight into allergic mechanisms, should also be considered. Based on the source

126

TABLE 9-1
Characteristics of the Six Types of Hypersensitivity Reactions

| | Early inflammatory reactions | | | | Late inflammatory reactions | |
| | Hematologic reaction | | | | | |
	Neutralization or inactivation	Cytotoxic or cytolytic	Atopic or anaphylactic	Arthus (toxic complex)	Delayed (cellular)	Granulomatous
Clinical state	Deficiencies, resistance to replacement therapy	Hemolysis, leukopenia, thrombocytopenia	Urticaria, hay fever, asthma	Serum sickness, glomerulonephritis	Tuberculosis, bacterial hypersensitivities, contact dermatitis	Tuberculosis, fungi, chronic granuloma
Sensitizing antigens	Hormones, clotting factors	Blood cells, drugs, haptens	Pollens, dander, haptens	Soluble proteins, carbohydrates, haptens	Bacteria, fungi viruses, proteins, haptens	Insoluble antigens
Antibody	Serum	Serum, complement-fixing, IgG, IgM	Serum, skin-fixing, nonprecipitable, IgE	Serum, precipitable, IgG, complement-fixing	Cellular	? Cellular
Transfer Skin reactions	Sera, cells	Sera, cells	Sera, cells; Wheal and flare: 5–15 min max.; fade 1–2 hr	Sera, cells; Arthus: 6 hr max.; fade 24 hr	Cells only; Delayed: 24–48 hr max.; nothing at 6 hr	Cells only; Delayed: weeks
Pathology, primary	Inactivation of biologically active molecules	Cell lysis by complement	Release of pharmacologically active substances	Perivascular poly infiltration	Perivascular and diffuse round-cell infiltration	Epithelioid cell, giant cell, granuloma
secondary	Metabolic or clotting abnormalities due to loss of active agents	Anemia, jaundice, hemosiderosis, infection, bleeding	Edema, smooth muscle contraction, eosinophilia	Thrombosis, fibrinoid necrosis	Parenchymal destruction associated with cellular infiltrate (necrosis)	Tissue replacement and distraction with granulomas

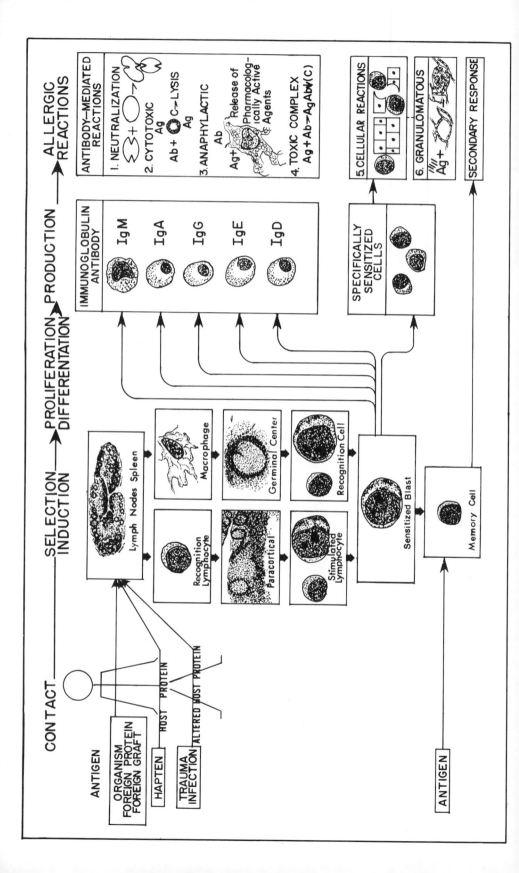

TABLE 9–2
Classification of Allergic Diseases According to Source of Antigen and Origin of Response

I. *Endogenous* immune response to *endogenous* antigens

   A. Circulating antibody
      1. Autoallergic hematologic diseases
      2. Antibodies to tissue antigens in human diseases
   B. Cellular (delayed) sensitivity
      1. Experimental autoallergic diseases
      2. Human counterparts of experimental autoallergic diseases

II. *Endogenous* immune response to *exogenous* antigens

   A. Circulating antibody
      1. Anaphylactic-type reactions
      2. Atopic reactions
      3. Arthus reactions
   B. Cellular (delayed) sensitivity
      1. Tuberculin reaction
   C. Granulomatous hyptersensitivity
      1. Berylliosis

III. *Exogenous* immune response to *endogenous* antigens

   A. Transfer of maternal antibody to fetus
      1. Erythroblastosis fetalis
      2. Neonatal leukopenia; thrombocytopenia
      3. Neonatal myasthenia gravis
   B. Experimental transfer of antibodies
      1. Masugi nephritis
   C. Experimental transfer of cells
      1. Graft-vs-host reaction

IV. *Exogenous* immune response to *exogenous* antigens

   A. Experimental transfer of antibodies and antigens
      1. Passive anaphylaxis (Prausnitz-Küstner reaction)
      2. Passive Arthus reaction
   B. Experimental transfer of cells and antigens
      1. Tuberculin reaction
      2. Contact dermatitis

V. *Endogenous* immune response to *complex* antigens (hapten-protein)

   A. Circulating antibody
      1. Drug-induced blood dyscrasias
      2. Drug-induced lupus erythematosus
   B. Cellular sensitivity
      1. Contact dermatitis

Modified from lecture notes of Frank J. Dixon, M.D.

Fig. 9–1. Immune response and immunopathologic mechanisms. Potential antigens (foreign material, haptens, or altered host material) induce immune reactivity. This reactivity is manifested by production of specifically reactive serum proteins (antibodies) or specifically modified cells (sensitized lymphocytes) capable of recognizing and reacting with antigen to which the individual is exposed. As a result of this process, the following allergic mechanisms may become manifest: 1) neutralization or inactivation of biologically active molecules, 2) cytotoxic or cytolytic reactions, 3) anaphylactic or atopic reactions, 4) Arthus (toxic complex) reactions, 5) delayed hypersensitivity (cellular) reactions, and 6) granulomatous reactions. Also produced is a population of cells with ability to cause more rapid and more intense response to second contact of immunizing antigen (memory cell). Mechanism of development of immune memory is poorly understood.

of antigen and the origin of the immune response in relation to the affected individual, this classification is presented in outline form in Table 9–2. A more complete understanding of the specific diseases discussed can be achieved by classifying each disease according to this table.

REFERENCE

1. Gell PGH, Coombs RRA: Clinical Aspects of Immunology, 2nd ed. Oxford, Blackwell, 1968

_____ 10 _____

Neutralization or Inactivation of Biologically Active Molecules

If an antibody is produced to an enzyme, hormone or other substance with a significant biologic function, and if this antibody essentially inactivates the enzyme or hormone, serious damage to the affected individual may occur (5). Antibody may neutralize or inactivate biologically active molecules by a number of different mechanisms (Fig. 10–1). In general these may be divided into two categories: 1) direct reaction with the biologically active molecule, resulting in some alteration of the molecule so that it is no longer active, and 2) interaction of the antibodies with the biologically active molecule in a way that may not directly inactivate the molecule, but allows the resulting antibody–antigen complex to be catabolized more rapidly in vivo, lowering the effective concentration of the biologically active molecules.

MECHANISMS OF ANTIBODY-MEDIATED INACTIVATION

DIRECT INACTIVATION

Biologically active molecules generally have one site that is necessary for biologic activity; a large portion of the molecule may not be directly involved. For example, an enzyme has an active site localized in a small area of the whole molecule. It is relatively simple to visualize that an antibody reacting with or near this active site would block the reaction of the enzyme with its substrate, however, this rarely occurs. Most antibodies that inactivate enzymes react with an antigenic site quite distant

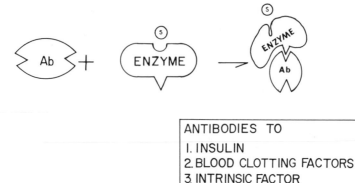

Fig. 10–1. Neutralization or inactivation of biologically active molecules. Reaction of antibody with enzyme or other biologically active molecule may result in loss of biologic function of both. The antigenic sites of an enzyme are usually located on a different part of the molecule than the substrate binding site. Inactivation occurs by alteration of the tertiary structure of the enzyme following reaction with antibody which affects the substrate binding site or activity of the enzyme molecules, or by increased catabolism of the enzyme–antibody complex. The biologic effect of neutralization depends upon the molecule neutralized.

from the biologically active site. Inactivation occurs by alteration of the tertiary structure of the enzyme due to its reaction with antibody (5). Not all such reactions result in inactivation. In fact, classic precipitin reactions with enzymes may occur with no apparent loss of activity in the precipitated enzyme, and at least one instance has been reported wherein reaction of an inactive form of the enzyme β-D-galactosidase with an antibody results in activation of the enzyme (16,23). Presumably reaction of the antibody with the inactive form of the enzyme results in an alteration of tertiary structure so that the active site becomes available.

Not only is the site of antibody reaction important in neutralization of a biologically active molecule, but the effect of the antibody also depends upon other characteristics of the antibody–antigen reaction, such as the ratio of antibody to antigen, the strength of antibody–antigen binding and the biologic properties of the antibody (e.g., complement fixation). Thus, inactivation may be induced by the antibodies formed in one individual, while the antibodies formed in another individual may react with the same enzyme, but not inactivate it (5).

INDIRECT INACTIVATION

Any discussion of the neutralizing properties of antibodies to biologically active molecules must take into account that the reaction occurs in vivo. It is well known that most antigen–antibody complexes formed in vivo are rapidly cleared by the reticuloendothelial system (32). A nonneutralizing antibody might effectively reduce the availability of an enzyme or hormone through this mechanism. However, not all antigen–antibody complexes are rapidly removed; some soluble complexes may continue to circulate. In some situations binding of antibody to a serum protein may actually produce a longer half-life as bound molecules are degraded more slowly than unbound molecules. This may lead to increased serum concentrations for material involved (13). The presence of such complexes may lead to particular clinical findings, some of which are described later (see Toxic Complex Glomerulonephritis, Chapter 13). Another complication may occur if antibodies to a given enzyme or hormone react with its antigen in the tissue before the release of the enzyme or hormone. This interesting possibility has not been fully investigated.

EXAMPLES OF ANTIBODY-MEDIATED INACTIVATION

Antibodies to biologically active molecules are generally found in three circumstances in man: 1) following transfusion, particularly when a given material is genetically lacking, such as anticlotting-factor antibodies in hemophiliacs; 2) in certain peculiar diseases associated with abnormalities of immune response, such as lupus erythematosus; and 3) following an allergic reaction to a drug, such as penicillin. The specific antibodies to biologically active molecules that will be considered in more detail here are 1) antibodies to insulin, 2) antibodies to blood clotting factors, 3) antibodies to intrinsic factor and erythropoietin, 4) the long-acting thyroid stimulator of Graves' disease, and 5) humoral factors associated with myasthenia gravis.

INSULIN

Banting and his group in 1938 observed an antibody-like neutralizer of insulin in a schizophrenic patient who had been receiving insulin shock treatments (22). Since that time, numerous accounts of "insulin resistance" have appeared. In many cases resistance to exogenous insulin derived from one source (ox) does not hold for insulin derived from another species (pig). However, in some cases resistance may occur to insulins of different origin because they contain some antigenic determinants in common and some determinants which are unique (22). Not all antiinsulins are neutralizing and not all insulins are neutralizable by the same antibody. The binding of insulin by antiinsulin in vivo usually causes retardation of the disappearance of insulin from the blood stream, i.e., a longer half-life. Insulin bonded to antibody is catabolized at the rate of the antibody (IgG) and not at the rate of insulin. Therefore, instead of reducing the half-life of insulin, antibody to insulin actually prolongs the half-life; the bound insulin is protected from degradation by insulinase in the liver (33). However, the antibody-bound insulin is prevented from exerting its biologic activity. The amount of insulin required to overcome the antibody depends upon the amount and binding affinity of the antibody, but a close correlation between antibody titers and insulin requirements is not seen (2). The insulin–antiinsulin reaction has been adapted to provide an extremely sensitive immunoassay for insulin (see Radioimmunoassay, Chapter 5). Acute skin reactions (19) and systemic anaphylactic shock (34) (see Chapter 12) may also occur if insulin is injected into a sensitive individual.

BLOOD CLOTTING FACTORS

The clotting system requires the interaction of up to 30 different factors (14). Antibodies that may inactivate these factors have been reported. Antibodies to antihemophilic globulin frequently appear in hemophiliacs (who genetically lack this globulin) treated with infusions containing antihemophilic globulin. The hemophiliac recognizes the antihemophilic globulin as foreign. Similarly, individuals who lack other clotting components may develop antibody to the appropriate component when transfused. For reasons which are poorly understood, individuals with diseases such as lupus erythematosus, tuberculosis, or hyperglobulinemia may also produce antibodies to clotting factors which complicates an already confusing clinical picture. Circulating anticoagulants have also been found in association with penicillin allergy. Finally, some individuals apparently produce circulating anticoagulants unassociated with any known disease. The exact mechanism of action of antibodies to clotting factors is poorly understood. The clinical effect depends upon the particular factor or factors affected.

INTRINSIC FACTOR

Pernicious anemia is a disease in which there is an abnormality in the absorption of vitamin B_{12}, which is required for the normal maturation of erythrocytes so that failure of B_{12} absorption leads to a deficit in production of mature erythrocytes and to an anemia. Absorption of B_{12} requires the action of a factor known as intrinsic factor secreted by the lining cells of the stomach (parietal cells) (7). Pernicious anemia is associated with at least two distinct antibodies (10). One reacts specifically with the parietal cells of the gastric mucosa, even the patient's own gastric mucosa; the presence of this antibody is almost invariably associated with a reduction in acid secretion and atrophic gastritis (10,11). The second, considered here, is antibody to intrinsic factor. This antibody was first observed because of an acquired resistance to intrinsic factor in patients being treated for pernicious anemia. This anti-intrinsic-factor antibody can be demonstrated to inhibit the binding of vitamin B_{12} to intrinsic factor and is associated with abnormalities of vitamin B_{12} absorption. Two types of anti-intrinsic-factor antibody have been observed: 1) blocking antibody, which prevents subsequent formation of vitamin B_{12}—intrinsic factor complexes and is associated with the presence of megaloblastic cells (28), and 2) binding antibody, which can be shown to bind to intrinsic factor but which does not prevent this bound intrinsic factor from subsequent combination with vitamin B_{12}. It has been postulated that intrinsic factor-blocking antibody plays a significant role in the pathogenesis of pernicious anemia.

ERYTHROPOIETIN

Erythropoietin is a biologically active material, believed to be produced by the kidney, which stimulates the production of erythrocytes in the bone marrow (9). Erythropoietic inhibitors have been identified in the plasma of patients with refractory anemia and it is possible that these patients may have an antibody that inhibits the action of erythropoietin (12), although the clinical significance of this antibody remains to be demonstrated.

LONG-ACTING THYROID STIMULATOR OF GRAVES' DISEASE

A serum protein with characteristics of an IgG antibody directed against a thyroid antigen is present in most patients with hyperthyroidism (Graves' disease). Although this long-acting thyroid stimulator (LATS) has properties consistent with antibody to thyroid microsomes, it is difficult to demonstrate because an inhibitor of LATS activity is present in normal serum, presumably in the albumin fraction. The exact relation of LATS, LATS inhibitor, and thyrotoxicosis remains to be clarified. However, there is evidence to support an in vivo activation of thyroid function by an autoantibody to thyroid tissue (15,17).

Rabbits that are immunized with thyroid components not only develop thyroiditis (see Chapter 14) but also produce a thyroid-stimulating globulin in their serum (25). This antibody has different properties than LATS of man (1). Therefore, hyperthyroidism may represent an autoallergic disease in which antibody produces an increase in the function of an organ but a cause and effect relationship of LATS and hyperthyroidism is not yet established.

MYASTHENIA GRAVIS

The etiology of myasthenia gravis is unknown, but there is evidence that a serum factor, perhaps an antibody, is responsible for inactivation of muscle function. The disease is characterized by muscle weakness and easy fatigue; weakness is most prominent in the muscles of the face and throat (3,31). The disorder appears to be due to a functional abnormality in which the conduction of nerve impulses from the motor nerve to the muscle fiber is impaired. Patients afflicted with this disease tire very easily; usually they awake with close to normal muscular function which deteriorates as muscle activity increases during the day (31). The clinical course is punctuated with remissions and exacerbations; total incapacitation and death from respiratory failure may occur (18). Therapy includes thymectomy and the use of anticholenesterase medication, which may temporarily reverse the muscle weakness, but little can be done if the disease progresses rapidly (18). The following associations implicate immune reactions in the etiology of myasthenia gravis: 1) Most myasthenics have a serum antibody that binds specifically to muscle fibers and epitheloid reticular cells of the thymus (26). However, the level of antibody does not always correlate to the severity of the disease and specific lesions that might be caused by an antibody-mediated mechanism (see Chapter 13) are not observed. These muscle-binding antibodies may be the cause, a secondary effect of the disease or only an associated finding. Support for a humoral factor as being responsible for myasthenia gravis also comes from the finding that newborn infants of mothers with myasthenia gravis may exhibit a temporary muscular weakness at birth due to the passive transfer of a humoral factor (?antibody) from the mother to the fetus (neonatal myasthenia gravis) (27). 2) Myasthenia gravis is frequently associated with a peculiar thymic hyperplasia in which germinal centers are found in the medulla of the thymus or with tumors of the thymus (4), and thymectomy may lead to an improvement in the clinical condition of selected patients (20). 3) Myasthenia gravis frequently occurs in patients who demonstrate other diseases of suspected allergic origin such as systemic lupus erythematosis, rheumatoid arthritis, Sjögren's syndrome, ulcerative colitis, pemphigus, pernicious anemia, and thyroiditis (6,18,24). 4) A variety of "autoantibodies" (see page 254) to organs other than thymus and muscle also occur frequently in the blood of patients with myasthenia gravis. These include antibodies to nuclear antigens, antithyroid antibodies and rheumatoid factor (24,29). 5) The most frequent lesion in the muscle is loss of fibers associated with focal collections of lymphocytes (lymphorrages) (3). These lesions might be caused by an infiltration of the muscle by specifically sensitized lymphocytes (see Chapter 14). 6) An experimental thymitis produced by immunization of animals with thymus extracts has been reported (8). Although it is claimed that animals with thymitis also have abnormalities in muscle function, others have been unable to confirm the experimental model (30). 7) Injection of rabbits with an acetylcholine receptor from an electric eel results in the production of precipitating antibody to the receptor and to a flaccid paralysis in the immunized animals that can be reversed by neostigmine (21), an agent that can also temporarily reverse the muscular weakness of patients with myasthenia gravis (18,31), thus supporting the contention of Simpson that myasthenia gravis might be caused by an autoallergic response to acetylcholine receptors (24). Therefore myasthenia gravis is included here as a possible neutralization or inactivation reaction by antibody of a biologically active molecule, such as the acetylcholine receptors leading to abnormalities of muscular function because of interference with acetylcholine-binding by its receptor.

NEUTRALIZING ANTIBODIES–CAUSE AND EFFECT

The presence of antibodies to a biologically active molecule in a patient with a given disease does not necessarily mean that the antibody actually causes the disease or is even responsible for any of the symptoms of the disease. For instance, there is no direct evidence that the antibodies found in patients with myasthenia gravis, hemophilia, pernicious anemia, diabetes or refractory anemia have any role in the etiology of the disease itself; they may occur secondarily to the primary disease process or to therapeutic events. However, the development of antibodies may cause resistance to therapy or secondary symptoms.

REFERENCES

1. Beall GN, Chopra IJ, Solomon DH, Pierce JG, Cornell JS: Neutralizing and nonneutralizing antibodies to bovine thyroid-stimulating hormone and its subunits. J Clin Invest 52:2979, 1973
2. Berson SA, Yalow RS: Quantitative aspects of reaction between insulin and insulinbinding antibody. J Clin Invest 38:1996, 1959
3. Buzzard EF: The clinical history and postmortem examination of five cases of myasthenia gravis. Brain 28:438, 1905
4. Castleman B: Pathology of the thymus gland in myasthenia gravis. In Thymectomy for Myasthenia Gravis. Viets HR, Schwab RS (eds). Springfield, Ill, Charles C Thomas, 1960

5. Cinader B (ed): Antibodies to Biologically Active Molecules. New York, Pergamon Press, 1967
6. Galbraith RF, Summerskill MA, Murray J: Systemic lupus erythematosis, cirrhosis and ulcerative colitis after thymectomy for myasthenia gravis. N Engl J Med 270:229, 1964
7. Glass GBJ: Gastric intrinsic factor and its function in the metabolism of B_{12}. Physiol Rev 43:529, 1963
8. Goldstein G, Hoffman WW: Electrophysiological changes similar to those of myasthenia gravis in rats with experimental autoimmune thymitis. J Neurol Neurosurg Psychiatry 31:453, 1968
9. Gordon AS, Cooper GW, Zanjani ED: The kidney and erythropoiesis. Semin Hematol 4:337, 1967
10. Irvine WJ: Immunologic aspects of pernicious anemia. N Engl J Med 273:432, 1965
11. Jeffries GH, Sleisenger MH: Studies of parietal cell antibody in pernicious anemia. J Clin Invest 44:2021, 1965
12. Jepson JH, Lowenstein L: Panhypoplasia of the bone marrow. I. Demonstration of a plasma factor with anti-erythropoietin-like activity. Can Med Assoc J 99:99, 1968
13. Levitt MD, Cooperband SR: Hyperamylasemia from the binding of serum anylase by an 11S IgA globulin. N Engl J Med 278:474, 1968
14. Margolius A, Jackson DP, Ratnoff OD: Circulating anticoagulants: A study of 40 cases and a review of the literature. Medicine 40:197, 1961
15. McKenzie JM: Humoral factors in the pathogenesis of Graves' disease. Physiol Rev 48:252, 1968
16. Melchers F, Messer W: The mechanism of activation of mutant β-galactosidase by specific antibodies. Eur J Biochem 35:380, 1973
17. Ochi Y, DeGroot LJ: Long acting thyroid stimulator of Graves' disease. N Engl J Med 278:718, 1968
18. Osserman KE: Myasthenia Gravis. New York, Grune and Stratton, 1958
19. Paley RG, Tunbridge RE: Dermal reactions to insulin therapy. Diabetes 1:22, 1952
20. Papatestas AE, Alpert LI, Osserman KE, Osserman RS, Kark AE: Studies in myasthenia gravis: Effects of thymectomy. Results on 185 patients with nonthymomatous and thymomatous myasthenia gravis, 1941–1969. Am J Med 50:465, 1971
21. Patrick J, Lindstrom J: Autoimmune response to acetylcholine receptor. Science 180:821, 1973
22. Pope CC: The immunology of insulin. Adv Immunol 5:209, 1966
23. Rotman MB, Celada F: Antibody-mediated activation of a defective β-D-galactosidase extracted from an Escherichia coli mutant. Proc Natl Acad Sci USA 60:660, 1968
24. Simpson JA: Myasthenia gravis: A new hypothesis. Scott Med J 5:419, 1960
25. Solomon DH, Beall GN: Thyroid-stimulating activity in the serum of immunized rabbits. II. Nature of the thyroid-stimulating material. J Clin Endocrinol Metab 28:1496, 1968
26. Strauss AJL, van der Geld HWR, Kemp PG Jr, Exum ED, Goodman HC: Immunological concomitants of myasthenia gravis. Ann NY Acad Sci 124:744, 1965
27. Strickroot FL, Schaeffer RL, Bergo HL: Myasthenia gravis occurring in an infant born of a myasthenic mother. JAMA 120:1207, 1942
28. Taylor KB, Roitt IM, Doniach D, Couchman KG, Shapland C: Autoimmune phenomena in pernicious anemia. Gastric antibodies. Br Med J 2:1347, 1962
29. van der Geld HWR, Feltkamp TEW, VanLoghem JJ, Oosterhuis HJGH, Biemond A: Multiple antibody production in myasthenia gravis. Lancet 2:373, 1963
30. Vetters JM, Simpson JA, Folkarde A: Experimental myasthenia gravis. Lancet 2:29, 1969
31. Viets HR: Myasthenia gravis. N. Engl J Med 251:97, 141, 1954
32. Weigle WO: Fate and biological action of antigen–antibody complexes. Adv Immunol 1:283, 1961
33. Yalow RS, Berson SA: Apparent inhibition of liver insulinase activity by serum and serum fractions containing insulin-binding antibody. J Clin Invest 36:648, 1957
34. Yasuna E: Generalized allergic reactions to insulin. J Allergy 12:295, 1940

11

Cytotoxic or Cytolytic Reactions

In this type of allergic response circulating antibody reacts with either an antigenic component of a cell or an antigen which has become intimately associated with a cell (40,42,44). As a result, a series of enzymatic reactions is usually activated (Fig. 11–1). The activation of this enzyme system causes the subsequent death or lysis of the target cell. The components of this enzymatic system are collectively called complement (23,24,25). The ultimate effect depends upon the type of cell involved and the severity of the allergic reaction.

IMMUNOHEMATOLOGIC DISEASES

REACTIONS TO ERYTHROCYTES

Disease conditions arising from the immune destruction of red blood cells result from loss of erythrocyte function or from the damaging effects of the released cell contents (hemoglobin) (7). These disorders include transfusion reactions, erythroblastosis fetalis, acquired autoallergic hemolytic diseases and hemolytic reactions to drugs (Fig. 11–2).

Transfusion Reactions

An immune reaction occurs when circulating antibody of host origin contacts erythrocytes from an incompatible donor. The antigen is exogenous, and the immune response is endogenous (Table 9–2). Some characteristics of the ABO blood group system are presented in Fig. 11–3 (41). An individual with blood type A has isoantibodies against type B erythrocytes. If this individual is transfused with type B blood, the anti-B antibodies react with B cells, causing them to agglutinate (30). These sensitized cells may then be lysed by complement or destroyed in the spleen. Over 14 human systems, which include over 60 different blood group factors, are now known (30,44). The ABO and Rh systems are most important

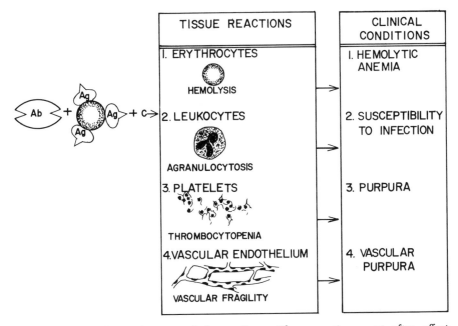

Fig. 11-1. Cytotoxic or cytolytic reactions. These reactions most often affect cellular elements in intimate contact with circulating plasma, such as erythrocytes, leukocytes, platelets or vascular endothelium. Circulating humoral antibody reacts with antigens present on cell membrane, activating the complement system. Through action of the complement system, integrity of cell membrane is compromised, then destroyed, because osmotic difference in intracellular and extracellular fluids causes release of intracellular fluids or because the altered cell is subject to phagocytosis. Such reactions may be observed experimentally with antibody to solid tissue cells, such as liver cells, when these cells are placed in suspension in appropriate antiserum and complement, indicating that this mechanism is not due to peculiarity in membranes of the affected cells but to availability of cell to action of antibody and complement.

to identify for routine transfusion service. The other antigens are rarely of importance clinically because of their infrequent occurrence. The possibility of such reactions is usually predictable from cross-match tests. It is not within the scope of this text to present further this complicated subject. (For more details the reader should consult references 30 and 44.)

Erythroblastosis Fetalis

A pregnant woman's blood may lack antigens present in the fetus contributed by paternal genes. An Rh— mother may become sensitized to Rh+ erythrocytes produced by the fetus. If the antibodies formed by the mother cross the placenta, they may destroy the fetal erythrocytes (Fig. 11-4).

The Rh antigenic system is a mosaic of genetically controlled specific antigenic determinants (44). The antigen in this situation is endogenous,

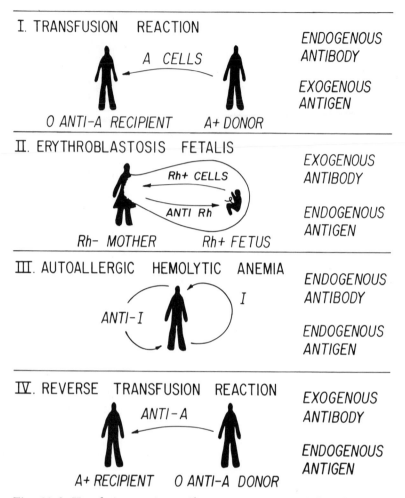

Fig. 11–2. Hemolytic reactions. Shown are 4 types of hemolytic reactions caused by antibody-mediated complement activation: **I)** Transfusion reactions. Erythrocytes from a donor (A+) which are antigenic for a recipient whose serum antibody to the donor's erythrocyte antigen (O anti-A) will be lysed immediately upon transfusion resulting in release of hemoglobulin and a clinic syndrome known as a transfusion reaction. Exogenous antigen and endogenous antibody. **II)** Erythroblastosis fetalis. Rh+ erythrocytes cross the placenta and stimulate the production of antibody to Rh if the mother is not Rh+. These antibodies will cross back through the placenta to attack fetal erythrocytes. Endogenous antigen and exogenous antibody. **III)** Autoallergic hemolytic anemia. An individual becomes sensitized to the antigens of his own erythrocytes (autoantibody). Endogenous antigen–endogenous antibody. **IV)** Reverse transfusion reaction. Antibodies are transfused from a donor to a recipient whose red cells contain the antigen. This passively transferred antibody causes lysis of recipient red cells. Endogenous antigen–exogenous antibody.

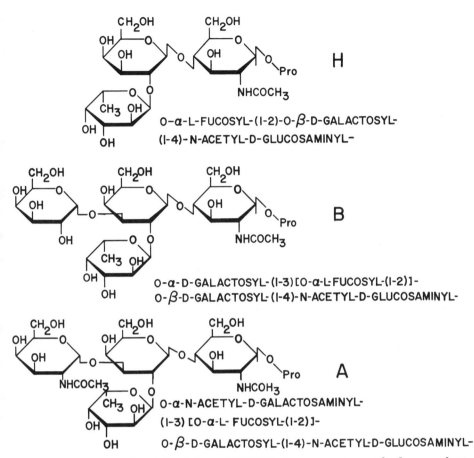

O-α-L-FUCOSYL-(I-2)-O-β-D-GALACTOSYL-
(I-4)-N-ACETYL-D-GLUCOSAMINYL-   **H**

O-α-D-GALACTOSYL-(I-3)[O-α-L-FUCOSYL-(I-2)]-
O-β-D-GALACTOSYL-(I-4)-N-ACETYL-D-GLUCOSAMINYL-   **B**

O-α-N-ACETYL-D-GALACTOSAMINYL-
(I-3)[O-α-L-FUCOSYL-(I-2)]-
O-β-D-GALACTOSYL-(I-4)-N-ACETYL-D-GLUCOSAMINYL-   **A**

Fig. 11–3. **Chemical relations of ABO blood group system.** Blood group identification depends upon presence of antigenic specificities on surfaces of red cells.
Blood group characteristics are inherited according to simple mendelian laws. ABO
blood group antigens have been characterized by analysis of purified blood group
substances obtained from secretions of ovarian cysts. Purified blood group substances contain about 85% carbohydrate and 15% amino acids. Peptide component contains 15 amino acids and is same for each blood group substance. Antigenic specificity is determined by carbohydrate moiety. Individuals with type O
blood, who do not have A or B group specificity, have a specificity now recognized
as H, which consists of three sugar groups attached to peptide. Addition of a
fourth sugar group to basic H structure produces A or B specificity. If additional
sugar is O-α-D-galactose, specificity is B; if it is O-α-N-acetyl-D-galactose, specificity
is A. Formation of H substance is controlled by a pair of alleles, H and h. H
gene gives rise to production of H specificity. H-active material is converted to
A- or B-active substances under influence of A or B genes. Rare individuals lack
A, B, and H reactivity, presumably due to inability to form normal precursor
for H substance. (Modified from Watkins WM: Science 152:172, 1966. ©
Copyright 1966 by the American Association for the Advancement of Science.)

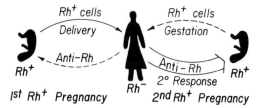

Fig. 11–4. Erythroblastosis fetalis. Rh— mother carrying an Rh+ fetus during first pregnancy in which sensitization occurs (**Top**). **Bottom,** subsequent pregnancy of a sensitized mother carrying an Rh+ fetus. During the first pregnancy, small numbers of Rh+ fetal erythrocytes, insufficient for sensitization, cross the placenta. However, at delivery a substantial number of Rh+ erythrocytes are released into maternal circulation. In a small percentage of Rh incompatible pregnancies, this is sufficient to immunize the mother. During a second pregnancy, the small number of erythrocytes that reach the maternal circulation will induce in the mother a secondary antibody response to the Rh antigen. The maternal antibody is IgG and crosses the placenta to the fetus where it acts on fetal erythrocytes, causing their destruction.

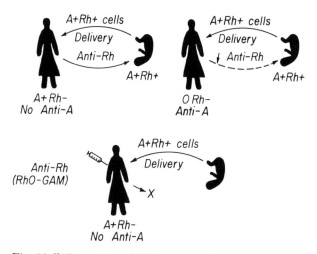

Fig. 11–5. Prevention of Rh Immunization by passive antibody. Top. Naturally occurring situation when an ABO and Rh incompatibility are combined; sensitization of the mother to Rh+ antigens is significantly less than where there is an Rh incompatibility but no ABO incompatibility. The presence of antibody to A in the non-A mother prevents sensitization to the Rh+ antigen, whereas the mother with no anti-A becomes sensitized to the Rh system. This observation was used as a rationale for passively transferring antibody to Rh to mothers who were Rh— and were carrying an Rh+ fetus. Administration of anti-Rh at delivery significantly reduces the incidence of sensitization of the mother to the Rh system, so that erythroblastosis fetalis has become a preventable disease through the application of immunoprevention.

and the immune response exogenous (Table 9–2). Because of the proliferation of cells by the fetus in an attempt to make up for the destruction of fetal erythrocytes in the erythrocyte series a characteristic morphologic picture of extramedullary hematopoiesis may be observed. The effect of high concentrations of hemoglobulin breakdown products during the immediate neonatal period may lead to brain damage (kernicterus).

Prevention of Rh Immunization

Clinical trials directed toward prevention of immunization of Rh— mothers carrying Rh+ fetuses have been successful (10). The observation that led to such a procedure was that protection against Rh immunization occurs if the fetus contains ABO blood group antigens not present in the mother (Fig. 11–5). Thus, if the fetus' blood is A Rh+ or B Rh+ and the mother's blood is O Rh—, the mother does not develop anti-Rh antibodies. In contrast, when the fetus' blood is O Rh+ and the mother's is O Rh—, when the fetus's blood is A Rh+ and the mother's is A Rh—, the mother does develop antiRh antibodies. Thus, the presence in the mother of antibodies to ABO group antigens on the fetal erythrocytes prevents immunization to Rh antigens if there is an Rh incompatibility as well. Fetal erythrocytes appear in the circulation of the mother at the time of delivery, and this is the time most Rh— mothers first become sensitized by Rh+ fetal cells. Because of the possibility that such sensitization could be prevented by passive transfer of anti-Rh antisera to Rh— mothers, trials were made on Rh— male volunteers. Passive transfer of anti-Rh serum along with Rh+ cells prevented immunization of these volunteers. Extensive trials have now been made in Rh— mothers, and the data clearly demonstrate that the incidence of Rh immunization in subsequent pregnancies can be greatly reduced by the passive transfer of anti-Rh sera (or globulin) to an Rh— mother at the time of delivery of an Rh+ fetus.

ABO Hemolytic Disease of Newborn

Hemolytic disease of the newborn due to ABO incompatibility rarely occurs even if the mother's blood contains high titers of anti-A or anti-B antibodies and the fetus' blood is A, B, or AB. This may be due to two reasons: 1) anti-A and anti-B antibodies are usually 19S and therefore do not cross the placenta, and 2) ABO blood group antigens are widely distributed in the fetal tissues and the placenta (38), so that the effect upon fetal erythrocytes of any 7S anti-A or anti-B antibodies that may cross the placenta is diluted out in the sense that the antibodies react with many other tissue sites. In contrast, the Rh specificity is unique for erythrocytes and the effect of anti-Rh antibodies that cross the placenta is concentrated on the fetal erythrocytes (38).

Acquired Autoallergic Hemolytic Disorders

Acquired autoallergic hemolytic disorders are caused in a given individual by formation of antibodies to antigens present on his own erythrocytes (7). It must be differentiated from congenital metabolic hemolytic disorders by careful testing. The major difference between allergic and congenital hemolytic diseases is that the erythrocytes are defective in the latter and do not usually survive in either the patient or a "normal" individual. In contrast, the erythrocytes are normal in patients with allergic hemolytic disease and survive better in a "normal" recipient than in the patient. Therefore, congenital disease demonstrates an *intra*corpuscular defect; allergic disease an *extra*corpuscular defect which is an autoantibody which can be demonstrated by the antiglobulin test of Coombs (see below). Two major forms have been identified: warm antibody mediated and cold antibody mediated (7,14).

Warm antibody disease is due almost always to IgG antibody which reacts with the patient's own red cells. In ⅔ of the cases, the antibody reacts with one of the Rh specificities (7). The antibody may appear as an isolated phenomena (idiopathic) but more frequently is associated with a collagen disease (see page 189) or with a lymphoproliferative disorder, particularly chronic lymphocytic leukemia. The patient's erythrocytes may be coated in vivo with IgG antibody, IgG and complement, or complement alone when tested by the Coombs' technique (7). The cells containing complement alone may have IgG when tested by more sensitive techniques (15). The action of antibody and complement leads to destruction of the erythrocyte's (hemolytic anemia)–usually by alteration of the cell membrane, and phagocytosis, which occurs principally in the spleen. Reaction of antibody and/or complement may alter the surface of the erythrocyte so that it is less likely to pass through phagocytic organs without being sequestered (34,35). Frank hemolysis by the complete complement sequence may also be observed. Treatment with corticosteroids may abort life-threatening acute hemolytic episodes. Splenectomy is of some temporary value, but usually the anemia recurs even after the spleen is removed indicating that the spleen is not necessary for red cell destruction. The reason for the production of the autoantibody is not clear.

Cold antibody hemolytic disease occurs in two forms: paroxysmal cold hemoglobinuria and cold agglutinin disease. In these disorders the antierythrocytic antibody is not capable of binding to the red cell at 37°C but will do so at lower temperatures. When cells that are coated by antibody in the cold are then warmed to body temperature, the complement components are fixed and the cells are susceptible to lysis. At warm temperatures the antibody comes off the cell so that complement may be detected on the affected cells in the absence of antibody. Hemolytic attacks occur on exposure to cold. The cold antibody binds to cells in the exposed areas of the body (skin). These cells are coated with complement and then are destroyed on entering the blood stream of warmer parts of the body. Paroxysmal cold hemoglobinuria refers to the production of dark urine due to the presence of hemoglobin from lysed red cells. The antibody responsible was first recognized in 1904 and is referred to as Donath-Landsteiner (DL) antibody (8). Demonstration of the antibody requires two steps: The patient's serum is mixed with erythrocytes at 4°C and the mixture then warmed to 37°C (17). Lysis occurs upon warming. This type of antibody is classically found in patients with syphilis, but may occur idiopathically or after a viral infection. The antibody is of the IgG class and the specificity is usually to blood group P (43). Cold agglutinin disease is similar but clear differences have been noted (20). Intense agglutination of red cells occurs in the cold, which is not the case with DL antibody. The IgG antibody is directed to the blood group I specificity, and is associated with mycoplasma infections, but rarely with lymphoproliferative diseases (7). Most patients with cold antibody hemolytic disease do well as long as they are kept warm and tolerate a chronic mild anemia with minimal disability. In fact, low titers of cold antibody are found in most normal adults and cause no apparent symptoms.

Hemolytic Reactions to Drugs

Hemolytic reactions to drugs may be activated by at least four mechanisms (Fig. 11-6). 1) Many drugs adhere to red cells and function as haptens. As such, the red cell–hapten complex induces an immune response, and cytotoxic reactions to the red cell or red cell–drug complex may occur (7). The exact mechanism of such a drug-induced hemolytic reaction depends upon the drug involved. Penicillin binds to red cells, and the antibody formed reacts with the penicillin bound to the cell. Antibody globulin can be demonstrated on the surface of affected cells by the indirect Coombs' test. 2) Quinidine binds only loosely to red cells. Antibody–quinidine complexes can dissociate from red cell surfaces and in complex form pass from one red cell to another. Destruction of red cells occurs as an "innocent bystander" reaction. Components of complement may be demonstrated on the affected cells in the absence of detectable antibody globulin. 3) α-Methyl dopa apparently induces alterations in red cells so that the affected cells become "autoimmunogenic." The antibody produced reacts with the patient's own red cells in the absence of bound drug. 4) Normal erythrocytes may also be destroyed during a hemolytic drug reaction because they bind activated complement components released from cells that have been antigenically altered and reacted with antibody and complement. In some cases of penicillin-induced hemolytic anemia, antipenicillin antibody lyses erythrocytes coated with penicillin. Activated complement components bind to normal nonpenicillin coated erythrocytes (21). In cases of hemolytic reactions to penicillin or quinidine, red cell destruction ceases soon after administration of the drug is stopped; α-methyl dopa hemolytic reactions may persist for as long as a year after the drug is stopped. In hemolytic reactions to drugs the source of the antigen is exogenous (or a complex of exogenous hapten and host red cell), and the origin of the allergic response is endogenous (Table 9-2).

REACTIONS TO LEUKOCYTES

Allergic responses similar to those described above for erythrocytes may also occur with polymorphonuclear leukocytes (14,40,42).

Neonatal Leukopenia

Destruction of fetal white blood cells may be accomplished by antibodies produced by antibodies produced by maternal immunization to fetal leukocyte antigens that cross the placenta.

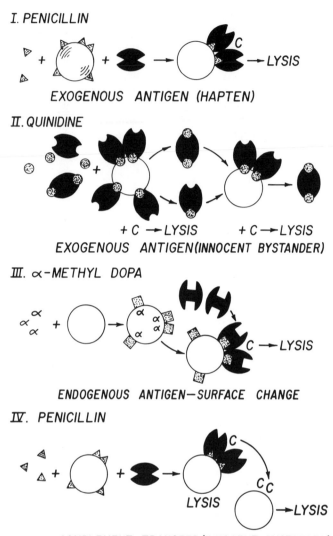

I. PENICILLIN

EXOGENOUS ANTIGEN (HAPTEN)

II. QUINIDINE

+ C → LYSIS   + C → LYSIS

EXOGENOUS ANTIGEN (INNOCENT BYSTANDER)

III. α-METHYL DOPA

C → LYSIS

ENDOGENOUS ANTIGEN—SURFACE CHANGE

IV. PENICILLIN

LYSIS   → LYSIS

COMPLEMENT TRANSFER (INNOCENT BYSTANDER)

Fig. 11–6. Hemolytic drug reactions. Hemolysis of red cells by drugs that act as inducing agents may occur via at least four mechanisms. I) Haptens on the cell surface that bind antihapten antibody. II) Immune complexes of drugs and antibody to the drug adhering to the cell and activating complement. III) Alteration of the cell surface due to metabolic effects producing a new cell surface antigen to which an antibody may react. IV) Transfer of activated complement from a cell with an antigenic surface that has reacted with antibody and activated complement.

Chronic Agranulocytosis

Destruction of a patient's own white blood cells may be caused by autoantibodies (40,42).

Acute Agranulocytosis

A loss of white blood cells may be caused by an allergic reaction to certain drugs that adhere to white blood cells and function as haptens. Sulfapyridine and aminopurine are two of the drugs that have been implicated. The consequence of leukocyte destruction is a decreased ability to defend against infection. In some situations drugs may have a direct nonimmune cytotoxic effect (idiosyncrasy), and some cases of agranulocytosis may be due to a congenital metabolic defect. In nonimmune agranulocytosis more than one line of leukocyte is usually involved; for instance, in some cases all leukocytes containing granules are destroyed or fail to develop.

REACTIONS TO PLATELETS

Allergic reactions to platelets may cause destruction of platelets with resulting purpura and other hemorrhagic manifestations (2). The word purpura (purple) is applied to hemorrhage into the skin and is easily recognized by the red or purple discoloration produced by the presence of red cells. The color is first red but becomes darker (purple) and fades to a brownish yellow as the red cells are destroyed or cleared from the site of hemorrhage. Since platelets function to prevent such hemorrhages, a loss of platelets permits purpuric lesions to develop. An antiplatelet antibody can be demonstrated in about 60% of the affected individuals. Thrombocytopenia may also occur congenitally or secondarily due to an increased splenic function (hypersplenism) or other nonimmune consumptive disorders.

Posttransfusion Thrombocytopenic Purpura

This occurs as a result of the production of autoantibody following repeated transfusions of allogeneic platelets (36).

Neonatal Thrombocytopenic Purpura

Neonatal thrombocytopenic purpura occurs as a result of maternal immunization by fetal platelet antigens, with thrombocytopenia occurring in the fetus when this antibody crosses the placenta (27).

Acute Idiopathic Thrombocytopenic Purpura

Acute idiopathic thrombocytopenic purpura is more common in children, and most affected individuals have a history of infection (e.g., rubella) occurring 1–2 weeks previously. The destruction of platelets may be due to antibodies to infectious antigens adherent to platelets, to antibody–antigen complexes adsorbed to platelets (innocent bystander), or to antibodies to platelets altered by the infectious process. Platelets are destroyed rapidly when transferred into an affected individual (18).

Chronic Idiopathic Thrombocytopenic Purpura

Chronic idiopathic thrombocytopenic purpura is caused by the production of autoantibodies against altered or naturally occurring platelet antigens and is more common in adults. The chronic form is frequently associated with systemic lupus erythematosus or a lymphoproliferative disorder (leukemia, myeloma).

Quinine (Sedormid) Purpura

Quinine purpura is an example of a reaction to a drug acting as a hapten on the platelet surface (1).

VASCULAR PURPURA

Hemorrhagic phenomena may occur due to sensitization to or destruction of vascular endothelium (42). A loss of integrity of small blood vessels permits blood cells to escape causing purpura and other hemorrhagic manifestations. The syndrome of anaphylactoid purpura is in this category. Clinically urticarial and hemorrhagic lesions are the most prominent features and tend to occur around joints. Variations in the clinical syndrome include 1) Abdominal involvement with edema and hemorrhage into the gastrointestinal tract (Henoch's syndrome); 2) joint involvement with effusion, swelling of the soft tissues, redness, and pain (Schönlein's syndrome); or 3) renal lesions of focal proliferative glomerulonephritis. Vascular purpura may be induced in experimental animals by the injection of heterologous antisera to endothelial antigens.

POSSIBLE ROLE OF CYTOTOXIC REACTIONS IN OTHER ALLERGIC CONDITIONS

Autoallergic Diseases

Cytotoxic antibody may produce damage in allergic thyroiditis, allergic aspermatogenesis and other autoallergic diseases, although it is generally believed that the primary mechanism of these diseases is delayed hypersensitivity (9,11,40).

Systemic Lupus Erythematosus

This is a syndrome characterized by a peculiar set of lesions, some of which may be caused in part by an autoantibody against nucleoprotein antigens present in the patient's own cells. This antibody, called LE factor, is revealed by incubation of the patient's serum with normal peripheral blood cells after mild agitation. The antibody reacts with the nuclei of lymphocytes; the nucleus–antibody complexes are phagocytized and may be seen within polymorphonuclear leukocytes in smears of blood buffy coat (see page 193).

Homograft Rejection

Stetson (37) and others have shown that specific antisera injected into a graft site may cause an acute "white" graft rejection. Although homograft rejection is usually mediated by sensitized cells (delayed sensitivity), antibody-mediated late rejection is now recognized. (See Chapter 14.)

Forssman Antigen

The Forssman antigen is a generic term for a family of antigens with overlapping specificities found in some plants (corn, spinach), some microorganisms (*Pneumococcus, Shiegella dysenteriae, Bacillus anthracis*), and some fish and animal tissues (carp, toad, chicken, horse, guinea pig, sheep, hamster, dog, cat, man). The injection of antiForssman serum into guinea pigs or chick embryos causes vascular damage and hemorrhage. The possibility of such a reaction occurring in humans is uncertain.

Acute Nephritis and Acute Endocarditis

The acute nephritis or acute endocarditis following streptococcal infection may be caused by the production of cytotoxic antibodies to antigens produced by the attachment of bacterial products to normal tissue components, by the production of antibodies to streptococcal antigens that cross-react with normal tissue antigens, or by the formation of antibody-streptococcal antigen complexes in vivo. However, such reactions are most likely mediated through the toxic complex reaction (see Chapter 13).

DEMONSTRATION OF CIRCULATING CYTOTOXIC ANTIBODIES

Demonstration in Vivo

The effect of the antibody may be produced by passive transfer of serum containing antibody into a normal recipient.

Demonstration in Vitro

The addition of the patient's serum to the target cells in a test tube, or the addition of the patient's serum to normal cells in the presence of the antigen, produces agglutination or lysis (complement present). In some cases antibody does not result in agglutination unless a second antibody is added. Such nonagglutinating antibodies are termed incomplete and may be detected by the Coombs' test (42,44). In the *direct Coombs' test*, target cells are already coated with incomplete antibody. The addition of an antiserum that reacts with the incomplete antibody than causes agglutination of the target cells. Thus, human Rh+ erythrocytes coated with incomplete anti-Rh antibody agglutinate when sheep antihuman-γ-globulin

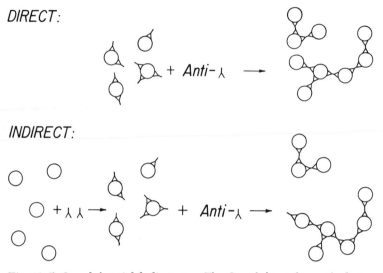

Fig. 11–7. Coombs' antiglobulin tests. The Coombs' test for antibody to erythrocytes is carried out in two forms: direct and indirect. **Direct:** cells taken from the patient are coated with antibody in vivo, and are agglutinated by the addition of anti-Ig which reacts with the antibodies coating the cells. **Indirect:** the patient's serum contains free antibody which binds to but does not agglutinate erythrocytes added in vitro. Agglutination is accomplished by addition of a second antibody which reacts with the first antibody (anti-Ig).

serum is added. In the *indirect Coombs' test*, the target cells are not coated with antibody but are mixed with a serum containing incomplete antibody to the target cells. The target cells are agglutinated by the addition of anti-γ-globulin serum. [Human Rh+ cells are added to human serum containing incomplete anti-Rh antibodies. These sensitized cells are agglutinated by sheep antihuman-γ-globulin serum (Fig. 11–7)]. In suspected Rh hemolytic disease, both the direct and the indirect Coombs' tests must be done to rule out the presence of incomplete Rh antibodies. The direct test is usually positive for fetal erythrocytes coated with maternal anti-Rh, when free antibody is not present in the fetal serum. On the other hand, the mother's serum will contain anti-Rh antibody detectable by the indirect test; maternal serum added to fetal cells results in coating of the fetal Rh+ cells which are then agglutinable by antibody to human IgG. Coombs' test may also be used to reveal agglutination of a patient's own cells in acquired hemolytic anemia, thus demonstrating an incomplete autoantibody.

Animal Experiments

The agglutination or lysis of all these cell types (erythrocytes, white blood cells, and platelets) has been duplicated in animal experiments in vitro using the appropriate antigen-antibody-complement system. The disease condition can be reproduced in vivo by passive transfer of the appropriate heterologous antibody.

THE COMPLEMENT SYSTEM

Complement-Mediated Cell Lysis

Complement consists of a system of at least 11 serum proteins found in different concentrations in normal serum. Components of the complement system (referred to as C1, C2, etc.) react with antigen–antibody complexes, and this reaction results in activation of components of the system which

TABLE 11-1
Sequence and Mechanism of Immune Hemolysis

Reaction	Biochemical event
$E + A \rightleftharpoons EA$	Reaction of erythrocyte and anti-erythrocyte antibody
$EA + C1 \xrightarrow{Ca++} EAC1q^*$	C1 attaches to antibody at a site on C1q and Fc portion of Ig antibody
$C1r \rightarrow C\overline{1r}$	Bound C1q* converts C1r to active form by cleavage of C1r
$C1s \rightarrow C\overline{1s}$	$C\overline{1r}$ activates C1s by cleavage of C1s
$C4 \rightarrow C\overline{4a} + C4b^*$ $C2 \rightarrow C2a^* + C\overline{2b}$	$C\overline{1s}$ cleaves C4 into $C\overline{4a}$ and C4b*, and C2 into C2a* and $C\overline{2b}$
$C4b^* + C2a^* \xrightarrow{Mg++} \overline{C4b2a}$	C4b* and C2a* combine to form C3 convertase
$C3 \rightarrow C\overline{3a} + C3b^*$	$\overline{C4b2a}$ cleaves C3 into $C\overline{3a}$ and C3b*, $C\overline{3a}$ is chemotactic for polymorphonuclear leukocytes
$C3b^* + C4b2a \rightarrow \overline{C4b2a3b}$	C3b* binds to activated bimolecular complex of C4b2a to form a trimolecular complex which is a specific enzyme for C5, C5 convertase. C3b* may also cause degradation of mast cells (anaphylatoxin)
$C5 \rightarrow C\overline{5a} + C5b^*$	C5 is cleaved into $C\overline{5a}$ and C5b* by C5 convertase; $C\overline{5a}$ has anaphylactic and chemotactic activity
$C\overline{5b}^* + C6789 \rightarrow \overline{C5b\text{-}9}$	C5b* reacts with other complement components to produce a macromolecular complex that has the ability to alter cell membrane permeability. $C\overline{8}$ is most likely the active component with $C\overline{9}$ increasing efficiency of effect of $C\overline{8}$ and producing maximal cell lysis.

E, erythrocyte.
A, antibody to erythrocyte.
$C\overline{1}$, $C\overline{4}$, etc., a line above the C number indicates the activated form of the component.
C4a, C4b, etc., the small letters indicate cleavage products of the parent complement molecule.
C4b*, C2a*, the asterisk indicates the cleavage product that contains an active binding site for other complement components.
Immunoelectrophoretic designation of some of the complement components:
C3, β1C-globulin (converted in free solution to 1G-globulin when cleaved by $C\overline{4b2a}$).
C4, β1E-globulin.
C5, β1F-globulin.
Modified from Cinader B (ed): Antibodies to Biologically Active Molecules. New York, Pergamon Press, 1967, p 9, and from the lectures of Hans Müller-Eberhard, Scripps Clinic and Research Foundation, La Jolla, California.

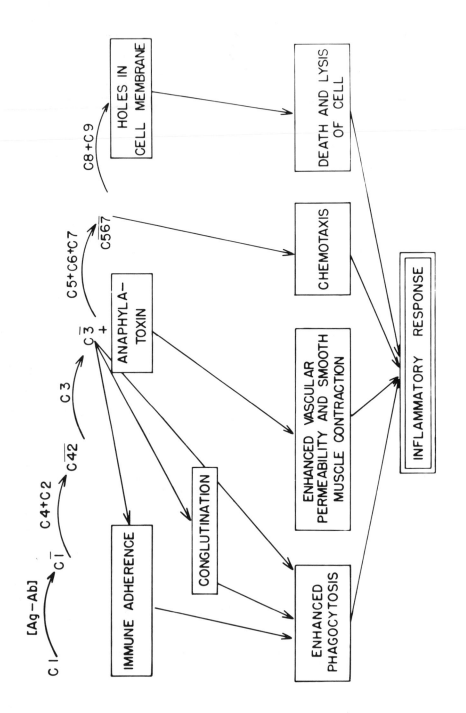

mediate cellular injury or inflammation (5,19,23,24,25,31,32). Complement components are usually necessary for the cytotoxic or cytolytic reactions, but may also play a role in reactions due to precipitating antibody [toxic complex reactions] (6). The sequence of events in complement-mediated immune hemolysis is given in Table 11–1, and other complement-mediated reactions are schematically illustrated in Fig. 11–8. The initial step in immune hemolysis is a reaction between the target cell and specific antibody (sensitization). The reaction sequence presented in Fig. 11–8 is then activated, with the eventual formation of discrete hole-like lesions (19) in the cell membrane through which intracellular components emerge, followed by lysis of the cell. C1 is a macromolecular complex consisting of three components, C1q, C1r and C1s. These components serve as a *recognition* unit and have the ability to bind to the Fc complement receptor of antibody complexed to antigens by a reversible ionic interaction. C2, C3, C4 and C5 serve as an enzymatic *activation* unit resulting in the production of a macromolecular assembly of C5, C6, C7, C8 and C9 which serves as an *adsorption* unit. C5–9 adheres to the cell surface, causing alteration of the permeability of the membrane. The altered membrane permeability permits excess fluid to enter the cell, eventually causing lysis of the cells.

COMPLEMENT-MEDIATED INFLAMMATION

C1 Fixation and Transfer Assay

A C1 fixation and transfer test may be used to quantitate the number of molecules of an antigen or an antibody on the surface of cells (3,4). Two IgG antibodies reacting in the form of a doublet on the surface of a cell will activate one molecule of C1. The C1 molecules can be transferred from the cell surface to sheep cells sensitized with C4 (EAC4). Upon

---

Fig. 11–8. Some immunopathologic mechanisms mediated by complement. Sequential steps of complement activation and recognized functions of activated components (see also Table 11–1). Prior to formation of activated C3 (C$\overline{3}$), little is known about biologic activity of complement system. C$\overline{3}$ is not only necessary for further activation of other stages of complement system but also produces recognized phenomena of immune adherence and conglutination (see text). The result is increased phagocytosis and pharmacologically active material, "anaphylatoxin," which causes increased vascular permeability and smooth muscle contraction by mechanisms involving histamine release. Activation of C5 + C6 + C7 complex results in ability of these complexes to attract and mobilize leukocytes, functions of complement system which have only recently been identified. For many years activity of complement system was assayed by ability of activation of all steps through C9 to cause death and lysis of appropriately sensitized cells. All above activities may play active role in inflammatory response due to mechanisms that activate complement. It is likely that future research will identify other activities in complement system and perhaps even additional components. (Adapted from Cinader B (ed): Antibodies to Biologically Active Molecules. New York, Pergammon Press, 1967, pp 1–24)

addition of C2 and subsequent complement components, the EACl4 sensitized red cells will be lysed. From the amount of hemoglobin released from the lysed cells and a conversion factor, the number of Cl molecules originally bound to the cells in question can be calculated (3).

Although the role of the complement system in immune cytolysis has been studied extensively, the possible role of complement in other tissue reactions has been recognized only recently (5,23,24,25). The activation of C3 enhances phagocytosis (opsonization) and is responsible for the in vitro reactions of immune adherence (the adherence of aggregates of antigen–antibody complexes to the erythrocytes of primates) and conglutination (massive aggregation of antibody-coated red cells in the presence of a heat-stable factor in normal bovine serum called conglutinin), and for the formation of a toxic product in vivo, anaphylatoxin, which causes increased vascular permeability and smooth muscle contraction. The term anaphylatoxin is used because C3b and C5a cause release of pharmacologically reactive substances from mast cells and produce effects similar to those of anaphylactic reactions (see Chapter 12). Activation of C5 + C6 + C7 results in an attraction for leukocytes (chemotaxis). The complement system may therefore have considerable effect in vivo prior to the final recognized step in the lytic sequence.

SERUM COMPLEMENT IN HUMAN DISEASES

Isolation of purified complement components (24,25) has permitted measurement of the separate components of complement in human serum. Low levels of total complement are found in a variety of diseases, including acute and chronic glomerulonephritis, systemic lupus erythematosus and congenital nephrosis, and during renal allograft rejection (31). Low serum levels of C1, C4, and C2 were noted in most patients in each of the situations listed above, although not consistently in chronic glomerulonephritis or congenital nephrosis. In acute inflammatory processes or after bleeding, a consistent increase in whole serum complement is noted. Hereditary deficiencies in the complement system have recently been recognized (24,25,33). Patients with hereditary angioneurotic edema (see Chapter 12) are deficient in a normal serum protein which inhibits the activated first component of complement, Cl esterase. A deficiency in C2 activity has been demonstrated in members of a family who also show defective in vitro immune adherence and bacteriolysis, although these individuals do not appear to have an increased susceptibility to infections. Individuals with documented C3 or C5 deficiencies have repeated bacterial infections and decreased phagocytosis, which is corrected by infusion of fresh plasma. C6-deficient rabbits have poor clotting of blood, although all known clotting factors are present in normal amounts (see page 312).

ALTERNATE PATHWAY OF COMPLEMENT ACTIVATION

In some types of inflammation, activation of the complement sequence occurs at C3 without participation of an antibody–antigen reaction, the C3 shunt (12,16). Cl activated by antibody may also activate C3 by bypassing C4 and C2 (22). This activation may be set off by a protein or system of blood proteins known as properdin (26), which in turn may be acted upon by endotoxin (12,13,28) or other microbial products, such as zymosan, a carbohydrate of yeast cell walls (26). The properdin system includes enzymes which assemble on a cell wall and activate the complement system beginning at C3 and/or C5. The properdin system may represent a nonimmune way of activation of a defensive mechanism. The role of the alternate pathway in disease is not clear but may be responsible for some cases of glomerulonephritis, hypocomplementemic glomerulonephritis (39), and certain skin diseases, such as bullous pemphigoid (29).

REFERENCES

1. Ackroyd JF: Sedormid purpura: An immunologic study of a form of drug hypersensitivity. Prog Allergy 3:531, 1952
2. Baldini M: Idiopathic thrombocytopenic purpura. N Engl J Med 274:1245, 1302, 1360, 1966
3. Borsos T, Colten HR, Spalter JS, Rogentine N, Rapp HJ: The C′1a fixation and transfer test. Examples of its applicability to the detection and enumeration of antigens and antibodies of cell surfaces. J Immunol 101:392, 1968
4. Borsos T, Rapp HJ: Hemolysin titration based on fixation of the activated first component of complement: Evidence that one molecule of hemolysin suffices to sensitize an erythrocyte. J Immunol 95:559, 1965
5. Cinader B, Lepow IH: The Neutralization of Biologically Active Molecules. In Antibodies to Biologically Active Molecules. Cinader B (ed). New York, Pergamon Press, 1967
6. Cochrane CG, Ward PA: The Role of Complement in Lesions Induced by Immunologic Reactions. In Immunology IV. Grabar P, Miesher P (eds). Basel, Schwabe, 1966
7. Dacie JV, Wolledge SM: Autoimmune hemolytic anemia. Prog Hematol 6:1, 1969
8. Donath J, Landsteiner K: Veber paroxysmale Hämoglolunurie. Munch Med Wochenschr 51:1590, 1904
9. Flax MH, Jankovic BD, Sell S: Experimental allergic thyroiditis in the guinea pig. I. Relationship of delayed hypersensitivity and circulating antibody to the development of thyroiditis. Lab Invest 12:119, 1963
10. Freda VJ, Gorman JG, Pollack W: Suppression of the primary Rh immune response with passive Rh IgG immunoglobulin. N Engl J Med 277:1022, 1967
11. Gell PGH, Coombs RRA: Clinical Aspects of Immunology, 2nd ed. Oxford, Blackwell, 1968
12. Gewurz H, Shin HJ, Mergenhagen SE: Interactions of the complement system with endotoxic lipopolysaccharide: Consumption of each of the six terminal complement components. J Exp Med 128:1049, 1968
13. Gilbert VE, Braude AI: Reduction of serum complement in rabbits after injection of endotoxin. J Exp Med 116:477, 1962
14. Gilliand BC, Evans RS: The immune cytopenias. Postgrad Med 54:195, 1973
15. Gilliand BC, Leedy JP, Vaughn JH: The detection of cell-bound antibody on complement coated human red cells. J Clin Invest 49:898, 1970
16. Götze O, Müller-Eberhard HJ: Lysis of erythrocytes by complement in the absence of antibody. J Exp Med 132:898, 1970
17. Hinz CF Jr, Picken ME, Lepow IH: Studies on immune human hemolysis. II. The Donath-Landsteiner reaction as a model system for studying the mechanism of action of complement and the role of C′1 and C′1 esterase. J Exp Med 113:193, 1961
18. Hirsch EO, Gardner FH: The transfusion of human blood platelets. J Lab Clin Med 39:556, 1952
19. Humphrey JH, Dourmashkin RR: The lesions in cell membranes caused by complement. Adv Immunol 11:75, 1969
20. Iwai J, Mei-Sai N: Etiology of Raynaud's disease. Jap Med World 5:119, 1925

21. Kerr R-O, Cardamone J, Dalmasso AP, Kaplan ME: Two mechanisms of erythrocyte destruction in penicillin-induced hemolytic anemia. N Engl J Med 287:1322, 1972
22. May JE, Frank MM: A new complement-mediated cytolytic mechanism—the C1 bypass activation pathway. Proc Natl Acad Sci USA 70:649, 1973
23. Mayer MM: The complement system. Sci Am 229:54, 1973
24. Muller-Eberhard HJ: Chemistry and reaction mechanisms of complement. Adv Immunol 8:1, 1968
25. Muller-Eberhard HJ: Complement. Annu Rev Biochem 38:389, 1969
26. Pensky J, Kinz CF, Todd EW, Wedgwood RJ, Boyer JT, Lepow IH: Properties of highly purified human endotoxin. J Immunol 100:142, 1968
27. Peterson OH, Larson P: Thrombocytopenic purpura in pregnancy. Obstet Gynecol 4:454, 1954
28. Wurz L: Properdin system and immunity. II. Interaction of the properdin system with polysaccharides. Science 122:545, 1955
29. Provost TT, Tomasi TB Jr: Evidence for complement activation via the alternate pathway in skin disease. I. Herpes gestationis, systemic lupus erythematosis and bullous pemphigoid. J Clin Invest 52:1779, 1973
30. Race RR, Sanger R: Blood Groups in Man. Philadelphia, Davis, 1962
31. Rapp HJ, Borsos T: Complement research: Fundamental and applied. JAMA 198:1347, 1966
32. Rosenberg LT: Complement. Ann Rev Microbiol 19:285, 1965
33. Ruddy S, Austen KF: Inherited abnormalities of the complement system in man. Prog Med Genet 7:69, 1970
34. Schreiber AD, Frank MM: Role of antibody and complement in the immune clearance and destruction of erythrocytes. II. Molecular nature of IgG and IgM complement-fixing sites and effects of their interaction with serum. J Clin Invest 51:583, 1972
35. Shohet SB: Hemolysis and changes in erythrocyte membrane lipids. N Engl J Med 286:577, 1972
36. Shulman NR, Aster RH, Leitner A, Hiller MC: Immunoreactions involving platelets. V. Post-transfusion purpura due to a complement-fixing antibody against a genetically controlled platelet antigen. A proposed mechanism for thrombocytopenia and its relevance in autoimmunity. J Clin Invest 40:1597, 1961
37. Stetson CA: The role of humoral antibody in the homograft rejection. Adv Immunol 3:97, 1963
38. Szulman AE: The histologic distribution of the blood group substances in man as determined by immunofluorescence. III. The A, B, and H antigens in embryos and fetuses from 18 mm in length. J Exp Med 119:503, 1964
39. Verroust PJ, Wilson CB, Cooper NR, Edgington TS, Dixon FJ: Glomerular complement components in human glomerulonephritis. J Clin Invest 53:77, 1974
40. Waksman BH: Cell lysis and related phenomena in hypersensitivity reactions, including immunohematologic diseases. Prog Allergy 5:340, 1958
41. Watkins WM: Blood group substances. Science 152:172, 1966
42. Wintrobe MM: Clinical Hematology, 5th ed. Philadelphia, Lea & Febiger, 1961
43. Worlledge SM, Rousso C: Studies of the serology of paroxysmal cold haemoglobinueria (P.C.H.) with special reference to its relationship with P Blood group system, Vox Sang 10:293, 1965
44. Zmijewski CM: Immunohematology. New York, Appleton, 1968

12

Atopic or Anaphylactic Reactions

The effects produced by atopic or anaphylactic reactions result from pharmacologically active substances released by the reaction of antigen with cells passively sensitized by antibody (Fig. 12–1). The mast cell (tissue) or basophil (peripheral blood) is responsible. Following the reaction with antigen, a number of substances are released or activated. These include histamine, heparin, bradykinin, slow-reacting substance, eosinophilic chemotactic factor, serotonin and acetylcholine (1,2,6,25).

The exact role of these anaphylactic mediators is unclear, although histamine and slow reacting substance appear to be the most important in man. These mediators may be differentiated by the fact that histamine causes a rapid constriction of smooth muscle, is active in the presence of atrophine and is ineffective in the presence of antihistamines. By contrast, slow reacting substance produces a delayed contraction of smooth muscles, is not affected by antihistamines and is blocked by atrophine (45). Eosinophils may also be active in anaphylactic reactions, and platelets appear to be the major carriers of pharmacologically active agents in the rabbit. The effects of these agents include contraction of smooth muscle, increased vascular permeability, early increase in vascular resistance followed by collapse (shock), and increased gastric, nasal, and lacrimal secretion. The type of lesion observed depends upon 1) the dose of antigen, 2) the route of contact with antigen, 3) the frequency of contact with antigen, 4) the tendency for a given organ system to react (shock organ), and 5) the degree of sensitivity of the involved individual (12). This final factor may be genetically controlled or may be altered by environmental conditions (temperature), unrelated inflammations (presence of a viral upper respiratory infection) or the emotional state of the individual. Some of the reactions seen clinically are urticaria (wheal and flare, hives), hay fever, asthma, eczema, angioneurotic edema and anaphylaxis.

Acute reactions (wheal and flare) and systemic shock are generally re-

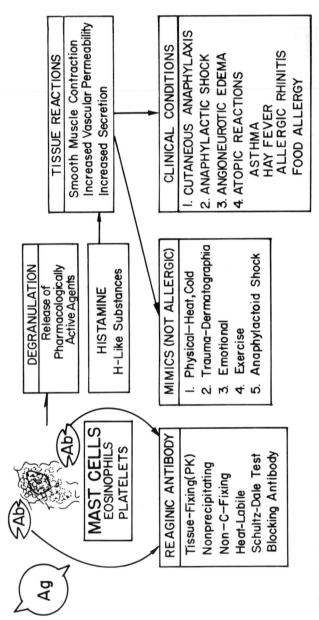

Fig. 12-1. Atopic or anaphylactic reactions. Reaction of antigen with particular type of antibody (reagin) capable of fixing to tissue (on mast cells that have cytoplasmic granules containing a variety of pharmacologically active mediators), results in release of pharmacologically active materials and degranulation of mast cells. Resulting tissue changes are caused by the pharmacologically active agents.

ferred to as anaphylactic; chronic recurring reactions (hay fever) are referred to as atopic. However, this distinction is not always made, and there is considerable overlap in the use of the terms. In the United States common usage has made the terms atopy and allergy essentially synonymous; in Britian allergy is used for all nonprotective immune reactions including toxic complex reactions and delayed hypersensitivity. An atopic individual is one who is prone to develop this type of allergic reaction. The antigen responsible for elicitation of an anaphylactic or atopic reaction is referred to as an allergen. The antibody involved is termed reagin.

REAGINIC ANTIBODY

Reaginic antibody has a special ability to bind to skin or other tissues (6,33,57). The term *atopic reagin* was adopted to refer to the particular tissue-fixing antibody found in the serum of patients with hay fever and asthma. The original use of the word reagin was to designate the reacting serum component responsible for the Wassermann reaction, the serologic test for syphilis. The Wassermann reagin is a peculiar serum reactant found in individuals infected with syphilis; it is demonstrable by its ability to combine with an antigen extracted from ungulate heart muscle and has no relation to anaphylactic or atopic reaction (7). It has been reported that reaginic antibody may be found in all the major immunoglobulin groups (IgA, IgG, IgM). However, in most cases reagin is found in a separate immunoglobulin class, IgE. In humans it may be assumed that atopic or anaphylactic reactions are almost always due to IgE antibody (12,33,45).

IgE antibody is termed *skin fixing* because it binds to mast cells in skin or basophils in the blood and sensitizes these cells to react to allergen. These IgE anaphylactic antibodies appear to be adapted to fit receptors of the tissue effector cell (mast cell in most species). The average number of IgE molecules on a basophil is 10,000–40,000 (34). The number of cell-bound IgE molecules does not depend upon the serum IgE concentration; even basophils taken from individuals with elevated serum IgE have some unoccupied receptors for IgE (34). It is not known how IgE is bound to basophils or mast cells but the Fc piece of IgE does bind to these cells. The number and affinity of cell bound IgE antibody molecules probably determines the sensitivity of basophils to allergen. However, the amount of mediators released from a given cell depends on enzyme systems which regulate the biochemical mechanisms of mediator release (see below). Clearly, antigen reacting with IgE or the cell surface initiates events leading to mediator release (42). Mediator release may also be initiated by reaction of anti-IgE with IgE on the cell surface (35).

The reaginic activity of an immunoglobulin is determined by its ability to fix to skin of the same species. If serum from a sensitive individual is passively transferred to the skin of a normal recipient, the classic wheal-and-flare reaction can be elicited at this site upon application of the antigen [Prausnitz-Küstner test] (50). Because the antibody fixes to the skin, the transfer site may be tested up to 45 days later and still elicit a positive reaction. In contrast, with local passive transfer of nonreaginic antibody (passive Arthus) the skin site must be tested within a few hours in order to obtain a positive reaction before the non skin-fixing antibody diffuses. The passive transfer of atopic or anaphylactic reactions may be accomplished by a variety of methods, all of which depend upon the ability of reagins or IgE antibodies to fix to tissue (mast) cells (6).

1. For the local passive cutaneous anaphylaxis transfer (Prausnitz-Küstner) test, antibody-containing serum is injected into the skin and after an appropriate period of time (usually several days) the same skin site is challenged with antigen.
2. For systemic passive cutaneous anaphylaxis, either the antibody is injected intravenously and the antigen intradermally (a method used only in experimental animals) or the antibody is injected intradermally and the antigen intravenously.
3. Transfer of a systemic reaction (passive systemic anaphylaxis) is best elicited by injection of the antibody intravenously followed by injection of the antigen intravenously 24 hours later.
4. Reverse passive cutaneous anaphylaxis may be elicited if the antigen fixes to skin; the antibody does not require tissue-fixing capacities. For reverse reactions the antigen is injected into the skin, and after a suitable period, the antibody is injected intravenously or at the same site. Reverse tests are useful for determining the skin-fixing properties of the immunoglobulins of one species for the skin of another species.

In most species studied the antibody that fixes to the skin of the same species (e.g., human reagin fixing to human skin) belongs to a special class of immunoglobulin with properties similar to human IgE. If a given antibody in a species fixes to the skin of individuals of the same species, it is termed homocytophilic. In some instances the immunoglobulins that fit tissue receptors of another species belong to a class other than IgE. For instance, human IgG antibodies may fix to guinea pig skin, but IgA, IgM or IgE does not fix to guinea pig skin. Immunoglobulins that fix to the skin of a species different from their source are termed heterocytophilic (6). Reagenic antibody has other properties different from usual antibody—it does not fix complement in the usual manner, and is heat-labile (56°C for 30 minutes). IgE antibody precipitates with antigen if sufficient amounts of antibody can be obtained. However, the amount of IgE antibody present in the serum of a sensitive individual is usually too small to be detected by precipitation, but can be detected by more sensitive techniques involving the anaphylactic response.

Because of the unusual properties noted above there is no simple test for reagin. The most commonly used clinical test is a skin test (12,50). Suspected allergins are injected into the skin of an individual to test for cutaneous anaphylaxis. In this way allergenic antigens may be identified. Skin testing must be done under careful supervision as systemic anaphylactic shock may be induced. Anti-anaphylactic drugs (i.e., epinephrine) must be kept on hand for rapid use if necessary. The local transfer of skin-fixing antibody may be used to demonstrate reaginic activity in serum (passive cutaneous anaphylaxis, Prausnitz-Küstner test (50).

In vitro tests include the Schultz-Dale test, histamine release by mast cells (degranulation) and the radioallergosorbent test (RAST). The

Schultz-Dale test utilizes organs containing smooth muscle (guinea pig intestine or rat uterus) in an organ bath (12). When the organ is taken from a sensitized animal or incubated with serum from a sensitized individual, contraction will occur when the specific antigen is added. The extent of this contraction may be measured with a kymograph. Contraction may also be induced by the addition of mediators (histamine, SRS). The release of histamine from mast cells in vitro may be induced by contact of sensitized mast cells with antigen (48). The amount of histamine release may be determined spectrophotometrically or by observation of mast cell degranulation. Mast cells may be passively sensitized by incubation with reagin-containing serum or the reactivity of sensitized mast cells to antigen inhibited by the addition of blocking serum (see below). The passive leukocyte-sensitizing (PLS) activity of a given serum is determined by incubating a reaginic serum with blood leukocytes from nonallergic donors for about 2 hours. The cells are then washed and treated with antigen for 1 hour. The amount of histamine present in the supernate is then determined photometrically. The extent of histamine release is used as an index of the serum reagin content. The PLS activity of ragweed-sensitive individuals is highest in the early fall (during the pollen season) and lowest in summer just prior to the pollen season (48).

The radioallergosorbent test (RAST) depends upon the binding of IgE antibody to specific antigen, and the subsequent binding of radiolabeled anti-IgE to the IgE antibody–antigen complex (12). The suspected antigen is first covalently chemically bound to insoluble particles. The insoluble antigen is then added to samples of serum. Those sera containing antibodies to the antigen will have antibody immunloglobulin bind to the insoluble antigen. Antibody of classes other than IgE may also bind so that excess insoluble antigen is used. The particles are washed and treated with a labeled antibody to IgE. The labeled anti-IgE will bind to the IgE antibody which is bound to the insoluble antigen. By determining the amount of labeled anti-IgE bound, an estimation of the IgE antibody to the specific antigen may be made. RAST-positive sera have approximately 70% correlation with positive skin tests.

MECHANISMS OF MEDIATOR RELEASE

Two types of mechanisms may operate for release of mediators from mast cells or basophils: *nonlytic*, in which mast cell lysosomal membranes fuse with each other and with the cell surface membrane, resulting in release of lysosomal contents (degranulation), and *lytic*, in which antibody–antigen complexes on the surface of mast cells bind complement components with subsequent cytolysis of the mast cell (8). Nonlytic release is the usual mechanism active in anaphylactic reactions involving reaginic antibody. The mast cell is not destroyed and granules re-form. Lytic release provides a mechanism whereby cytolytic allergic reactions mediated by IgG or IgM may produce anaphylactic symptoms.

The mechanism by which reaction of antigen with reaginic antibody on mast cells or basophils causes the release of mediators is unknown (1). For atopic reactions to occur, the antibody must be fixed to the tissue.

Only minute amounts of antibody are required. A secretory response involving microtubules is suspected. Colchicine, which inhibits microtubule function, blocks mediator release (41). An intermediate proteolytic enzyme system may be activated as normal metabolic activity of the cells involved is necessary. Recent evidence indicates that activation of an enzyme system responsible for mediator release involves decreasing cellular levels of cyclic AMP (45). (See Control of Atopic and Anaphylactic Reactions below.)

CUTANEOUS ANAPHYLAXIS

Cutaneous anaphylaxis (urticaria, wheal and flare, hive) is elicited in a sensitive individual by skin test (scratch or intradermal injection of antigen). Grossly visible manifestations are erythema, itching, a wheal, pseudopods, and a spreading flare, reaching a maximum in 15–20 minutes and fading in a few hours (12). Histologically there is edema, with essentially no cellular infiltration. The major cause of the swelling and "edema" may actually be related to the appearance of intracellular vacuoles in epidermal cells, not interstitial edema. The mechanism is the same as in systemic anaphylaxis, but the reaction is localized because of antibody fixation in the skin and release of histamine or histamine-like substances into the skin with local changes in vascular permeability. Cutaneous anaphylaxis should be differentiated from the Arthus reaction in terms of both time of appearance and morphology of the reaction.

SYSTEMIC ANAPHYLAXIS

Anaphylaxis or anaphylactic shock is a generalized reaction elicited in a sensitized animal by the intravenous injection of antigen (6). However, in highly sensitive individuals, a severe systemic reaction to small doses of the allergen placed on the skin (scratch or patch test) may occur. For this reason, the clinical allergist must be prepared to administer adrenalin or epinephrine to any patient during skin testing. These drugs counteract the systemic effects of the systemic anaphylactic reaction. The nature of the systemic reaction is species-dependent. In all species smooth muscle contraction is prominent, with increased permeability of small vessels, leukopenia, fall in temperature, hypotension, incoagulability of blood, slowing of heart, and decreased serum complement levels (6).

Guinea Pig

Death occurs in 2–5 minutes, with prostration, convulsions, respiratory embarrassment, involuntary urination, defecation, itching, sneezing and coughing. At autopsy the lungs are inflated due to bronchiolar contraction with air trapping. This reaction is similar to human asthma.

Rabbit

Death occurs in minutes; the course is similar in other respects to that in the guinea pig, except for little respiratory difficulty. Autopsy shows right heart failure attributed to pulmonary circulatory obstruction.

Dog

Death occurs after 1–2 hours. There is profound prostration with vomiting and bloody diarrhea. Liver engorgement due to hepatic vein obstruction is revealed at postmortem.

Rat

Death occurs in 30 minutes to 5 hours. There is congestion of the small intestine and midzonal and periportal necrosis of the liver.

Man

Man exhibits a combination of the above reactions. Circulatory shock with dizziness and faintness may be the only manifestation, but collapse, unconsciousness, and death can occur. In six reported cases death occurred in 16–120 minutes (36). There was obstruction and edema of the upper respiratory tract, laryngeal edema, and increased eosinophils in sinusoids of spleen and liver. Acute systemic anaphylaxis in man is usually iatrogenic, produced by injection of drugs (penicillin), but can occur naturally, e.g., following insect (bee, wasp) stings.

ANGIONEUROTIC EDEMA

Angioneurotic edema is an hereditary condition in which edema and swelling are more extensive than the localized hive (10). The lesion may involve the eyelids, lips, tongue, and areas of the trunk. Involvement of the gastrointestinal tract may produce symptoms of acute abdominal distress, but the symptoms almost always disappear in a few days without surgical intervention. The only significant life-threatening complication is severe pharyngeal involvement, which may lead to asphyxia. The pathologic alteration is firm, nonpitting edema of the dermis and subcutaneous tissue, differentiated from a wheal-and-flare reaction by the absence of erythema. In addition, antihistamines have no effect upon angioneurotic edema, and the lesions cause a burning or stinging sensation rather than itching. Urticaria may accompany angioneurotic edema, but is clearly a separate lesion.

Angioneurotic edema is inherited as a non sex-linked dominant autosomal trait. Biochemically, there is a deficiency of C1 esterase inhibitor or C1 esterase inhibitor is present in an inactive form. C1 esterase is the active form of the first component of complement. During attacks the C4 and C2 levels in the serum are decreased, indicating that activation of the complement system is important in this phenomena. The injection of C1 esterase into the skin of normal individuals produces a wheal-and-flare reaction, but the injection of C1 esterase into the skin of patients with angioneurotic edema produces a firm, nonpitting induration with no flare (localized angioneurotic edema). Thus, production of the lesions of angioneurotic edema must involve factors other than lack of C1 esterase inhibitor (10). The kinin system (see page 281) may be activated by tryptic enzymes. C1 esterase inhibitor is also an inhibitor of the kinin system

(55). Thus, interactions of different inflammatory systems may be responsible for the clinical picture observed.

It has been claimed that attacks of angioneurotic edema may be terminated by the injection of fresh frozen plasma from normal individuals, presumably owing to the presence of C1 esterase inhibitors in such preparations (9). However, this observation has not been generally reproducible.

URTICARIA

Giant urticaria is manifested by the widespread development of firm, raised wheal-like lesions over large areas of the skin. They are superficial, erythematous and intensely pruritic with raised serpiginous edges and blanched centers. Individual lesions last about 48 hours, but new eruptions may appear for an indefinite period. Although allergic mechanisms may be operative, identification of an eliciting allergen is not possible in most instances and nonimmunologic stimuli such as heat, cold or sunlight frequently initiate urticarial lesions (55). However, in some instances the lesions of cold urticaria can be transferred with serum factors—either IgM (63), suggesting the involvement of a cryoimmunoglobulin (see page 198), or IgE—indicating that an IgE-mediated reaction can cause giant urticaria.

ATOPIC ALLERGY

Atopic allerpy is a term applied to a group of human allergies to natural antigens; it includes asthma, hay fever, allergic rhinitis, urticaria (hives), eczema, serous otitis media, conjunctivities and food allergy (12,49). Similar reactions may be found in some other species (other primates, dogs, seals). The mechanisms are essentially the same as those involved in systemic and cutaneous anaphylaxis. Anaphylaxis is included by many under the general term of Atopy.

CHARACTERISTICS OF ATOPIC ALLERGY

The clinical features of atopic allergy are itching and whealing, sneezing, and respiratory embarrassment. The pathologic features include edema, smooth muscle contraction, and leukopenia. The pharmacologic characteristics are histamine release and partial protection by antihistamines.

FACTORS AFFECTING CLINICAL REACTION

The type of reaction seen clinically depends upon four factors, described below (12).

Route of Access of Antigen

If contact occurs via the skin, hives (wheal and flare) predominate; if contact is via respiratory mucous membranes, asthma and rhinitis occur; if contact occurs via the eyes, conjunctivitis will predominate, or if through the ears serous otitis; if contact occurs via the gastrointestinal tract, food allergy, with cramps, nausea, vomiting, and diarrhea results.

Dose of Antigen

The rarity of death from atopic allergy, in contrast to anaphylaxis, is most likely due to the dose and route of access of the antigen. In systemic anaphylaxis, large doses of antigen are given intravenously; in atopic allergy, the doses are low and contact is across mucous membranes. Such a conclusion is justified by the observation that anaphylactically sensitized guinea pigs exposed to small amounts of antigen by inhalation develop typical asthmatic symptoms.

The Shock Organ

Individual differences in reactivity depend upon individual idiosyncrasy, pharmacologic abnormality of the target tissue (increased histamine content) or increased susceptibility of a given organ due to nonspecific irritation or inflammation. Many affected individuals commonly have an atopic reaction involving one organ system (asthma) with sparing of other organs.

Familial Susceptibility

Members of an atopic family have an increased incidence of atopic type reactions. This phenomenon may be due to a tendency to form a particular type of antibody (IgE). The serum IgE concentrations of pairs of monozygotic twins are significantly more similar to each other than are the levels of otherwise comparable pairs of dizygotic twins (4). In addition, genetic control of basal IgE levels in man is supported by statistical analysis of serum IgE levels in normal adults (29). It is possible, although not yet established, that genetic control of the immune responses by immune response cistrons (see page 52) may extend to the IgE immunoglobulin class; certain individuals inherit cistrons that select an IgE antibody response to a given antigen rather than a response with another immunoglobulin class (40). Elevated serum IgE levels during the first year of life frequently occur in infants who develop atopic disease later, suggesting the early expression of a genetically controlled propensity of atopic individuals to produce IgE immunoglobulin (46).

ASTHMA

Even though everyone knows at least one individual with asthma and the characteristic symptoms have been known since the fifteenth century (65), it is difficult, if not impossible, to find a definition of asthma with which everyone will agree (2). Asthma presents clinically as repeated acute attacks of respiratory distress due to airway obstruction, presumably caused mainly by constriction of the smooth muscles of the small bronchi. There are at least two forms of asthma: one clearly mediated by the anaphylactic mechanism and one which is not mediated by known allergic reactions. The allergically mediated form is caused by the activation of effector cells (mast cells) sensitized by IgE antibody. In many cases of allergic asthma, the antigen responsible can be identified. Allergic asthma is termed "extrinsic" because of the clear identification of an exogenous eliciting antigen in most cases. The mechanism of activation of the nonallergic form of asthma is not well understood but is probably due to an imbalance of the physiologic control of smooth muscle tone (see Control of Atopic and Anaphylactic Reactions below). Immune mechanisms are not believed to be involved and a specific eliciting antigen cannot be identified. Constriction of bronchial smooth muscle may be triggered by a variety of nonimmune mechanisms including chemical irritation, change in temperature, physical activity and emotional stress, as well as by a variety of respiratory infections. The nonimmune form of asthma is termed intrinsic because no exogenous eliciting antigen can be identified. One possible explanation is that intrinsic asthma is caused by sensitivity to a chronic infecting organism, but proof of this hypothesis is lacking. Allergic asthma is usually seasonal although it is year-round in parts of the world where pollen allergens are present for most of the year, i.e., Bermuda grass pollen in Southern California; or if nonpollen allergens, such as animal dander, are responsible. Intrinsic asthma occurs throughout the year without exception. A condition of intrinsic asthma may evolve from a background of seasonal asthma or from a nonatopic background of chronic bronchitis.

A number of pathologic changes have been found in the lungs of patients with either type of asthma. In the acute attack, which may be fatal because of acute asphyxiation, there is marked constriction of the bronchi and occlusion of the bronchi with a particularly thick mucous secretion (mucous plugs). In a chronic asthmatic the pulmonary changes are 1) marked thickening of the basement membrane of the bronchial mucosa, 2) hypertrophy of the bronchial smooth muscle, 3) hypertrophy of the bronchial mucous glands, 4) chronic inflammatory cells in the bronchial wall with a substantial increase over normal in the number of mast cells, and 5) the presence of mucous in the bronchi containing large numbers of eosinophilic leukocytes. The thickened basement membrane may contain deposits of IgG or IgM, but IgE has not often been detected. Other stigmata of chronic inflammation and airway obstruction, including focal fibrosis and scarring, emphysema and atelectasis, may be found in the periphery of the lung. Since repeated asthma attacks are also associated with increased susceptability to pulmonary infections, some of the pathologic changes may be due to repeated bronchopneumonia.

Therapy for asthma depends on whether or not a specific eliciting antigen can be identified. If it can the best treatment is avoidance of the antigen. Immunotherapy by injection of the antigen in a manner that will change the reactivity of the patient may also be successful (see Hyposensitization, Desensitization and Tolerance below). Drugs that produce bronchodilation or that alter the state of activation of effector mast cells may be effective in both extrinsic and intrinsic allergy (see Control of Anaphylactic Reactions below), and prompt administration by aerosal or injection may be required to prevent death in an acute attack. Psychotherapy may be effective in some cases as the extent of a given attack may be increased by anxiety; the frequency of asthma is higher for individuals in emotional distress. Special breathing exercises may reduce symptoms, especially in growing children. Steroid therapy is of limited value because of undesirable side effects but will produce dramatic relief of asthmatic symptoms.

An acute form of infective asthma may occur in persons with Aspergillus infection. These individuals are allergic to Aspergillus, a mold, which may cause a pulmonary infection. A small number of individuals with pulmonary aspergillosis develop allergy to the infecting agent which causes obstruction of the involved bronchi with mucous plugs (31). Bronchopulmonary impaction and aspergillosis hypersensitivity is an example of a true intrinsic allergic reaction.

HAY FEVER (SEASONAL ALLERGIC RHINITIS)

Seasonal upper respiratory reactions to pollen are commonly referred to as hay fever. The eliciting antigens represent a variety of air-born plant pollens which effect a reaction in the nasal passages and eyes of affected individuals. Symptoms include sneezing, nasal congestion, watery discharge from the eye, conjunctival itching and cough with mild bronchoconstriction. Pathologic changes are not extensive. Usually there is edema of the submucosal tissue with an infiltration of eosinophils which is entirely reversible. The degree of reaction and severity of symptoms are directly related to the amount of exposure to the allergen responsible. Treatment consists of avoidance, antihistamines or specific immunotherapy (31). Again, psychological factors may considerably determine the degree of discomfort. Hay fever may progress to asthma, but usually the severity of symptoms gradually diminishes with aging.

NASAL POLYPS

Nasal polyps are tumor-like masses that form in the nasal air passages causing chronic airway obstruction and rendering nasal breathing very difficult or impossible. These masses can be removed surgically but usually recur promptly. The relationship between nasal polyps and allergic rhinitis (inflammation of the nasal mucous membranes due to atopic reactivity) is uncertain, although some observers feel that sinusitis and polyps may be caused by bacterial allergy. Nasal polyps characteristically show marked edema, swelling of hydrophilic ground substance and scattered eosinophilic infiltration. Eosinophilic polymorphonuclear leukocytes are associated with severe persistent allergic rhinitis, and it has been suggested that persistent contact with small amounts of antigen leads to the characteristic picture. The prolonged nature of the swelling may be explained by continued production of hydrophilic ground substance by tissue fibroblasts.

FOOD ALLERGY

Ingestion of allergens may lead to remarkable gastrointestinal reactions known collectively as food allergy (52). The relationship of the GI reaction to atopic sensitivity is not clear, as many individuals with positive skin reactions to an allergen do not react to ingestion of the allergen, whereas individuals with repeated episodes of vomiting or diarrhea which occur on eating a given food do not produce a skin reaction to the food. Allergy to cow's milk is the most frequently suspected GI reaction to food (21). Milk contains over 16 proteins that might be allergenic and skin reactions to a number of these proteins occur in some sensitive children (24). In addition, unsuspected bovine food additives, such as penicillin, may be present in milk and elicit allergic reactions (64). Food allergy may lead to hypoproteinemia due to loss of protein in the GI tract and persistent diarrhea (62). Other manifestations of food allergy are extensive skin eruptions (urticaria or eczema) or systemic shock (23). Avoidance of the allergen is the primary therapy and artificial diets are sometimes required to prevent food allergy reactions (52).

ASPIRIN INTOLERANCE

Aspirin, one of the world's most widely used drugs, is generally thought to be almost completely devoid of undesirable effects when used within a therapeutic dose range. However, it is now known to be responsible for a variety of atopic and anaphylactic reactions, including asthma, rhinitis, nasal polyps (14,54) and even anaphylactic shock (16,61). A strong plea has been made to reevaluate the widespread uncontrolled use of aspirin (15).

Aspirin is a chemically active molecule which acetylates serum proteins, including human serum albumin, so that it is possible that chronic aspirin intolerance may be caused by alteration in the antigenicity of albumin (30) or by aspirin acting as a hapten. On the other hand, an idiosyncratic effect of aspirin in disruption of the physiologic control of smooth muscle and mucous secretion has also been proposed as responsible for aspirin intolerance (53). Aspirin intolerance may develop in children (14) or appear in adults with no previous history of atopy (53). Aspirin intolerance manifested by asthma represents a minority of asthmatic children; the onset is later and less sudden than asthma that is not related to aspirin (14).

In adults the symptoms of aspirin intolerance appear suddenly with a watery rhinorrhea followed by development of nasal polyps, chronic asthma and in some cases even shock reactions to ingestion of aspirin (54). The chronic asthma related to aspirin intolerance responds well to drug therapy, but, of course, avoidance of aspirin is the obvious treatment. This is easier said than done as aspirin is included in many drug mixtures where its presence is unsuspected and other cross-reacting haptens may elicit reactions in aspirin sensitive individuals. Yellow food color #5 contains such a related hapten.

INSECT ALLERGY

Atopic or anaphylactic reaction to contact with insects may be divided into three groups: 1) inhalent or contact reactions to insect body parts or products, 2) skin reactions (wheal and flare) to biting insects, and 3) systemic shock reactions to stinging insects (20,56). Asthmatic or hay fever-like reactions may occur on air-borne exposure of a sensitive individual to large numbers of insects or their body parts (17). This occurs outdoors to insects that periodically appear in large numbers, such as locusts or grasshoppers, and indoors more chronically to beetles, flies, spiders, etc. Biting insects may produce delayed hypersensitivity or acute wheal-and-flare skin reactions. In a given individual a delayed reaction may convert with age to an anaphylactic one (18). The common reaction to a mosquito or flea bite is a localized cutaneous anaphylactic reaction. There is a very limited toxic effect of the saliva introduced by the insect bite; the reaction is an allergic one. An individual who has little or no reaction to a mosquito bite may not have developed an allergic response or may be tolerant to the allergen (38). Among the author's children, one has essentially no reaction to mosquito bites; one produces large delayed hypersensitivity skin reactions; a third has large wheal-and-flare reactions; while the fourth produces a small limited wheal with no flare. Serious effects of a reaction to biting insects may occur in parts of the world where large numbers of mosquitos appear in waves; multiple mosquito bites to a sensitive individual may produce systemic effects. Immunotherapy is warranted in a highly sensitive individual who risks extensive exposure (19). Fatalities occur more frequently from stinging insects, such as bees and wasps. More people die each year as a result of being stung by an insect than from being bitten by a snake (3). Deaths from stinging insects are due to systemic anaphylaxis and usually occur within one hour of being stung. Therefore, immediate therapy is required. This may be provided by injection of epinephine (see page 174). Immunotherapy may prevent subsequent severe reactions. People who raise bees may permit a bee to sting them and limit the amount of venom injected; by increasing the amount on subsequent stings, it is claimed that the degree of reaction to a larger dose is less.

It is not clear why these acute allergic reactions to insect bites and stings develop, although it has been postulated that the reaction induces immediate avoidance behavior and may limit the exposure of a bitten individual to a dose of a toxic venom that could be even more damaging (58). On the other hand, a systemic anaphylactic reaction to an insect sting may be interpreted as an immune mechanism which should be protective, but is instead deleterious and potentially fatal.

ATOPIC ALLERGENS

Atopic reactions may occur to very unusual antigens. Systemic anaphylactic reactions have been unleashed by ingestion of beans, rice, shrimp, fish, milk, cereal mixes, potatoes, Brazil nuts and tangerines (23). Men have complained about being allergic to their wives, but usually they are reacting to some component of makeup, hair spray or other cosmetic agent. Halpern, from France, has reported the case of a young wife who developed systemic anaphylactic symptoms shortly after intercourse; appropriate tests demonstrated that she was extremely anaphylactically sensitive to her husband's seminal fluid (27). Many individuals who work with laboratory animals develop anaphylactic reactions to the dander from these animals. The incidence of such sensitivity increases with the amount of contact with the animals. During the days of cavalry many officers and troops had to be discharged or moved to different tasks because of an allergic reaction to horse dander. As many as 20% of the cavaliers were involved.

Documentation of allergic reactions of horses to humans has not been found.

ATOPIC ECZEMA–ATOPIC DERMATITIS

This is a chronic skin eruption of varied etiology which usually occurs in young individuals who develop atopic reactions (hay fever) at a later age. The pathologic changes in the skin are consistent with those of a severe contact dermatitis (see below). Erythema, papules, and vesicles are accompanied by intense pruritus. There is perivascular accumulation of mononuclear cells, followed by infiltration into the epidermis with epidermal spongiosis. As the affected child becomes older, thickening of the skin of the affected areas occurs (lichenification). Identification of an antigen that elicits the eczema is very difficult, but in some cases there is evidence that the antigens are those that also elicit atopic reactions (pollen, house dust, animal dander). Atopic eczema is morphologically more like a reaction of cellular or delayed hypersensitivity, but is discussed here because of its association with atopic conditions. An allergic etiology of all eczema must be questioned since typical eczema may occur in children with severe combined immunologic deficiency (32). Therefore, although proven eczema of atopic allergic origin exists, eczema-like (eczematoid) skin lesions can be produced in other ways.

IMMUNOTHERAPEUTIC MODIFICATION OF ATOPIC ALLERGY: DESENSITIZATION, HYPOSENSITIZATION AND TOLERANCE

Atopic or anaphylactic conditions may be treated by starting with the injection of small amounts of the offending allergen and increasing the amount of antigen over a protracted period of time (1,12,44,48). This injection immunotherapy (Fig. 12–2) may result in a significant decrease in allergic symptoms. The mechanism of this beneficial effect is not always clear. In some cases injection therapy results in the production of non-IgE antibody to the injected allergen. It appears that by careful immunization with the offending allergen it may be possible to induce the formation of nonreaginic, precipitating IgG antibody. Since the precipitating antibody reacts with the same antigen as the reaginic antibody, the precipitating antibody will compete with the reaginic antibody in the reaction with antigen and help prevent atopic symptoms. The formation of precipitating antigen–antibody complexes may also produce tissue damage, but many more molecules of precipitating antibody reacting with antibody are needed to produce a reaction of clinical significance than molecules of reaginic antibody (48). Such blocking antibody may be demonstrated in vitro by its ability to inhibit the release of anaphylactic mediators from sensitized mast cells upon exposure to antigen. The production of blocking antibody is referred to as hyposensitization. In some individuals who have had a beneficial response to injection therapy, no blocking antibody is demonstrable. The decrease in sensitization of such individuals may be due to the induction of tolerance [no longer produce IgE antibody] (37) or to neutralization of the IgE antibody with excess antigen (desensitization, see Chapter 7). Desensitization may be produced by providing enough antigen in small

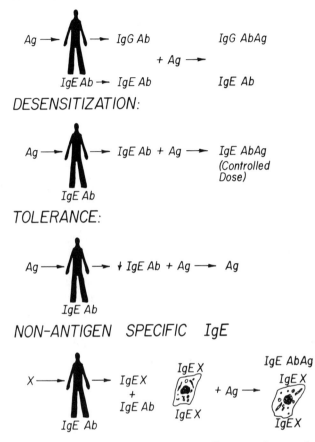

HYPOSENSITIZATION:

DESENSITIZATION:

TOLERANCE:

NON-ANTIGEN SPECIFIC IgE

Fig. 12–2. **Immunotherapy of Atopic Allergies.** Immunotherapy of atopic reactions by injection of the specific allergen is known to be effective, particularly for alleviation of the symptoms of hay fever. The mechanism of reduction of allergic symptoms is unclear. At least three possibilities include: 1) hyposensitization, production of IgG blocking antibody, 2) desensitization, consumption of IgE antibody by repeated small doses of allergen and 3) tolerance, a loss or significant decrease in IgE antibody production to the allergen. Another possible mechanism not yet identified as occurring due to specific immunotherapy is the production of nonspecific IgE that might block the effector cell receptors for IgE allergen-specific antibody (5,28).

doses to combine with the IgE antibody so that the IgE antibody is not available for reactive tissue sites. Desensitization may occur with injection therapy for hay fever. Frequently a series of injections is required preceding each hay fever season, suggesting that injections of allergen bind the available antibody as it is produced without producing significant symptoms. With cessation of injections, continued IgE antibody production is able to overcome the antigen and become available for tissue sensitization (12).

The presence of high concentrations of an IgE that does not bind a particular antigen (nonantibody IgE) might saturate mast cell binding sites and prevent the functional sensitization of mast cells by IgE with specific antibody activity. This would be an IgE "blocking" effect, i.e., nonantibody IgE blocking IgE antibody. Support for this concept comes from the observations that individuals with high IgE serum concentrations secondary to worm infestations or leprosy may have a decreased incidence of "allergic" reactions (5,28).

ANAPHYLACTOID REACTIONS

Any event causing histamine release may cause atopic symptoms which may be confused with a true allergic reaction. Anaphylactoid shock is produced in normal (nonimmune) animals by injection of a variety of agents capable of releasing histamine, without the mediation of an antigen–antibody reaction. The clinical, physiologic and pathologic picture resulting is virtually indistinguishable from true anaphylaxis, but is not produced by an immune reaction. Physical agents (heat, cold), trauma (dermatographia), emotional disturbances or exercise may evoke pharmacologic mechanisms which mimic allergic reactions. Dermatographia is most likely caused by the release of anaphylactic mediators from mast cells by a degree of physical trauma that does not induce a reaction in normal individuals. Such a reaction may confuse the results of skin testing as a wheal may result from insertion of a needle alone (11,26). In some patients a reaction to a physical agent may actually have an immune basis. A physical agent may cause release or production of altered tissue antigens to which a patient is sensitive. Reactions to light (photo allergy) may be caused by agents activated by sunlight that are applied to the skin to form haptens (13). Such reactions are usually contact dermatitis reactions (see page 217). Cholinergic urticaria is believed to be produced by an abnormal response to acetycholine released from efferent nerves after exposure to emotional stress, physical activity or trauma. Cholinesterase levels of the skin may be reduced in cholinergic urticaria leading to prolonged survival of acetylcholine which may act to release histamine from tissue mast cells.

The clinical findings in an atopic reaction are often confused by associated nonimmune factors. Thus, asthma is frequently complicated by infection or bronchiectasis which may overshadow the allergic condition. The severity and duration of asthmatic attacks may be greatly influenced by psychologic conditions, and typical attacks may occur due to emotional stress, with no known contact with an allergen. These anaphylactoid reactions may be mediated by nonimmunologic mediator release, an imbalance of the sympathetic nervous system or hyperreactivity of end organ smooth muscle (see below).

CONTROL OF ATOPIC AND ANAPHYLACTIC REACTIONS

The severity of reaction by an anaphylactically sensitized individual upon exposure to the specific allergen depends not only upon the amount of allergen and reaginic antibody, but also upon the reactivity of mast cells, the excitability of the end organ (smooth muscle) and the effect of the autonomic nervous system (Fig. 12–3). Imbalance of these homeostatic control mechanisms for atopic and anaphylactic reactions explains how exposure to nonimmunologic stimuli, such as heat, cold, physical exercise or light, may in some individuals serve to excite physiologic reactions that mimic allergic reactions (anaphylactoid reactions). The concept of cyclic nucleotides as "second messengers" in controlling cellular responses (51,59) has led to a theoretic appreciation of the mechanisms controlling anaphylactic reactions (2,25).

Mast Cells

It has been suggested that control or sensitivity of mast cells to allergen (i.e., the amount of mediators released by sensitized mast cells following contact with allergen) is accomplished by balanced adrenergic receptors (α- and β-receptors) which control the cellular level of a postulated enzyme system, the activation of which leads to mediator release (45). Contact of the sensitized mast cell with antigen causes activation of the enzyme system via an, as yet, unknown mechanism. The amount of enzyme available is determined by the cellular level of cyclic AMP, which in turn is controlled by the stimulation of the α- and β-receptors. Stimulation of the β receptor activates adenyl cyclase and causes an increase in cyclic AMP (decreased enzyme) while activation of the α receptor results in decreased cyclic AMP (increased enzyme). Cyclic AMP is normally broken down to 5' AMP by phosphodiesterase, so that inhibition of phosphodiesterase leads to increased cyclic AMP and decreased enzyme. The extent of reaction of mast cells to antigen may be controlled by stimulating or blocking the controlling receptors. α- and β-adrenergic receptors may be stimulated or blocked with various drugs. Norepinephrine stimulates α-receptors which results in a decrease in cellular cyclic AMP (increased enzymes and senitivity to allergen) while isoproteranol stimulates β-receptors (decreased sensitivity to allergen). Phenoxyzbenzamine blocks α-receptors and propranolol blocks β-receptors. Epinephrine stimulates both α- and β-receptors, but selective stimulation may be achieved by the use of epinephrine combined with one of the blocking drugs. Methylxanthines (theophylline) inhibit phosphodiesterase and thus prevent cyclic AMP breakdown (decreased sensitivity to antigen). Two new drugs apparently will block the release of mediators after contact of sensitized mast cell with allergen. The way that these drugs, diethylcarbamazine and disodium chromoglycate, inhibit histamine release is not known (45,47,49). Specific desensitization of sensitized cells occurs as patients treated with sodium cromolyn and challenged with antigen remain refractory to subsequent challenge with the same antigen but not a different antigen when retested after 5 hours (39).

End Organ Sensitivity

It has been theorized that the unleashing of severe atopic reactions also depends upon a loss of a balance between homeostatic α and β end

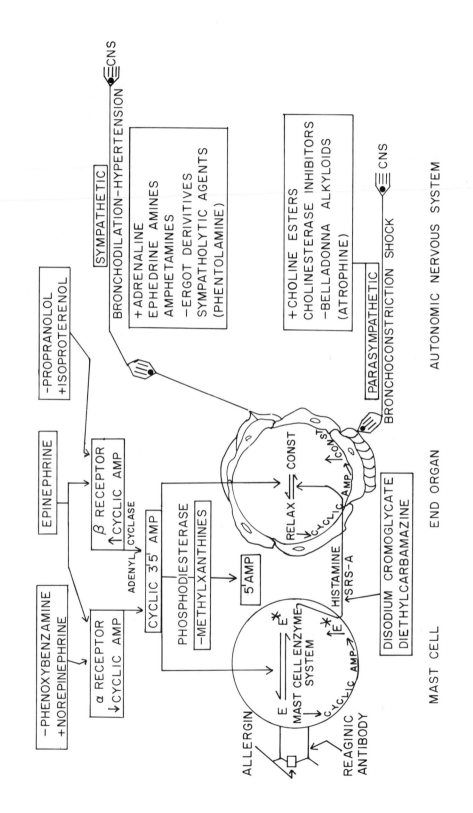

organ (smooth muscle) adrenergic receptors (60). It is postulated that the end organ effect of the pharmacologically active agents released by IgE sensitized mast cells upon contact with antigen is through stimulation of α-adrenergic receptors, similar to those discussed above for the mast cell. A decrease in the amount of cyclic AMP, is the key to activation of end organ cells. Stimulation of α-receptors leads to blocking of cyclic AMP. On the other hand, activation of β-receptors causes an increase in adenylcyclase activity which increases production of cyclic AMP from adenosine triphosphate (ATP). This gives the opposite effect of α-receptor activation leading to relaxation of smooth muscle cells and bronchodilation. The β-adrenergic theory states that atopic individuals do not have the normal adrenergic end organ homeostatic mechanism (60). Activation of α-receptors in normal nonatopic individuals does not produce significant anaphylactic symptoms because such activation is counterbalanced by activation of the β-adrenergic system. Thus, in the terms of this theory, bronchial asthma is not primarily an immunologic disease but is due to an abnormality in the β-adrenergic end organ system.

The cyclic AMP levels of the end organ cells may be controlled in a similar manner as described above for mast cells. Thus, stimulation of α-receptors leads to a decrease in cyclic AMP and increased anaphylactic effects; stimulation of β-receptors leads to increased cyclic AMP and decreased end organ effects. The marked beneficial effect of epinephrine upon anaphylactic symptoms is due to its apparent stimulation of end organ β-receptors and not because of its effect on mast cells.

The Autonomic Nervous System

The excitability of the end organ smooth muscle (bronchial muscles, arterioles, gastrointestinal muscles) is also controlled by the autonomic nervous system and is maintained by a balance of sympathetic (adrenergic) and parasympathetic (cholinergic) effects. In general, parasympathetic effects are similar to anaphylactic effects (bronchial constriction, increased gastrointestinal peristalsis, dilatation of bladder sphincter, dilatation of

---

Fig. 12–3. Control of atopic–anaphylactic reactions. The end result of unleashing an anaphylactic reaction depends upon the sensitivity of the mast cell to stimulation and the state of excitability of the end organ. Mast cell sensitivity depends upon amount of IgE receptor available and level of cyclic AMP; cyclic AMP levels are decreased by stimulation of α adrenergic receptors and increased by stimulation of β adrenergic receptors. Decreased cyclic AMP causes formation of active enzyme which increases sensitivity of mast cell for release of mediators, while increased cyclic AMP lowers mast cell sensitivity. Similar receptors control cyclic AMP and level of excitability of organ smooth muscle. The magnitude of an anaphylactic reaction may be controlled by drugs which affect α and β adrenergic receptors. The excitability of the end organ is also controlled by the autonomic nervous system which provides an additional point at which drugs may be used to influence anaphylactic reactions and a mechanism whereby emotions, via CNS connections with the autonomic nerves, may modulate anaphylactic reactions. (For further discussion, see text.)

arteries, pupil constriction) while sympathetic effects are the opposite (bronchial and pupil dilatation, arterial and sphincter constriction). In a normal individual the effects of the two components of the autonomic system are usually in balance with a tendency to sympathetic dominance (22). It is known that certain situations may result in a temporary imbalance of these systems. Thus, stimulation of the parasympathetic system by injection of mecholyl or acetylcholine in a normal individual results in a temporary drop in blood pressure. Immediately after this effect the individual may be hyperresponsive to sympathetic stimulation, so-called sympathetic tuning (22). A permanent imbalance may be produced in experimental animals by producing lesions in the pituitary. For instance, ablation of areas of the anterior pituitary which reduces parasympathetic discharge protects against the lethal effects of anaphylaxis (43). Anaphylactically sensitized individuals may have a permanent imbalance of autonomic control that predisposes them to increased reactivity to mediator release. The shock organ effect may be explained by a local imbalance of autonomic effects. Anaphylactoid reactions may be overreactions of this balancing system induced by physiologic change. Because the autonomic nervous system is indirectly connected through neuronal synapses to higher areas of the brain, it is possible for emotional conditioning to affect the autonomic balance. Thus, emotional states may lead to parasympathetic tuning with resultant atopic or anaphylactic symptoms (cholinergic urticaria).

An imbalance of any or all of three levels, mast cell, end organ or autonomic nervous system, may explain the increased sensitivity of atopic individuals to anaphylactic mediators. Atopic individuals injected with small doses of histamine have a much greater reaction than nonatopic individuals (22,60). It has been shown that the lymphocytes of atopic individuals have a decreased ability to respond to certain stimuli by increased cyclic AMP levels. Thus, atopic individuals may be unable to balance the effects of α-stimulation or allergen contact (decreased cyclic AMP).

TREATMENT OF ATOPIC ALLERGY

Therapeutic procedures to prevent or decrease atopic reactions may be applied at the various levels of the reaction: contact with antigen, IgE receptor, sensitivity of the mast cell to stimulation, degranulation of mast cell, mast cell mediator activity, sensitivity of end organ cell, autonomic nervous system balance and emotional state of the reactive individual.

1. Avoidance of contact with the allergen is the most effective means of preventing atopic allergic reactions, thus removing antigen stimulation of the IgE receptor. Avoidance is not always feasible and other methods must be used.
2. The availability of the IgE receptor may be reduced by hyposensitization, desensitization or tolerance as the result of injection therapy (see above).
3. The sensitivity of the mast cell upon reaction of IgE receptors with allergen may depend upon the amount of cyclic AMP available. This level may be controlled by the drugs indicated in Fig. 12–3. If mast

cell cyclic AMP can be increased by the methods indicated above, the extent of mast cell mediator release upon reaction of sensitized cells with allergen may be decreased and atopic symptoms controlled.

4. Two new drugs, diethylcarbamazine and disodium chromoglycate, significantly decrease the release of mediators from mast cells upon contact with allergen (47,49). Their mechanism of action is unknown.

5. The effect of mast cell mediators may be partially controlled by drugs that interfere with histamine activity (antihistamines). The fact that antihistamines are only partially effective in decreasing atopic symptoms indicates that other mediators play an important role. However, antihistamines compete with tissue receptors for histamine so that it may be impossible for antihistamines to compete effectively enough to provide complete relief of symptoms.

6. The sensitivity of the end organ (smooth muscle) to atopic mediators also depends upon cellular cyclic AMP levels. If end organ cyclic AMP can be increased as indicated in Fig. 12–3, then atopic symptoms should be decreased.

7. Sympathetic stimulation or parasympathetic blockade may also have a significant beneficial effect upon atopic reactions through the effect of the autonomic nervous system upon end organ excitability (Fig. 12–3).

8. It is well known that the severity of atopic reactions (particularly asthma) depends upon the emotional state of the individual. Anxious or insecure patients have more severe symptoms than more secure or stable patients. Thus, the emotional state of the reactive individual should be evaluated and treated with psychotherapy, if necessary.

REFERENCES

1. Austen KF, Humphrey JH: In vitro studies of the mechanism of anaphylaxis. Adv Immunol 3:1, 1963
2. Austen KF, Lichtenstein LM (eds): Asthma: Physiology, Immunopharmacology and Treatment. New York, Academic Press, 1973
3. Barr SE: Allergy to hymenopteria stings—Review of the world literature: 1953–1970. Ann Allergy 29:49, 1971
4. Bazaral M, Orgel HA, Hamburger RN: Genetics of IgE and allergy: Serum IgE levels in twins. J Allergy Clin Immunol 52:211–244, 1974
5. Bazaral M, Orgel HA, Hamburger RN: The influence of serum IgE levels of selected recipients, including patients with allergy, helminthiasis and tuberculosis, on the apparent P–K titer of a reaginic serum. Clin Exp Immunol 14:117, 1973
6. Block KS: The anaphylactic antibodies of mammals including man. Prog Allergy 10:84, 1967
7. Coca AF, Grove EF: Studies on hypersensitiveness. XIII. A study of the actopic reagins. J Immunol 10:445, 1925
8. Cochrane CG: Immunologic tissue injury mediated by neutrophilic leukocytes. Adv Immunol 9:97, 1968
9. Cohen G, Peterson A: Treatment of hereditary angioedema with frozen plasma. Ann Allergy 30:690, 1972
10. Donaldson VH, Ratnoff OD, DaSilva WD, Rosen FS: Permeability-increasing activity in hereditary angioneurotic edema plasma. J Clin Invest 48:642, 1969
11. Ebken RK, Bauschard FA, Levine MI: Dermatographism: Its definition, demonstration, and prevalence. J Allergy 41:338, 1968
12. Ellis EF: Immunologic basis of atopic disease. Adv Pediatr 16:65, 1969

13. Epstein JH: Photoallergy, A review. Arch Dermatol 106:741, 1972
14. Falliers CJ: Aspirin and subtypes of asthma: Risk factor analysis. J Allergy Clin Immunol 52:141, 1973
15. Farr RS: Presidential message. J Allergy 45:321, 1970
16. Fein BT: Aspirin shock associated with asthma and nasal polyps. Ann Allergy 29:589, 1971
17. Feinberg AR, Feinberg SM, Benaim-Pinto C: Asthma and rhinitis from insect allergies. J Allergy 27:437, 1956
18. Feingold BF, Banjamini E, Michaeli D: The allergic responses to insect bites. Annu Rev Entomol 13:137, 1968
19. Frazier CA: Biting insect survey: A statistical report. Ann Allergy 32:200, 1974
20. Frazier CA: Insect Allergy. St. Louis, Green, 1969
21. Frier S, Kletter B: Clinical and immunological aspects of milk protein intolerance. Aust Paediatr J 8:140, 1972
22. Gellhorn E: Autonomic Imbalance and the Hypothalamus. Minneapolis, University of Minnesota Press, 1957
23. Golbert TM, Patterson R, Pruzansky JJ: Systemic allergic reactions to ingested antigens. J Allergy 44:96, 1969
24. Goldman AS, Sellars WA, Halpern SR, Anderson DW, Furlow TE, Johnson CH: Milk allergy. II. Skin testing of allergic and normal children with purified milk proteins. Pediatrics 32:572, 1963
25. Goodfriend L, Sehon AH, Orange RP (eds): Mechanisms in Allergy: Reagin-mediated Hypersensitivity. New York, Marcel Dekker, 1973
26. Grolnick M: An investigative and clinical evaluation of dermatographism. Ann Allergy 28:395, 1970
27. Halpern BN, Ky T, Robert B: Clinical and immunological study of an exceptional case of reaginic type sensitization to human seminal fluid. Immunology 12:247, 1967
28. Hamburger RN, Fernandez-Cruz E, Arnaiz A, Perez B, Bootello A: The relationship of the P–K titer to the serum IgE level in patients with leprosy. Clin Exp Immunol 17:253, 1974
29. Hamburger RN, Orgel HA, Bazeral M: Genetics of hyman serum IgE levels. In Mechanisms in Allergy. Goodfriend L, Sehon AH, Orange RP (eds). New York, Marcel Dekker, 1973, p 131.
30. Hawkins D, Pinckard RN, Crawford IP, Farr RS: Structural changes in human serum albumin induced by ingestion of acetylsalicylic acid. J Clin Invest 48:536, 1969
31. Hinson RFW, Moon AJ, Plummer NS: Bronchopulmonary aspergillosis. Thorax 7:317, 1952
32. Hitzig WH: The Swiss type of agammaglobulinemia. In Immunologic Deficiency Diseases in Man. Good RA (ed). New York, National Foundation Press, 1968, p 82
33. Ishizaka K, Ishizaka T, Hornbrook MH: Physico-chemical properties of human reaginic antibody. IV. Presence of a unique immunoglobulin as a carrier of reaginic activity. J Immunol 97:75, 1966
34. Ishizaka T, Ishizaka K: IgE molecules and their receptor sites on human basophil granulocytes. In Mechanisms in Allergy. Goodfriend L, Sehon AH, Orange RP (eds). New York, Marcel Dekker, 1973, p 221
35. Ishizaka T, Ishizaka K, Johansson SGO, Bennich H: Histamine release from human leukocytes by anti- E antibodies. J Immunol 102:884, 1969
36. James LP, Austen, KF: Fatal systemic anaphylaxis in man. N Engl J Med 270:597, 1964
37. Katz DH, Hamaoka T, Benacerraf B: Induction of immunological tolerance in bone-marrow-derived lymphocytes of the IgE antibody class. Proc Natl Acad Sci USA 70:2766, 1973
38. Killby VA, Silverman PH: Hypersensitive reactions in man to specific mosquito bites. Am J Trop Med Hyg 16:374, 1967
39. Kolotkin BM, Lee CK, Townley RG: Duration and specificity of sodium cromolyn on allergen inhalation challenges in asthmatics. J Allergy Clin Immunol 53:288, 1974
40. Levine BB: Genetic controls of reagin production in mice and man: Role of Ir genes in ragweed hayfever. In Mechanisms in Allergy. Goodfriend L, Sehon AH, Orange RP (eds). New York, Marcel Dekker, 1973, p 97

41. Levy DA, Carlton JA: Influence of temperature on the inhibition by colchicine of allergic histamine release. Proc Soc Exp Biol Med 130:1333, 1969
42. Lichtenstein LM, Osler AG: Studies on the mechanisms of hypersensitivity phenomena. IX. Histamine release from human leukocytes by ragweed pollen antigen. J Exp Med 120:507, 1964
43. Luparello JJ, Stein M, Park CD: Effect of hypothalamic lesions on rat anaphylaxis. Am J Physiol 207:911, 1964
44. Norman PS: Specific therapy in allergy. Med Clin North Am 58:111, 1974
45. Orange RP, Austen KF: Chemical mediators of immediate hypersensitivity. Hosp Pract 6:79, 1971
46. Orgel HA, Hamburger RN, Bazarel M, Gorrin H, Groshong T, Lenoir M, Miller JR, Wallace W: Development of IgE and allergy in infancy. J Allergy Clin Immunol (in press)
47. Orr TSC, Pollard MC, Gwilliam J, Cox JSG: Mode of action of disodium cromoglycate: Studies on immediate type hypersensitivity reactions using "double sensitization" with two antigenically distinct rat reagins. Clin Exp Immunol 7:745, 1970
48. Osler AG, Lichtenstein LM, Levy DA: In vitro studies of human reaginic allergy. Adv Immunol 8:183, 1968
49. Pepys S: Hypersensitivity Disease of the Lungs Due to Fungi and Organic Dusts. In Monographs in Allergy. Vol. 4. Kallós P, Hašek M, Interbitzen TM, Miescher P, Waksman BH (eds). Basel, Karger, 1969
50. Prausnitz C, Küstner H: Studies on sensitivity. Zentralbl Bakteriol (Orig) 86:160, 1921. English trans. in Gell PGH, Coombs RRA: Clinical Aspects of Immunology. Philadelphia, Davis, 1963, p 808
51. Robinson GA, Butcher RW, Sutherland EW: Cyclic AMP. New York, Academic Press, 1971
52. Rowe AH, Rowe A Jr: Food Allergy. Springfield, Ill., Charles C Thomas, 1972
53. Sampter M: Intolerance to aspirin. Hosp Pract 8:85, 1973
54. Sampter M, Beers RF Jr: Intolerance to aspirin. Ann Intern Med 68:975, 1968
55. Sheffer AL, Austen KF, Gigli I: Urticaria and angioedema. Postgrad Med 54:81, 1973
56. Shulman S: Insect allergy: Biochemical and immunochemical analyses of the allergens. Prog Allergy 12:246, 1968
57. Stanworth DR: Reaginic antibodies. Adv Immunol 3:181, 1963
58. Stebbings JH Jr: Immediate hypersensitivity: A defense against arthropods. Perspect Biol Med 17:233, 1974
59. Sutherland EW, Robinson GA, Butcher CW: Cyclic AMP. Circulation 37:279, 1968
60. Szentivanyi A: The beta adrenergic theory of the atopic abnormality in bronchial asthma. J Allergy 42:203, 1968
61. Van Dellen RG, Peters GA: Acute anaphylactic reactions and aspirin allergy. Postgrad Med 49:197, 1971
62. Waldmann TA, Wochner RD, Laster L, Gordon RS Jr: Allergic gastroenteropathy: A cause of excessive gastrointestinal protein loss. N Eng J Med 276:761, 1967
63. Wanderer AA, Maselli R, Ellis DF, Ishizaka K: Immunologic characterization of serum factors responsible for cold urticaria. J Allergy Clin Immunol 48:13, 1971
64. Wicher K, Reisman RE, Arbesman CE: Allergic reaction to penicillin present in milk. JAMA 208:143, 1969
65. Willis T: Second part, Sect. 1, Chapt. 12. Pharmaceutic Rationalis on the Operations of Mechanics in Humane Bodies. London, Dring, 1684, pp 78–85

13

Arthus (Toxic Complex) Reaction

Toxic complex reactions may be caused by immunoglobulin antibody reacting directly with tissue antigens or by complexes of soluble antibody and antigen. This latter reaction is initiated when antigen in the tissue spaces reacts with precipitating antibody, forming microprecipitates in and around small vessels, or when antigen in excess in the blood stream reacts with potentially precipitating antibody and these complexes lodge in the blood vessel walls causing local inflammation [Fig. 13–1] (106). The antigen–antibody complexes fix complement with activation of C3a, C5a and C567 (chemotactic factor). This results in the accumulation of neutrophilic polymorphonuclear leukocytes, which in turn release lysosomal enzymes that cause destruction of the elastic lamina of arteries (serum sickness), basement membrane alterations (glomerulonephritis), or dissolution of the walls of small vessels [Arthus reaction] (5,19–21). The alternate pathway for complement activation, entering by activation of C3 [the C3 shunt (44), see page 154] and bypassing antibody–antigen reaction and C1, 4, and 2, has been demonstrated to be active in the pathogenesis of some types of lesions which are identical to immune complex-mediated lesions (76,102). Activation of this pathway also results in activation of C567, production of complement chemotactic factor, accumulation of polymorphonuclear cells and destruction of the tissue.

CLASSIC ARTHUS REACTION

The Arthus reaction (5) is a dermal inflammatory response caused by the reaction of precipitating antibody with antigen placed in the skin. The reaction consists of edema, erythema and hemorrhage which develop over a few hours, reaching a maximum in 2–5 hours or even later if the reaction is severe. Histologically there are edema, hemorrhage, vascular

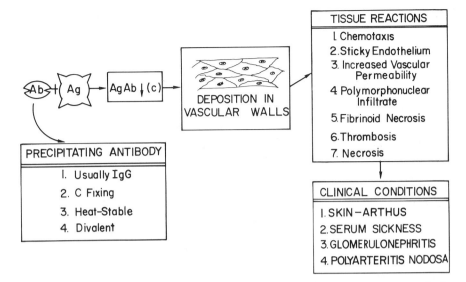

TISSUE REACTIONS

1. Chemotaxis
2. Sticky Endothelium
3. Increased Vascular Permeability
4. Polymorphonuclear Infiltrate
5. Fibrinoid Necrosis
6. Thrombosis
7. Necrosis

PRECIPITATING ANTIBODY

1. Usually IgG
2. C Fixing
3. Heat-Stable
4. Divalent

CLINICAL CONDITIONS

1. SKIN—ARTHUS
2. SERUM SICKNESS
3. GLOMERULONEPHRITIS
4. POLYARTERITIS NODOSA

Fig. 13–1. Arthus (toxic complex) reactions. Reaction of circulating antibody with soluble antigen to form soluble antigen–antibody complex which fixes complement is a primary feature of toxic complex reactions. These toxic complexes appear to localize in walls of small arteries, where complement system is activated. Of particular importance is chemotactic component of complement, with resultant accumulation of polymorphonuclear leukocytes, release of lysosomal enzymes of these polymorphonuclear leukocytes, and destruction of tissue by released leukocytic enzymes. If tissue reaction, particularly that involving affected vessel wall, is severe, fibrin and white cell thromboses occur with ischemic necrosis of affected site. Toxic complex reaction is mediated by complement-fixing precipitating antibody, usually of IgG class.

fibrinoid necrosis and massive emigration of neutrophils and eosinophils. If the reaction is severe, polymorphonuclear and platelet thrombosis occurs, with resulting ischemic necrosis. The mechanism of this type of reaction is the formation of intradermal antigen–antibody complexes, with localization of antigen–antibody complexes in vessel walls, and fixation of complement leading to cell clumping, damage to vascular endothelium, and followed by blockage of flow in small vessels and capillaries and ischemic necrosis (19). The Arthus reaction may be inhibited in varying degrees by decreasing the number of circulating leukocytes by nitrogen mustard administration or irradiation, decreasing the level of platelets; administering heparin, which interferes with the clotting mechanism; or administering nonprecipitating antibody, which competes with precipitating antibody for antigen [monovalent antibody fragments] (19,20). The presence of antigen and antibody may be demonstrated in vascular subendothelial deposits by the fluorescent antibody technique. Typical lesions, produced by interaction of preformed antigen–antibody complexes, are similar histologically to polyarteritis nodosa in man—a segmental vascular fibrinoid necrosis with exudation of neutrophils and eosinophils. The lesions produced by this technique are usually distributed in vessels throughout the body, with involvement of any vascular organ including stomach, kidney, liver, brain, joints, or heart. A severe joint inflammation (arthritis) may be produced by direct injection of antibody–antigen complexes into the joint fluid.

SERUM SICKNESS

The syndrome of serum sickness was first recognized by von Pirquet and Schick in 1905 (104). It classically consisted of arthritis, glomerulo-nephritis and vasculitis appearing 10 days to 2 weeks following passive immunization with horse serum (horse antitetanus toxin). The disease was the result of the production by the treated individual of circulating precipi-tating antibody to the injected horse serum. Rich (78) produced the disease by injections of large amounts of bovine serum albumin (BSA) into rabbits. Dixon et al. (27), by following the elimination of radiolabeled BSA, demon-strated that the lesions appeared at the time of immune elimination of the labeled antigen when *soluble complexes* in antigen excess could be demonstrated in the serum. By a continuous infusion of BSA, they were able to identify three types of immune responses in rabbits: 1) some animals did not respond (immune paralysis, a type of tolerance), did not make antibody to BSA or produced antibody in such low amounts that it was overwhelmed by the massive doses of antigen, and did not develop serum sickness; 2) some animals produced large amounts of antibody which formed complexes with antigen in antibody excess that were rapidly cleared from the blood stream and did not induce lesions; 3) most animals produced a moderate amount of antibody; antigen–antibody complexes were formed in *antigen excess*, and these animals developed typical lesions of serum sickness. Complexes formed in vitro and injected into animals may also produce lesions, but only if the complexes are formed in antigen excess.

Horse serum contains at least 30 different, separate antigens, so that complexes of one or more of these antigens may be present in the circulation even though there may be present at the same time excess antibody to other antigens. Therefore, demonstration of circulating antibody to some components does not rule out the presence of complexes from another antigen–antibody system. In addition, some individuals may produce reaginic antibodies or a state of delayed hypersensitivity to some of the antigens in horse serum, resulting in a very complicated clinical symptom.

GLOMERULONEPHRITIS

Inflammation of the glomeruli of the kidney is known as glomerulo-nephritis, and is caused by humoral antibody-mediated reactions either by deposits of antibody–antigen complexes formed elsewhere or by direct reaction of antibody with tissue antigens.

TOXIC COMPLEX GLOMERULONEPHRITIS

One of the features of serum sickness is acute glomerulonephritis (29,98) caused by the formation of large amounts of soluble antibody–antigen complexes (antigen excess) which become lodged on the epithelial side of the glomerular basement membrane and appear as lumpy deposits of antigen–antibody complex when examined by immunofluorescence. Following this localization, there is fixation of complement components resulting in the production of the complement chemotactic factor, the attraction of polymorphonuclear leukocytes and the proliferation of endothelial cells. These events lead to destruction of the glomerulus. Experimentally, this processs may be produced by 1) an appropriate host antibody response to an exogenous antigen (serum sickness) 2) the passive transfer of exogenous antigen and exogenous antibody, or 3) the injection of preformed soluble antigen–antibody complexes.

A chronic form of toxic complex glomerulonephritis may be produced by repeated injections of small amounts of antigen into an appropriately immunized animal or by repeated injections of soluble complexes (98). The lesion is a chronic membranous glomerulonephritis with a variable amount of polymorphonuclear leukocyte infiltration and endothelial proliferation which may lead to scarring and destruction of the glomerulus. It is believed that this type of mechanism is operative in the production of glomerulonephritis associated with various human diseases such as lupus erythematosus (DNA–anti-DNA), diabetes mellitus (insulin–antiinsulin), and thyroiditis (thyroglobulin–antithyroglobulin) in which antitissue antibodies are found (Table 14–3). In addition, the deposition of toxic complexes of antibody and viral antigens is responsible for some cases of human glomerulonephritis; deposits of the tumor antigen, carcinoembryonic antigen (CEA, see page 333) and antibody to CEA have been identified as being responsible for renal damage in a patient with colonic carcinoma, and rare instances of glomerulonephritis due to depositions of IgE antibody–antigen complexes may occur in atopic individuals (73).

EXPERIMENTAL ALLERGIC GLOMERULONEPHRITIS

Experimental glomerulonephritis may be induced by injection of animals with heterologous or homologous glomerular basement membrane extract in complete Freund's adjuvant (98). This injection results in the production of antibody to glomerular basement membrane. This antibody then localizes on the capillary side of the basement membrane and may be observed by immunofluorescence as a diffuse thin layer along the membrane (in contrast to the location and form of the toxic complex deposition described above). The reaction of this antibody with the basement membrane results in the binding of complement, polymorphonuclear leukocyte infiltration, and basement membrane destruction. A transient form of the experimental disease may be transferred with serum from an affected sheep injected into a normal sheep if the affected sheep is nephrectomized several days prior to transfer (66). Many attempts to transfer the disease with either cells or serum were without effect until nephrectomy was included. This step is necessary because the nephritogenic antibody is absorbed both in vivo and in vitro by the sheep glomerular tissue. Experimental allergic glomerulonephritis is an example of an autoallergic disease involving the toxic complex reaction.

NEPHROTOXIC SERUM (MASUGI) NEPHRITIS

Experimental glomerulonephritis may also be produced in animals by the injection of heterologous antisera to glomeruli (98). For example, if a rabbit is immunized with rat glomeruli, the passive transfer of this rabbit anti-rat-glomerulus serum to rats causes nephrotoxic serum nephritis. The nephritis observed following the injection of heterologous antisera to kidney consists of a biphasic response: 1) an acute transient proteinuria is observed in rats injected with rabbit antiserum to rat glomerulus as a result of the formation of complexes of rabbit antibodies and antigens present in rat glomerulus; 2) after 10 days to 2 weeks, a potentially fatal chronic proliferative glomerulonephritis may develop. This second lesion is caused by the production of host (rat) antibodies to donor (rabbit) γ-globulin. These rat antibodies react with the rabbit antiglomerular antibodies localized on the rat glomeruli, causing the second-phase lesions (98).

POSTSTREPTOCOCCAL GLOMERULONEPHRITIS

The occurrence of acute glomerulonephritis in humans may be associated with exposure to a few strains of group A β-hemolytic streptococci (98). Such streptococcal strains have been termed nephritogenic. There is a characteristic latent period following the onset of infection during which no significant renal symptoms are observed. The acute glomerulonephritis is characterized by the onset of proteinuria and hematuria. The occurrence of these alterations corresponds in time with the appearance of a host immune response to streptococcal antigens as evidenced by the appearance of circulating antibodies. Immunofluorescence examination of affected kidneys reveals a morphologic alteration similar to that of toxic complex glomerulonephritis (described above). Complement, γ-globulins and streptococcal antigens may be found bound to glomeruli. Although several immune mechanisms have been invoked to explain the pathogenesis of acute glomerulonephritis, the findings are most consistent with a toxic complex inflammatory reaction (112).

There are several observations worthy of further comment. One question has been why only certain strains of streptococci are nephritogenic. The answer is not known. It is possible to produce an acute experimental glomerulonephritis by infecting animals with nonnephritogenic organisms or even by injecting them with killed organisms, and acute glomerulonephritis may occur in humans with severe infections of various types. However, poststreptococcal glomerulonephritis, as the name implies, may occur after all other clinical evidence of infection is gone. It was once thought that certain streptococcal antigens, namely, streptococcal M protein, might have an unusual affinity for the glomerulus. If an appropriate antibody–antigen complex between streptococcal M protein and host antibody could be produced, this complex would be selectively bound to the glomerulus. The fixation to the glomerulus of this complex could be followed by the binding of complement and the attraction of polymorphonuclear leukocytes, leading to glomerular inflammation. The existence of such a glomerular-binding antigen has not been demonstrated. It is also possible that these nephritogenic streptococci have antigenic specificities that cross react with some human tissue antigens and that circulating antibody produced to these streptococcal antigens react with glomerular antigens (111). If this were the case, immunofluorescence examination would reveal linear lesions such as are seen in experimental allergic glomerulonephritis, rather than the lumpy-bumpy deposits which are usually found. In addition, convincing demonstration of such cross-reacting antigens is lacking.

ANTI-BASEMENT-MEMBRANE GLOMERULONEPHRITIS

There is evidence that direct anti-basement-membrane antibodies are responsible for some cases of human glomerulonephritis. The recurrence of glomerulonephritis in patients who have received transplants for renal failure caused by the disease demonstrates that recipients who have glomerulonephritis may produce an antibody that reacts with the glomeruli of the transplanted kidney. Immunofluorescence examination of such kidneys reveals immunoglobulin deposition in a linear pattern on the basement membrane. It has been postulated that the reaction to the original infectious agent (streptococcus, virus) has caused destruction and dissolution of the host basement membrane and that the host produces an antibody to this material that reacts with the remaining basement membrane. Potential basement membrane antigens are present in the circulation of normal individuals (98) and it is more likely that streptococcal or viral infections may provide an adjuvant function for such antigens. However, only 5–10% of patients with glomerulonephritis appear to develop such an autoantibody.

HYPOCOMPLEMENTEMIC GLOMERULONEPHRITIS

Nonimmune activation of complement via the alternate pathway may lead to deposition of complement in renal glomeruli and produce glomerulonephritis (107). Toxic complexes may initiate the deposition of complement but be undetectable when the complement components are still active (102). In either situation the deposits of complement components without detectable immunoglobulin is associated with lowering of the serum complement and is termed hypocomplementemic glomerulonephritis (107).

CLINICAL—IMMUNOPATHOLOGIC CORRELATIONS
IN GLOMERULONEPHRITIS

Glomerulonephritis may be caused by deposition of immune complexes formed elsewhere, by reaction of antibody directly with glomerular basement membrane antigens or by the activation of complement by the alternate pathway. Each of these mechanisms may produce an identical clinical picture or pathologic lesion (Fig. 13–2). Clinically glomerulonephritis is a syndrome with markedly variable expression; but the disease can be classified generally into acute, subacute and chronic (101). The acute disease may include gross hematuria, oliguria or anuria, edema, azotemia and death because of renal failure. However, recovery from the acute disease occurs in over 99% of the cases. Adults may develop a more per-

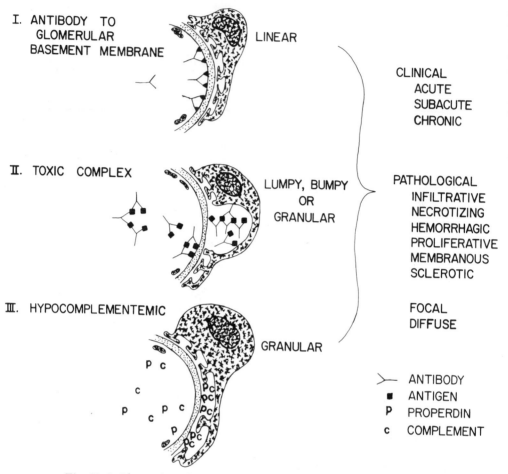

I. ANTIBODY TO
   GLOMERULAR
   BASEMENT MEMBRANE   LINEAR

                                        CLINICAL
                                          ACUTE
                                          SUBACUTE
                                          CHRONIC

II. TOXIC COMPLEX
                            LUMPY, BUMPY   PATHOLOGICAL
                                OR   INFILTRATIVE
                            GRANULAR   NECROTIZING
                                                HEMORRHAGIC
                                                PROLIFERATIVE
                                                MEMBRANOUS
                                                SCLEROTIC

III. HYPOCOMPLEMENTEMIC
                                                FOCAL
                                                DIFFUSE
                            GRANULAR

                                        >—   ANTIBODY
                                        ▪   ANTIGEN
                                        P   PROPERDIN
                                        c   COMPLEMENT

Fig. 13–2. Glomerulonephritis– clinical-pathologic correlations. The three pathologic mechanisms of glomerulonephritis illustrated may produce a varied clinical
and pathologic picture. No single mechanism produces a particular type of clinical
picture or pathologic lesion, although hypocomplementemic glomerulonephritis is
usually of the chronic variety. A capillary lumen, basement membrane endothelial
cell foot plates and an epithelial cell are illustrated. I) Antiglomerular basement
membrane antibody reacts with antigens on the lumen side of the glomerular
basement membrane and produces a linear deposition when examined by immunofluorescence. II) Toxic complexes found elsewhere pass through the glomerular
basement membrane and lodge on the epithelial side producing lumpy-bumpy
or granular deposits. III) Complement in the absence of immunoglobulin may
be detected as granular deposit. Hypocomplementemic glomerulonephritis may
be caused by a preceding immunoglobin deposit or by the action of properdin,
both of which may activate complement. (Modified from illustration of C. Wilson.
Scripps Clinic and Research Foundation, La Jolla, California)

sistent subacute or chronic progression and acute exacerbations, with proteinuria, hematuria and other evidence of renal failure. Pathologically, a
variety of lesions may be seen in the glomeruli. During the acute stage,
the lesions may be necrotic (death of glomerular cells), infiltrative or exu-
dative (glomeruli full of polymorphonuclear leukocytes), or hemorrhagic
(red blood cells in glomeruli). Subacute glomerulonephritis is associated
with proliferative (increased number of glomerular cells) or embolic (fibrin
thrombi in glomerular capillaries) lesions. Chronic glomerulonephritis features membranous (thickening of glomerular basement membrane), or
sclerotic (scarring of glomeruli) changes. Of course, intermediate stages
of the disease usually demonstrate an overlap of lesions.

Each of the above lesions may be produced by one of the three immunopathologic mechanisms. The pathologic type of lesion depends upon the
degree of injury produced in a given period of time and not upon the
immunopathologic mechanism. Thus the deposit of large amounts of
toxic immune complexes, or antibody to the basement membrane causing
acute complement activation, will lead to infiltration of the glomerulus
with a large number of polymorphonuclear leukocytes and extensive dissolution of the basement membrane. The dissolution permits proteins of
large molecular weight to pass through the basement membrane (detected
clinically as proteinuria). If large segments of the basement membrane
are destroyed, larger blood components such as erythrocytes will pass
through the basement membrane, producing hematuria. The loss of protein
leads to hypoproteinemia, decreased intravascular osmotic pressure, edema
and heart failure—the clinical picture of acute glomerulonephritis. The
deposit of small amounts of immune complex over long periods of time
produces a build-up on the basement membrane of undigested protein
leading to thickening of the basement membrane and a gradual loss of
the filtering capacity of the glomeruli (membranous glomerulonephritis)
which causes retention of nitrogen (azotemia) and gradual renal failure.
Thus the pathologist cannot identify the immunopathologic mechanism
responsible for a given case of glomerulonephritis by defining the histo-
pathologic lesion. Identification of the mechanism requires immunofluorescent studies, serologic work-up and careful clinical documentation
of the course of the disease (102).

GOODPASTURE'S DISEASE

The combination of pulmonary hemorrhage and glomerulonephritis
is known as Goodpasture's syndrome (7). In severe cases there is extensive
intraalveolar hemorrhage and marked proliferative glomerulonephritis.
Immunoglobulin and complement may be identified in the basement membranes of pulmonary alveoli and renal glomeruli. Antibody eluted from
the kidneys of such patients binds to lung tissue, and antibody eluted
from lung tissue binds to kidney, indicating the presence of cross-reacting
antigens in lung and kidney basement membranes (70). Antibody to lung
tissue induces pulmonary hemorrhage and glomerulonephritis when injected
into animals (26). Glomerulonephritis may be induced in animals by immunization with human lung tissue, and antibody eluted from involved
kidneys demonstrates strong binding to human lung and kidneys (88).

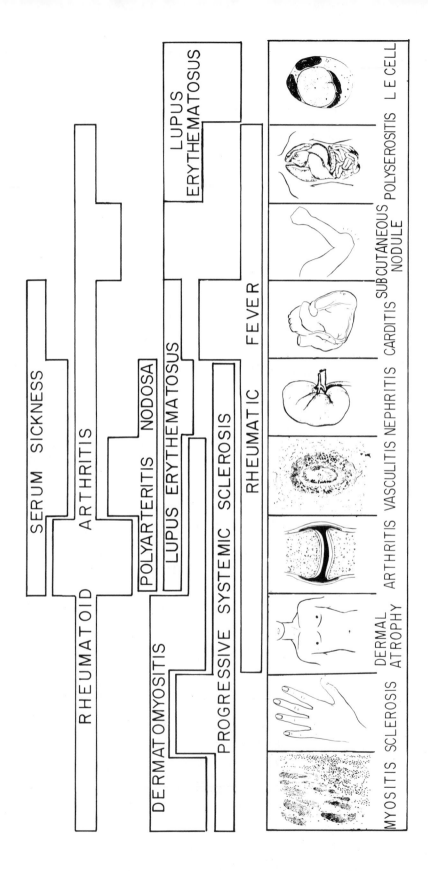

EXPERIMENTAL ALLERGIC INTERSTITIAL NEPHRITIS

Immune injury to renal tubules may be induced by immunization of experimental animals with whole kidney (57) or an antigen from the basement membrane of the renal tubule (65). The lesion begins as a polymorphonuclear infiltrate but progresses to a chronic mononuclear infiltrate with atrophy and degeneration of the tubules. Linear deposits of IgG may be detected along the basement membrane of the proximal tubules (65). Immune-mediated interstitial nephritis may occur in association with collagen diseases (56) or renal graft rejection in humans (109).

COLLAGEN DISEASES

A number of disorders are grouped together as collagen diseases because they have in common a morphologically similar lesion in connective tissue (58). The characteristic lesion is fibrinoid necrosis—an increase in ground substance with swollen, fragmented collagen fibers and necrosis, resulting in a structureless eosinophilic area resembling fibrin in appearance. The collagen diseases include polyarteritis nodosa, systemic lupus erythematosus (SLE), dermatomyositis, progressive systemic sclerosis (scleroderma), thrombotic thrombocytopenic purpura, rheumatic fever and rheumatoid arthritis. While there is no unequivocal evidence that allergic reactions cause all collagen diseases, most of the lesions observed may be explained by immune complex-mediated mechanisms. Toxic complexes are almost certainly responsible for most of the lesions of polyarteritis nodosa, rheumatoid arthritis and lupus erythematosis. The toxic complexes responsible for the latter two diseases are formed by autoantibodies to the patient's own tissues.

The collagen diseases vary markedly in their clinical features, time course, location of lesions, pathologic picture and immune findings. As depicted in Fig. 13–3, there is considerable overlap of pathologic features within the collagen disease group. The incidence of collagen diseases is increased in association with the autoallergic and granulomatous diseases discussed in Chapters 14 and 15. Many individuals with a collagen disease have angiitis or glomerulonephritis, immunoglobulin abnormalities, and autoantibodies with varied specificity of reactivity including falsely positive tests

---

Fig. 13–3. Pathologic features of collagen diseases.   The lesions associated with collagen diseases (bottom). Relative frequency with which each lesion is associated with each disease (top). Serum sickness is included because, although it is an iatrogenic disorder, it is an allergic reaction of the toxic complex type and its characteristic lesions (vasculitis, glomerulonephritis, myocarditis and arthritis) are associated with naturally occurring collagen diseases. This relation suggests a role for toxic complex reaction in collagen disease, but this reaction alone cannot explain all of the observed lesions. Tests for antinuclear antibodies have replaced the LE cell test in clinical practice.

for syphilis. Some of the protean manifestations of syphilis, which are not unlike many of the features of the collagen diseases, may be the result of autoallergic reactions caused by alteration of host tissue or allergic reactions to the infecting organisms located in host tissue. Similarly, the lesions seen in the collagen diseases may result from allergic reactions to as yet undetected infectious agents (?L-forms, viruses, episomes).

The inconsistent clinical and pathologic features of the collagen diseases may be the result of the operation of different types of allergic reactions with different degrees of severity at different times, directed toward different antigenic specificities with different tissue locations. The interplay of these variables could produce varying clinical pictures during the course of a disease in a given individual. It is within the scope of this text to cover only some of the clinical and pathologic features of these diseases. For further information the reader is referred to the standard textbooks of medicine and pathology.

NZB MICE

Before consideration of the human collagen diseases, a discussion of the immunopathology of NZB mice is warrented. New Zealand black (NZB) and NZB/NZW F_1 hybrid mice have been studied extensively from an immunologic standpoint because they spontaneously develop lesions similar to human collagen diseases, in particular, lupus erythematosis (53). The NZB inbred mouse strain was developed by Marianne Bielchowsky in New Zealand in the 1950s for cancer research (9). These mice were found to respond quite differently from other mouse strains. After immunization with a variety of exogenous antigens, NZB mice produce abnormally high humoral antibody responses but less intense, delayed (cellular) hypersensitivity (15,92). These mice spontaneously develop a number of immunopathologic abnormalities including a Coombs' positive hemolytic anemia, LE and rheumatoid-like factors, hypergammaglobulinemia and glomerulonephritis (53). The thymi of NZB mice develop germinal centers with aging (12); germinal centers are not normally found in the thymus, but sometimes occur in humans with myasthenia gravis (page 135). The development of these immunologic abnormalities occurs after about 4–6 months of age; young mice do not have immune abnormalities and female mice develop more severe abnormalities than male mice at an earlier age (53). Neonatal thymectomy causes the immune abnormalities to appear earlier and in a more severe form (29). Repeated grafting of young syngeneic thymi to growing NZB mice delays the appearance of the immune abnormalities (62). With aging, the peripheral lymphoid tissues of NZB mice are depleted of thymus-derived (T) cells more rapidly than the organs of other mouse strains (89,105). An antibody that is cytotoxic for T cells appears early in life and may contribute to the loss of T cell function (85). It is postulated that NZB mice demonstrate a genetic abnormality of lymphoid cell control; suppressor T cell activity becomes depleted with aging, leading to uncontrolled responses by humoral antibody-forming B cells (93). Further evidence for loss of control lymphoid cell proliferation is the development of lymphoid cell tumors and hypergammaglobulinemia in NZB mice. The high incidence of lymphoid cell proliferative disease and monoclonal hypergammaglobulinemia suggests an uncontrolled growth of B cells leading to immunoglobulin-producing tumors (90).

In the absence of T cell suppressor control, an abnormal antibody response to a chronic viral infection is the most likely explanation for the immune-mediated abnormalities in NZB mice. A viruslike agent was identified in the tissues of NZB mice and the inoculation of cell-free filtrates from the tissues of NZB mice with severe lesions can induce renal and hemolytic disease in mice of an unrelated strain (71). Either a chronic virus infection causes antigenic alteration of normal tissue and autosensitization or antibody-viral-antigen complexes produce toxic complex lesions. The lupuslike lesions of NZB mice are increased in NZB mice that are experimentally infected at birth with viruses (96). The glomerular lesions are consistent with immune complex deposition and antinucleic acid antibody (probably directed to viral antigens) has been found in affected glomeruli (63). However, the incidence and severity of the Coomb's positive hemolytic anemia is not affected by chronic viral infection (96). Therefore humoral antibody to both viral and self antigens may play an immunopathogenic role in the lesions of NZB mice. These mechanisms for lesion production are suspected to be operative in many of the collagen diseases of man.

POLYARTERITIS NODOSA

This disease consists of multiple foci of localized infarcts affecting almost any organ or combination of organs in the body (2,61,80). Inflammation of small arteries results in thrombosis and obstruction to blood flow, leading to many small areas of necrosis and scarring (69). The arterial lesion is similar to that seen in serum sickness arteritis, and γ-globulin may be identified in the areas of fibrinoid necrosis (80). The role of this γ-globulin in the production of the lesion is unclear (2,27). The γ-globulin may be antibody which is reacting with antigen that is part of the vessel wall; it may be part of an antigen–antibody precipitate formed elsewhere in the circulation and deposited in the vessel wall, or the γ-globulin may be nonspecifically absorbed to an arterial lesion evoked by an unrelated mechanism. Acute glomerulonephritis similar to that observed after streptococcal infections may be found associated with polyarteritis nodosa. The glomeruli in such cases also contain γ-globulin.

Complexes of viruses and immunoglobulin probably cause half of the cases of polyarteritis nodosa (99). A substantial number of patients with polyarteritis nodosa also have Hepatitis B antigenemia (42), suggesting that polyarteritis occurring naturally may be due to an immune response to viral hepatitis infection with HB antigen release (see page 243). The association of polyarteritis with drug administration also suggests that some cases of polyarteritis may be caused by an immune response to drugs administered for therapy of other diseases.

Only about half of the cases of histologically proven polyarteritis nodosa survive over five years. Early and vigorous treatment with corticosteroids significantly improves the prognosis, but it is only partially effective and long term therapy is required to suppress symptoms or prevent exacerbations (36).

SYSTEMIC LUPUS ERYTHEMATOSUS

Systemic lupus erythematosus (SLE) is a complex syndrome caused by autoantibodies produced to a wide variety of the patient's own cellular antigens–particularly nuclear antigens (59,87,91). This disease appears most frequently in women of childbearing age and characteristically involves many different tissues. The fatal form is a rapidly advancing systemic disease featuring high fever, skin rash, nephritis, polyarthritis, polyserositis (pleural, pericardial, and peritoneal effusions), and central nervous system symptoms. With recent diagnostic techniques (mainly tests for antinuclear antibodies), milder forms of SLE have been recognized which may include only a remitting myalgia and malaise. Degrees of severity between these extremes are common, and the clinical course usually is characterized by spontaneous remissions and exacerbations. The diagnosis and classification of SLE in a given patient is based on the results of a series of clinical findings and laboratory tests (23).

The pathologic changes of SLE include 1) a membranous glomerulonephritis which may result in formation of so called wire-loops, hyaline thrombosis and hematoxylin bodies; 2) a periarteriolar fibrosis in the spleen; 3) a scattered focal thickening, necrosis and fibrosis of medium-sized arterioles in many different organs; and 4) a patchy atrophy of the epidermis and collagen degeneration of the dermis, both of which occur more frequently in areas of the skin exposed to sunlight.

A principle diagnostic finding has been the presence of the LE cell, a polymorphonuclear neutrophil which has phagocytized nuclear material (49). Its formation depends upon the presence of an antibody capable of reacting with DNA. When peripheral blood from a patient with SLE is incubated in vitro, this antibody presumably reacts with the nuclei of lymphocytes (60). The swollen nuclear material is then phagocytized by polymorphonuclear neutrophils in the peripheral blood, and LE cells are formed (Fig. 13–4).

A variety of antinuclear antibodies has been identified in the sera of patients with SLE, and identification of these has largely replaced the LE cell test in the clinical laboratory. These include anti-DNA, antinucleoprotein, antihistones, antiacidic nuclear proteins, antinucleolar RNA and antibodies to fibrous or particulate nucleoprotein (94). Of particular interest is the type of immunofluorescent staining pattern observed when serum from a patient with SLE is allowed to bind to tissue nuclei and the localization of the bound immunoglobulin is determined by addition of fluorescent-labeled antibody to immunoglobulin [indirect fluorescent antibody test] (68,94). Four major patterns are seen: nuclear rim (anti-DNA or antinucleoprotein), speckled (antiacidic nuclear proteins), nucleolar (antinucleolar RNA), and diffuse (not antigenically specific). The clinical significance of these different staining patterns is not yet fully understood, as specific staining patterns are not clearly diagnostic of a given disease (Table 13–1).

Patients with SLE may have a number of serologic abnormalities in addition to the antibodies responsible for the formation of the LE cell. These include a positive reaction to the Coombs' test (antibody to red blood cells), antibodies to blood clotting factors, a falsely positive reaction

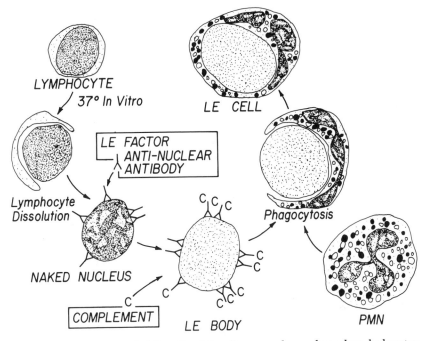

LYMPHOCYTE
37° In Vitro
LE CELL
LE FACTOR
ANTI-NUCLEAR
ANTIBODY
Lymphocyte
Dissolution
Phagocytosis
NAKED NUCLEUS
COMPLEMENT
LE BODY
PMN

Fig. 13–4. Formation of LE cell. LE cells are polymorphonuclear leukocytes that have phagocytized the nuclei of lymphocytes due to coating of the nuclei with antibody. This takes place at 37°C upon incubation of the whole blood of a patient with SLE who has antibody to DNA or other nuclear antigens. Lymphocytes break up and lymphocyte nuclei become coated with antibody (LE factor), swell and are phagocytized by polymorphonuclear leukocytes.

to the Wassermann test and antibodies to cytoplasmic antigenic components (60). These antibodies are most likely responsible for most of the SLE lesions. The lesions are pathologically consistent with the toxic complex mechanism. The membranous glomerulonephritis of SLE may contain deposits of immunoglobulin and DNA (59); both granular and linear deposits of Ig have been observed. Immunoglobulin and complement may also be

TABLE 13–1
Nuclear Staining Patterns Observed In Patients with SLE

Staining pattern	Disease association	Specificities of antibody
Rim	SLE	DNA or nucleoprotein
Speckled	SLE; scleroderma; other connective tissue diseases	Ribonucleoprotein
Nucleolar	Scleroderma; Sjögren's syndrome	4–6S RNA
Diffuse	SLE; Sjögren's syndrome; rheumatoid arthritis	Nucleoprotein; unknown

detected in the vascular lesions of the spleen and other organs, in the basement membrane of the skin (76) and in the choroid plexis of the brain (64). (The latter may explain the predominance of CNS symptoms even in the absence of significant vasculitis.) Immunoglobulin deposits may be found along the basement of grossly normal appearing skin (positive lupus band test) and is associated with a high incidence of renal disease (38).

The etiology of naturally occurring SLE remains unsolved, but two major theories are offered:

1. SLE is a virus-induced disease. Antibodies to viral antigen (74,99) and intracellular tubular inclusions consistent with viral particles are frequently found in patients with SLE (72,83). Although a specific virus responsible for SLE has not been identified, a virus infection could account for some cases of SLE.
2. There is an imbalance of humoral and cellular immunity similar to that described for NZB mice (see above). This leads to abnormal antibody formation to a variety of antigens, including host molecules, as well as formation of toxic complexes or autoantibodies, and LE syndrome (99).

The most acceptable explanation at the present time is a combination of the above, i.e., an abnormal humoral antibody response to a chronic viral infection (92) and significant autoantibody formation.

In recent years the features of SLE have appeared in patients receiving certain drugs (87). The important difference between this disorder and naturally occurring SLE is that the drug-induced symptoms generally disappear upon discontinuation of the drugs. The drugs incriminated include diphenylhydantoin, isoniazid, hydralazine, and procainamide—used for the treatment of epilepsy, tuberculosis, hypertension, and cardiac arrythmias, respectively. Other drugs produce LE-like syndromes less frequently (10).

The mechanisms of induction of LE-like syndromes are not yet fully understood. Possible mechanisms include 1) formation of toxic complexes of antibody and drug, 2) production of autoimmunogens by binding of drug to host molecules as a hapten, and 3) alteration of host cell surfaces or nucleoprotein by chemical action of drug-producing immunogenic denatured host molecules. Patients with hydralizine-induced LE may have antibodies to hydralizine as well as antibodies to native DNA (48). In contrast, procainamide induces antibodies to denatured DNA presumably due to complexes of the drug and host DNA; antibodies to native DNA or to procainamide alone are not produced (11). Procainamide acts by stabilization of cell membranes. It may bind to erythrocyte surfaces, alter red cell membrane and produce immunogenic membrane fragments that lead to autoantibody formation and a Coombs' positive hemolytic anemia (10). Hydralizine and isoniazid may form active radicals which inactivate and alter DNA (35), producing immunogenic DNA fragments. Thus the induction of autoantibodies or formation of drug–antibody toxic complexes results in drug-induced LE-like syndromes; different drugs may act by different mechanisms.

Treatment of SLE is generally designed to reduce both the inflammatory reaction of the disease and the amount of pathogenic antibodies (50). Two agents are used for life-threatening episodes: corticosteroids and immunosuppressive drugs (aziothioprine), and in some cases a combination of the two (28). Corticosteroids suppress acute exacerbations of SLE and prolong life (50). Since the severe acute episodes are potentially fatal, physicians have been unwilling to withhold treatment of an affected individual; therefore, no well controlled double-blind study has been done. Nevertheless it is clear that steroid therapy not only prolongs the lives of patients with SLE but also significantly changes the character of the syndrome. Prior to steroid therapy, patients frequently died of an acute crisis; now the disease is more protracted, and chronic renal or neurologic problems cause death (17). Lower doses of steroids and antiinflammatory drugs may control symptoms in patients with less severe disease. Effective therapy reduces the acute symptoms (fever, joint pain, etc.) and reverses the immunologic abnormalities. The intensity of therapy depends upon the severity of the disease and the degree of response, which may vary considerably from patient to patient. Complications of intensive therapy must be controlled, the major effect being reduction of the production of blood cells (agranulocytosis) and decrement in defensive reactions resulting in susceptibility to a variety of infections (see Secondary Immune Deficiencies, page 313). Although the present therapy considerably improves the prognosis and condition of patients with SLE, it is far from satisfactory. Over 50% of those with renal or neurologic involvement die within 10 years of the onset of symptoms.

DERMATOMYOSITIS

Symptoms of this disease complex include an erythematous skin rash, mild arthritis and progressive muscular weakness, each of which may occur with a different degree of severity. The primary lesion is in muscle and consists of a degeneration of muscle fibers associated with a varying degree of infiltration of mononuclear cells (1). Many patients have polymyositis—inflammatory lesions in the muscle—without a skin rash. The causes of the disease are quite varied and several clinical subdivisions have been suggested. The characteristic symptom is muscle weakness of insidious onset. The incidence of dermatomyositis is increased in association with malignant tumors, the lymphoproliferative syndromes, and certain autoallergic diseases. Females are affected twice as commonly as males. The diagnosis is most often confirmed by muscle biopsy, and the activity of the disease process may be followed by detection of enzymes released from affected muscle tissue. An experimental disease, experimental allergic myositis, may be produced in animals by immunization with xenogeneic muscle tissue in complete Freund's adjuvant (25). This experimental disease is more like a delayed hypersensitivity reaction than an antibody-mediated inflammation. The inflammatory lesions in the muscles of patients with myositis are also more consistent with a delayed hypersensitivity reaction, and are similar to those of myasthenia gravis (51). This suggests that more than one type of allergic reaction may be responsible for the disease of dermatomyositis. The disease frequently has remissions and exacerbations, but the natural course is progressive. Corticosteroid therapy may provide effective relief, but death from progressive muscular weakness producing respiratory failure usually occurs when the patient becomes refractory to therapy. Immunosuppressive drugs have been reported to induce remissions in some steroid-resistant cases (47).

PROGRESSIVE SYSTEMIC SCLEROSIS (SCLERODERMA)

This degenerative disease, primarily involving the skin, is characterized by fibrotic thickening (sclerosis) of connective tissue in association with mild to moderate mononuclear cell infiltration (97). Scleroderma refers to scarring of the skin, the only lesion in some cases; but systemic involvement of synovia, gastrointestinal tract, kidneys, heart, and lungs may occur and lead to maladsorption, cardiac or renal failure. Females are affected approximately twice as frequently as males. Skin thickening is usually first noted on the fingers, then on the upper extremities and upper torso. The skin loses its flexibility and becomes taut and shiny. The dermis of the skin or the muscular wall of the gastrointestinal tract is replaced with compact bundles of collagen. Inability to move fingers and difficulty in swallowing may be prominent symptoms. Arthralgia is usually present. Joint lesions show focal collections of chronic inflammatory cells; the appearance may essentially be identical to that of early rheumatoid arthritis or may take the form of thickening of collagen. Renal failure and hypertension may occur. The kidneys have concentric thickening of small renal arteries, and sometimes fibrinoid necroses of the arterial wall (32), and a membranous glomerulonephritis. The course of the disease may be rapidly progressive or slowly evolving over a number of years. A variety of serologic abnormalities occur including the presence of LE factors, antinuclear antibodies, rheumatoid factors and a variety of other autoantibodies (81). No satisfactory treatment is known. For more details on progressive systemic sclerosis, see references 79 and 110.

THROMBOTIC THROMBOCYTOPENIA PURPURA

This syndrome consists of thrombocytopenia (decreased number of blood platelets), hemolytic anemia, and hemorrhagic skin lesions [purpura] (4). Autopsy reveals widespread thrombotic occlusion of arterioles and capillaries by hyaline masses that are usually located beneath the endothelium. Central nervous system symptoms may occur, presumably due to microvascular occlusions. The anemia is microangiopathic—secondary to mechanical destruction of erythrocytes by physical trauma of contact with the altered vascular walls. The etiology of the vascular lesions is unknown, but they may be caused by a form of toxic complex or autoantibody deposits leading to focal fibrinoid necroses and hyaline scarring, or by activation of the clotting mechanism by toxic complexes.

RHEUMATIC FEVER

Rheumatic fever is an acute systemic disease that includes inflammation of the heart (carditis), joints (polyarthritis), involuntary movements of muscles (chorea, St. Vitus' dance), inflammation of the skin (erythema marginatum) and the development of subcutaneous nodules. These findings occur in a variety of combinations that together are evaluated to permit the diagnosis of rheumatic fever (31).

Rheumatic fever occurs as an inconsistent sequel to group A streptococcal infections. There is a cross-reacting antigenic specificity between certain streptococcal proteins and cardiac muscle (111). Antibodies with this cross-reacting specificity appear in the sera of patients with rheumatic fever. It is possible that these antibodies react with heart tissue and are responsible for the production of lesions.

The cardiac lesion consists of a focus of fibrinoid necrosis, usually in perivascular areas in the myocardium (46). These areas of fibrinoid necrosis contain variable numbers of mononuclear inflammatory cells and peculiar oval cells with striated nuclei (Anitschkow's myocytes) that appear to arise from the inflamed myocardium (46). The composite of fibrinoid necrosis and cellular reaction has a characteristic microscopic appearance and is called an Aschoff body. The affected areas evolve into thick fibrous tissue so that old Aschoff bodies appear as focal perivascular scars. The endocarditis may be extensive, with formation of Aschoff bodies in the valve leaflets. This leads to vascularization, fibrosis, fusion and distortion of the valve leaflets. Loss of function of affected heart valves may lead to chronic cardiac failure, with the type of failure depending upon the cardiac valve involved. Variable degrees of polyarthritis, vasculitis and glomerulonephritis may be associated with rheumatic carditis, and subcutaneous nodules histologically identical to those seen in rheumatoid arthritis may occur. Erythema marginatum, a red, flat topped lesion with a pale center is a skin manifestation of the vasculitis associated with rheumatic fever.

The natural course of rheumatic fever is now understood fairly well and has been changed by recognition of the relationship of a preceding group A streptococcal infection and development of the disease (31). Refinement of the diagnosis of streptococcal infection and prompt introduction of measures to eliminate the infection, usually by intensive therapy with penicillin, significantly reduces the occurence of cardiac sequelae (43). The most important prognostic finding is evidence of carditis during an acute attack of rheumatic fever. If carditis is present, subsequent development of significant disease is likely; if carditis is not present, then development of rheumatic heart disease, even if subsequent attacks of rheumatic fever occur, is unlikely.

RHEUMATOID ARTHRITIS

Rheumatoid arthritis is a syndrome in which inflammation of the joints caused by autoantibodies is the major feature.

The precise diagnosis of mild rheumatoid arthritis is difficult, as evidenced by the arbitrary criteria established by a Committee of the American Rheumatism Association for classic, definite, and possible rheumatoid arthritis (3). The most common symptoms include a symmetric arthritis usually involving the knee joints or the small joints of the hands (86). The arthritis is the result of an inflammatory synovitis which begins as a chronic inflammatory infiltration but usually proceeds to destructive granulomatous inflammation (pannus) eroding the articular surface. The synovia becomes hyperplastic and filled with lymphocytes and plasma cells.

Muscle wasting and the formation of subcutaneous nodules are found in about 20% of rheumatoid patients. The subcutaneous nodules consist of a stellate center of fibrinoid necrosis surrounded by a palisade of mononuclear cells and a variable amount of fibrous tissue. Serositis, myocarditis, vasculitis and peripheral neuropathy may also be found.

One of the features of rheumatoid arthritis is rheumatoid factor—a circulating antibody with reactivity to certain components of immunoglobulins (6). The specificity of its reaction is variable. Three general reactive specificities are recognized: 1) to xenogeneic immunoglobulins (rabbit, horse), 2) to allogeneic immunoglobulins (denatured human IgG), or 3) to autologous immunoglobulins (the patient's own IgG). Rheumatoid factor usually is an IgM (19S) antibody which reacts with one or more of the above antigens, although 7S rheumatoid factors have been described. The formation of rheumatoid factor is the result of an immune reaction by the host to one or more specific antigenic determinants present in his own γ-globulins (6). Rheumatoid factor is usually detected by agglutination of particles (erythrocytes, latex) coated with γ-globulins; it also reacts with antigen–antibody complexes. Investigations of its reactive specificities have suggested that rheumatoid factor reacts with antigenic groupings of IgG that are usually buried in the native molecule. These antigenic specificities may be revealed by unfolding of the IgG molecule due to various denaturing processes or to the reaction of IgG antibody with antigen. The presence of 22S complexes of 19S rheumatoid factor and 7S IgG in the sera of patients indicates that reaction of rheumatoid factor with IgG occurs in vivo. Such a reaction may be responsible for some of the toxic complex lesions associated with rheumatoid arthritis (vasculitis, glomerulonephritis). Necrotizing arthritis is especially likely to evolve in patients with high titers of rheumatoid factor.

In most cases rheumatoid factor (anti-IgG) forms large soluble complexes with IgG in vivo. These complexes appear to be cleared from the circulation with no further tissue damage by the reticuloendothelial system. In rare cases the rheumatoid factor–immunoglobulin complexes are soluble at body temperature but can be precipitated from the patient's serum by cooling (cryoglobulins) (45). Patients with cryoglobulins are more apt to develop secondary lesions (vasculitis), presumably due to the presence in vivo of soluble circulating complexes. Some cryoimmunoglobulins are not immune complexes but abnormal Igs found in the sera of patients with collagen diseases and patients with lymphoproliferative disorders. These "monoclonal" cryoimmunoglobulins do not cause the significant vascular and glomerular lesions found with the immune complex (mixed) cryoimmunoglobulins (99).

The relation of rheumatoid factor in serum to the arthritis remains obscure. Pertinent findings are that 1) rheumatoid factor is found in some normal individuals, 2) rheumatoid arthritis may occur in agammaglobulinemic individuals, 3) the infusion (transfer) of large amounts of rheumatoid factor to a normal individual causes no noticeable lesions, and 4) there is an increased incidence of rheumatoid factor in relatives of patients with rheumatoid arthritis. However, the serum levels of rheumatoid factor do correlate well with the appearance of subcutaneous nodules, the presence of deforming arthritis and the incidence of systemic disease. It is possible that rheumatoid factor represents antibodies to antigen–antibody complexes found in vivo during the course of the disease (37). Rheumatoid factor may also react with genetically controlled isoantigens (allotypes) located on immunoglobulins (see Chapter 5).

Although most of the serologic findings do not support an etiologic role for rheumatoid factor in the pathogenesis of rheumatoid arthritis, observations on synovial fluid (the fluid of the articular cavity) support a toxic complex autoallergic mechanism for the inflammation of rheumatoid arthritis (113–115). The synovial fluid aspirated from patients with active rheumatoid arthritis may contain demonstrable immune complexes and the polymorphonuclear leukocytes in such fluids have complexes of rheumatoid factor and IgG in their cytoplasm. There is also a selective lowering of complement components in the synovial fluid during attacks of rheumatoid arthritis. It is postulated that an as yet unidentified antigen (infectious agent, host autoantigen) present in the joint cavity stimulates the production of an antibody (Fig. 13–5). Antigen–antibody complexes are formed which produce an alteration in the tertiary structure of the antibody revealing new or buried antigenic determinants. These determinants in turn stimulate the production of another antibody, rheumatoid factor, (usually IgM) which can react with IgG in the absence of the original antigen. IgM–IgG complexes form in the synovial fluid which activate complement components which attract polymorphonuclear leukocytes. A proliferation of lymphocytes and plasma cells in the synovial lining tissue converts the synovium into a lymphoid organ which produces rheumatoid factor that is released into the synovial fluid (114). Through this process a chronic cycle of arthritis is produced. Hyperplasia of granulation tissue and inflammatory cells occurs and extends as a mass (pannus) over the articular cartilage, which is destroyed by the action of polymorphonuclear leukocyte enzymes. This pannus produces a scar in the joint which may eventually lead to complete immobilization of the joint (113). Polymorphonuclear leukocytes containing phagocytized immune complexes may be demonstrated in the synovial fluid. The synthesis of complement components by synovial inflammatory tissue may also contribute to the severity of the arthritis (82).

The clinical cause of rheumatoid arthritis is quite variable (86); rapid progression to severe disability or a prolonged benign course with little or no joint deformity. Spontaneous remissions and exacerbations occur frequently and make evaluation of therapy difficult. Rheumatoid arthritis does not usually shorten life, but can lead to total disability in about 10% of the cases. Inflammation of the heart, great vessels and lung (diffuse interstitial pulmonary fibrosis) is infrequent but may occur and is believed to be part of the rheumatoid process.

Therapy is directed toward controlling pain with mild drugs and preventing severe deformities by active physical therapy or orthopedic surgery. Corticosteroids may provide temporary relief of pain but do not control the disease. Salicylates have a beneficial effect and along with low doses of steroids are the drugs of choice in most cases (34). The complications of long-term high dose steroid therapy outweight therapeutic advantages.

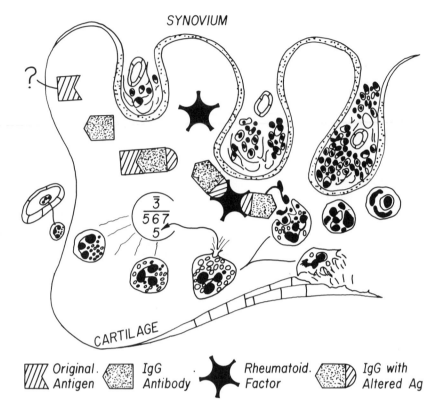

Original. Antigen   IgG Antibody   Rheumatoid. Factor   IgG with Altered Ag

Fig. 13–5. Pathogenesis of rheumatoid arthritis. The activation of complement by immune complexes of rheumatoid factors and host immunoglobulin leading to the attraction of polymorphonuclear leukocytes which release lysosomal enzymes that in turn cause destruction of articular cartilage is believed to be the primary pathogenic mechanism (see text and reference 115).

SKIN DISEASES

A variety of skin lesions are believed to be caused by allergic reactions, primarily antibody-mediated immunopathologic reactions. This includes erythema margination, discussed under rheumatic fever and the skin lesion of SLE, as well as erythema nodosum, pemphigus and pemphigoid, and erythema multiforme. Some of these, such as pemphigus, pemphigoid and SLE lesions, may be due to action of antibody directly upon the target cells while others, such as erythema nodosum and erythema multiforme require the mediation of inflammatory cells for full expression.

ERYTHEMA NODOSUM

The lesions of erythema nodosum are painful red nodules that appear bilaterally on the shins (30). The lesions occur predominately in women in the fall and winter months. Their appearance is usually associated with an infection, a collagen disease or a reaction to a drug. The major pathologic finding is a subcutaneous vasculitis featuring a polymorphonuclear infiltrate of small veins or arterioles. It is generally believed that erythema nodosum is caused by a toxic complex allergic reaction. The skin reactions usually fade and do not require treatment.

PEMPHIGUS AND PEMPHIGOID

Pemphigus and pemphigoid are skin lesions caused by denudation of the epidermis. In pemphigus the epidermis separates above the basal layer resulting in either formation of large fluid filled spaces (pemphigus vulgaris) or stripping of the upper (horny and granular) layers of epidermis (pemphigus foliaceus). In pemphigoid, separation occurs between the basal layer of the epidermis and the dermis, leading to the formation of subepi-dermal bullae. Antibodies to intracellular substances specific to the stratified epithelium are found in the sera of patients with pemphigus; in contrast, antibodies to the subepidermal basement membrane are found in patients with pemphigoid (8). Thus pemphigus antibodies attack the epithelial cells in the stratified layers leading to their separation from each other, cell death and bullae formation, while pemphigoid antibodies attack the basement membrane separating the epidermis from the dermis and produc-ing subepidermal bullae. Evidence that antiepithelial autoantibodies cause the lesions includes: 1) the patient's own immuno–globulin binds to his skin cells, 2) both IgG and complement are demonstrable in the lesions, 3) the site of the lesion, intraepithelial or subepithelial, is directly related to the site of Ig binding in pemphigus and pemphigoid (8). Several clinical courses are recognized, from rapidly fatal to relatively benign. Corticoster-oid and immunosuppressive therapy are highly efficacious in severe cases. Successful therapy not only reverses the skin lesions but also causes a reduction in the titer of autoantibodies (16).

ERYTHEMA MULTIFORME

Erythema multiforme may vary from a mild skin eruption consisting of erythematous or edematous flat lesions to widespread eruptions with bullous formation and extensive sloughing of the surface of the skin, in-volvement of internal organs with mucous membranes and rapid progression to death (Stevens-Johnson syndrome) (18). The skin lesions consist of large circular macules or papules with a central blue depression and an elevated red periphery. The variety of types of lesions is reflected in the term erythema multiforme. Vesicles and bullae may occur and new crops of lesions may appear in the center of fading plaques, resulting in a target-like appearance. These eruptions usually resolve in a few weeks but a mortality rate of up to 20% occurs with the more severe form of the disease (33). Lesions begin in the dermal vessels with an extensive lymphocytic infiltrate; edema fluid accumulates, leading to formation of a cavity of fluid and inflammatory cells lying between the dermis and epidermis, i.e., a subepidermal bullae. The occurrence of the disease is associated with infections and the use of certain drugs. Evidence of an allergic reaction includes: 1) a latency period of 10–21 days between initial exposure to a drug and development of the disease; 2) the lesions may appear in a few hours on second exposure to the drug; 3) recurrence of the disease consistently occurs after subsequent exposure to the offending drug (95); 4) the changes in the small blood vessels are consistent with an allergic vasculitis (1); and 5) skin tests with a suspected antigen have elicited the cutaneous lesion (14,84). No circulating autoantibodies to epidermal or dermal antigens have been demonstrated and Ig and complement are not present in the lesions. Therefore, it is suspected that erythema multiforme is a type of allergic skin reaction, perhaps a toxic complex reaction, but the mechanism of production of this disease is still unclear. Severe cases are benefited by corticosteroid treatment.

AMYLOIDOSIS

Amyloidosis is a disease in which there is an extracellular deposition of a hyalin, microscopically amporphorus, material which stains with dyes such as congo red that usually stain only linear polysaccharides—hence the name amyloid [starch-like] (77). It is now known to be a hydrophilic proteinateous substance containing numerous fibrils (22). Its protein content is heterogeneous (13); both fibril and plasma protein components are present. Although the lesion of amyloidosis is different from those of the collagen diseases listed above, amyloidosis is included here because it may be found associated with collagen diseases. The etiology of amyloidosis is unknown.

The deposition of amyloid is found in a variety of forms (22): 1) primary familial, 2) primary sporadic, 3) secondary, 4) localized, 5) senile, and 6) associated with multiple myeloma.

1. Primary familial amyloidosis is characterized by its appearance in families, but the clinical manifestations depend upon the organ mainly involved.

2. Primary sporadic amyloidosis is the most common form of amyloidosis. It appears in individuals with no familial tendency. Infiltrations of amyloid are usually located around small blood vessels and are found in the heart, kidney, spleen, liver, tongue, gastrointestinal tract and other organs.

3. Secondary amyloid occurs in association with a prolonged inflammatory disease (such as tuberculosis or rheumatoid arthritis). Deposits are found in many organs but most often in kidney, liver and spleen. Separation of primary and secondary on the basis of the organs involved (i.e., primary: heart and tongue; secondary: liver, spleen and kidney) no longer appears to be valid.

4. Localized amyloid may be seen in tumor-like masses, primarily in the upper respiratory tract and frequently in association with neoplastic masses.

5. Senile amyloid deposits are frequently ($\sim$30%) seen in the hearts of individuals over sixty years of age. No apparent clinical manifestations result.

6. Amyloidosis may be found in 10–20% of patients with plasma cell

neoplasia (multiple myeloma), suggesting a relationship to increased γ-globulin production.

The symptoms observed in patients with amyloidosis depend upon the organ involved. Enlargement of the spleen and liver is frequent. Cardiac or renal failure may occur and localized neurologic symptoms may be found as amyloid deposition impinges upon nerve fibers. Until recently the diagnosis of amyloidosis was infrequently made prior to death, but now the diagnosis may be apparent upon microscopic examination of tongue biopses.

The origin of amyloid remains obscure. At least two chemically distinct classes of amyloid fibrils have been demonstrated (41). One of these is a component of the immunoglobulin light chain. It is found in primary amyloidosis and amyloid associated with multiple myeloma (40). Amyloid depositions contain immunoglobulin when stained by specific fluorescent-labeled antibody (100), and amino acid sequence analysis indicate an homology between amyloid fibril proteins and immunoglobulin light chains (40). The other type of fibril is also seen in familial amyloidosis and in secondary amyloidosis (75). This second fibril has a unique amino acid composition and antigenic specificity not related to any known protein (67). The immunoglobulin form of amyloid is associated with increased immunoglobulin production (multiple myeloma). The presence of immunoglobulin in amyloid depositions and its relationship to immunoglobulin light chains has suggested that amyloid deposition results from increased synthesis or decreased catabolism of immunoglobulin in the affected tissue sites. Fiber structures similar to amyloid may be formed from immunoglobulin light chains (Bence-Jones proteins) by protolytic digestion under physiologic conditions (39). Therefore these amyloid depositions may represent incompletely catabolized immunoglobulins. Early investigators suggested that antibody–antigen complexes might contribute to amyloid, particularly in secondary amyloidosis. Although this hypothesis remains unproven, it is consistent with the recent observations listed above, but is an unlikely explanation for those amyloid depositions that do not have homology with immunoglobulins (67).

An experimental amyloidosis may be produced in mice by repeated injections of endotoxin (108), casein (54) or bacterial products (52) that stimulate the reticuloendothelial system. However, passive infusions of serum from a donor mouse with hypergammaglobulinemia does not cause amyloidosis in the recipient mouse (54). Therefore, hyperglobulinemia alone is not sufficient for amyloid deposition. On the other hand, the passive transfer of cells, cell products or serum from mice with experimental amyloidosis may cause amyloid deposition in recipient mice associated with the reticuloendothelial cells of the recipient (55). How this is accomplished in the recipient animal is not known.

REFERENCES

1. Adams RD, Denny-Brown D, Pearson CM: Diseases of the Muscle: A Study in Pathology. 2nd ed. New York, Harper & Row, 1962
2. Alarcon-Segovia D, Brown AL: Classification and etiologic aspects of necrotizing

204 IMMUNOPATHOLOGY

angiitides: An analytical approach to a confused subject with a critical review of the evidence for hypersensitivity in polyarteritis nodosa. Mayo Clin Proc 39:205, 1964

3. American Rheumatism Association: On criteria for rheumatoid arthritis: Review of the rheumatic diseases. JAMA 171:1213, 1959
4. Antes EH: Thrombotic thrombocytopenic purpura: A review of the literature with a report of a case. Ann Intern Med 48:512, 1958
5. Arthus M: Injections repetées de serum de cheval chez le lapin. C R Soc Biol (Paris) 55:817, 1903
6. Bartfeld H, Epstein WV: Rheumatoid factors and their biologic significance. Ann NY Acad Sci 168:1, 1969
7. Benoit FL, Rulon DB, Theil GB, Doolan PD, Watten RH: Goodpasture's syndrome: A clinicopathologic entity. Am J Med 37:424, 1964
8. Beutner EH, Jordon RE, Chorzelski TP: The immunopathology of pemphigus and bullous pemphigoid. J Invest Dermatol 51:63, 1968
9. Bielschowsky M, Goodall CM: Origin of inbred NZB mouse strains. Cancer Res 30:834, 1970
10. Blomgren SE: Drug-induced lupus erythematosis. Semin Hematol 10:345, 1973
11. Blomgren SE, Condemi JJ, Vaughan JH: Procainamide-induced lupus erythematosis. Am J Med 52:388, 1972
12. Burnet FM, Holmes MC: Thymic changes in mouse strain NZB in relation to the autoimmune state. J Pathol Bacteriol 88:229, 1964
13. Cathcart ES, Skinner M, Cohen AS: Immunogenicity of Amyloid. Immunology 20:945, 1971
14. Cavendish A: A case of dermatitis from 9-bromofluorene and a peculiar reaction to a patch test. Br J Dermatol 52:155, 1940
15. Carottini J-C, Lambert P-H, Dixon FJ: Comparison of the immune responsiveness of NZB and NZB × NZW F₁ hybrid mice with that of other strains of mice. J Exp Med 130:1093, 1969
16. Chorezelski TP, Von Weiss JF, Lever WF: Clinical significance of autoantibodies in pemphigus. Arch Dermatol 93:570, 1966
17. Chzatum DE, Hurd ER, Strunk SW, Ziff M: Renal histology and clinical course of systemic lupus erythematosis. A prospective study. Arthritis Rheum 16:670, 1973
18. Claxton RC: Review of 31 cases of Stevens-Johnson syndrome. Med J Aust 50:963, 1963
19. Cochrane CG: Mediators of the Arthus and related reactions. Prog Allergy 11:1, 1967
20. Cochrane CG: Immunologic tissue injury mediated by neutrophilic leukocytes. Adv Immunol 9:97, 1968
21. Cochrane CG, Ward PA: The Role of Complement in Lesions Induced by Immunologic Reactions. In Immunology IV. Graber P, Miesher P (eds). Basel, Schwabe, 1966
22. Cohen AS: Amyloidosis. N Engl J Med 277:522, 1967
23. Cohen AS, Canoso JJ: Criteria for the classification of systemic lupus erythematosis. Arthritis Rheum 15:540, 1972
24. Costanza ME, Pinn V, Schwartz RS, Nathanson L: Carcinoembryonic antigen–antibody complexes in a patient with colonic carcinoma and nephrotic syndrome. N Engl J Med 289:520, 1973
25. Dawkins RL: Experimental myositis associated with hypersensitivity to muscle. J Pathol Bacteriol 90:619, 1965
26. DeGowin RL, Oda Y, Evans RH: Nephritis and lung hemorrhage: Goodpasture's syndrome. Arch Intern Med 111:62, 1963
27. Dixon FJ, Vasquez JJ, Weigle WO, Cochrane CG: Pathogenesis of serum sickness. Arch Pathol 65:18, 1958
28. Donadio JV, Holley KE, Wagoner RD, Ferduson RH, McDuffie FC: Treatment of lupus nephritis with prednisone and combined prednisone and azathioprine. Ann Intern Med 77:829, 1972
29. East J, DeSousa MAB, Parrott DMV, Jaquet H: Consequences of neonatal thymectomy in New Zealand black mice. Clin Exp Immunol 2:203, 1967
30. Epstein WL: Erythema Nodosum. In Immunological Diseases. Sampter M (ed). 2nd ed. Boston, Little, Brown and Co, 1971, p 944

31. Feinstein AR: A new look at rheumatic fever. Hosp Pract 2:71, 1968
32. Fennel RH Jr, Reddy CRRM, Vasquez JJ: Progressive systemic sclerosis and malignant hypertension. Arch Pathol 72:209, 1961
33. Fletcher MWC, Harris RC: Erythema exudativum multiforme (Mebra)–bullous type. J Pediatr 27:465, 1945
34. Freemont-Smith K, Bayles TB: Salicylate therapy in rheumatoid arthritis. JAMA 192:1123, 1965
35. Freese E, Sklarow S, Freeze EB: DNA damage caused by anti-depressive hydrazines and related drugs. Mutat Res 5:343, 1968
36. Fronhert PP, Sheps SG: Long-term follow-up study of periarteritis nodosa. Am J Med 43:8, 1967
37. Gell PGH, Kelus AS: Anti-antibodies. Adv Immunol 6:461, 1967
38. Gilliam JN, Cheatum DE, Hurd ER, Stastny P, Ziff, M: Immunoglobulin in clinically uninvolved skin in systemic lupus erythematosis. Association with renal disease. J Clin Invest 53:1434, 1974
39. Glenner GG, Ein D, Eanes ED, Bladen HA, Terry W, Page DL: Creation of "amyloid" fibrils from Bence-Jones proteins in vitro. Science 174:712, 1971
40. Glenner GG, Terry W, Harada M, Isersky C, Page D: Amyloid fibril proteins: Proof of homology with immunoglobulin light chains by sequence analyses. Science 172:1150, 1971
41. Glenner GG, Terry WD, Isersky C: Amyloidosis: Its nature and pathogenesis. Semin Hematol 10:65, 1973
42. Gocke DJ, Hsu K, Morgan C, Bombardieri S, Lockshin M, Christian CL: Association between polyarteritis and Australia antigen. Lancet 2:1149, 1970
43. Gordis L: Effectiveness of comprehensive-care programs in preventing rheumatic fever. N Engl J Med 289:331, 1973
44. Götze O, Müller-Eberhard HJ: The C3 activator system: An alternate pathway of complement activation. J Exp Med 134:905, 1971
45. Grey HM, Kohler PF: Cryoimmunoglobulins. Semin Hematol 10:87, 1973
46. Gross L, Ehrlich JC: Studies on the myocardial Aschoff body. I. Descriptive classification of the lesions. Am J Pathol 10:467, 1934
47. Haas DC: Treatment of polymyositis with immunosuppressive drugs. Neurology 23:55, 1973
48. Hahn BH, Sharp GC, Irvin WS, Kantor OS, Gardner CA, Bagby MK, Perry HM, Osterland CK: Immune responses to hydralazine and nuclear antigens in hydralazine-induced lupus erythematosis. Ann Intern Med 76:365, 1972
49. Hargraves MM, Richmond H, Morton R: Presentation of 2 bone marrow elements: The "tart" cell and the "LE" cell. Mayo Clin Proc 23:25, 1948
50. Holman HR: Systemic Lupus Erythematosis. In Immunological Diseases. Sampter M (ed). Vol 2. New York, Little, Brown and Co, 1971, p 995
51. Housley J: Muscle in Allergic Disease: Myasthenia Gravis. In Clinical Aspects of Immunology. Gell PGH, Coombs RRA (eds). 2nd ed. Oxford, Blackwell, 1968, p 1020
52. Howes EL Jr, Incus T, McKay DG, Christian CL: A model for amyloidosis. Arthritis Rheum 6:278, 1963
53. Howie JB, Helyer BJ: The immunology and pathology of NZB mice. Adv Immunol 9:215, 1968
54. Jaffee RH: Amyloidosis produced by injections of proteins. Arch Pathol Lab Med 1:25, 1926
55. Janigan DT, Druet RL: Experimental immune amyloidosis in x-irradiated recipients of spleen homogenates or serum from immunized donors. Am J Pathol 52:381, 1968
56. Klassen J, Andres GA, Brennan JC, McClusky RT: An immunologic renal tubular lesion in man. Clin Immunol Immunopathol 1:69, 1972
57. Klassen J, McClusky RT, Milgrom F: Non-glomerular renal disease produced in rabbits by immunization with homologous kidney. Am J Pathol 63:333, 1971
58. Klemperer P: The concept of collagen diseases in medicine. Am Rev Resp Dis 83:331, 1961
59. Koffler D, Schur PH, Kunkel HG: Immunological studies concerning the nephritis of systemic lupus erythematosus. J Exp Med 126:607, 1967
60. Kunkel HG, Tan EM: Autoantibodies and disease. Adv Immunol 4:351, 1964

61. Kussmaul A, Maier R: Ueber eine bisher nicht beschriebene eigenthümliche Arterienerkrankung (Periarteritis Nodosa), die mit Morbus Brightii und rapid fortschreitender allgemeiner Muskellähmung einhergeht. Dtsch Arch Klin Med, 1:484, 1866
62. Kysela S, Steinberg AD: Increased survival of NZB/W mice given multiple syngeneic young thymus grafts. Clin Immunol Immunopath 2:133, 1973
63. Lampert PH, Dixon FJ: Pathogenesis of the glomerulonephritis of NZB/W mice. J Exp Med 127:507, 1968
64. Lampert PW, Oldstone MBA: Host immunoglobulin G and complement deposits in the choroid plexis during spontaneous immune complex disease. Science 180:408, 1973
65. Lehman DH, Wilson CB, Dixon FJ: Interstitial nephritis in rats immunized with heterologous tubular basement membrane. Kidney Internatl 5:187, 1974
66. Lerner RW, Dixon FJ: Transfer of ovine experimental allergic glomerulonephritis (EAG) with serum. J Exp Med 124:431, 1966
67. Levin M, Pras M, Franklin EC: Immunologic studies of the major non-immunoglobulin protein of amyloid. I. Identification and partial characterization of a related serum component. J Exp Med 138:373, 1973
68. Luciano A, Rothfield NF: Patterns of nuclear fluorescence and DNA-binding activity. Ann Rheum Dis 32:337, 1973
69. McCombs RP: Systemic "allergic" vasculitis: Clinical and pathological relationships. JAMA 194:1059, 1965
70. McPhaul JJ, Dixon FJ: Characterization of human anti-glomerular basement membrane antibodies eluted from glomerulonephritic kidneys. J Clin Invest 49:308, 1970
71. Mellors RC, Huang CY: Immunopathology of NZB/Bl mice. V. Virus-like (filtrable) agent separable from lymphoma cells and identifiable by electron microscopy. J Exp Med 124:1031, 1966
72. Morton WL: Endothelial inclusions in active lesions of systemic lupus erythematosis. J Lab Clin Med 74:369, 1969
73. Nagai T, Tadao T, Ogino K, Kith T: IgE deposits in glomeruli with membranes nephropathy and marked asthematic predisposition in humans. Jap Circ J 37:1227, 1973
74. Phillips PE, Christian CL: Virus antibodies in systemic lupus erythematosis and other connective tissue diseases. Ann Rheum Dis 32:450, 1973
75. Pras M, Reshef T: The acid soluble fraction of amyloid–a fibril-forming protein. Biochim Biophys Acta 271:193, 1972
76. Provost TT, Tomasi TB Jr: Evidence for complement activation via the alternate pathway in skin diseases. I. Herpes Gestations, systemic lupus erythematosis, and bullous pemphigoid. J Clin Invest 52:1779, 1973
77. Puchtler H, Sweat F: A review of early concepts of amyloid in context with contemporary chemical literature from 1839 to 1859. J Histochem Cytochem 14:123, 1965
78. Rich AR, Gregory JE: The experimental demonstration that polyarteritis nodosa is a manifestation of hypersensitivity. Bull Johns Hopkins Hosp 72:63, 1943
79. Rodnan GP: Progressive Systemic Sclerosis (Diffuse Scleroderma). In Immunological Diseases. Sampter M (ed). 2nd ed. Boston, Little, Brown and Co, 1971
80. Rose GA, Spencer H: Polyarteritis nodosa. Q J Med 26:43, 1957
81. Rothfield MF, Rodnan GP: Serum anti-nuclear antibodies in progressive systemic sclerosis (scleroderma). Arthritis Rheum 11:607, 1968
82. Ruddy S, Colten HR: Rheumatoid arthritis. Biosynthesis of complement components by synovial tissue. N Engl J Med 290:1284, 1974
83. Schaff Z, Barry DW, Grimley PM: Cytochemistry of tuboreticular structure in lymphocytes from patients with systemic lupus erythematosis and in cultured human lymphoid cells. Comparison to a paramyxamius. Lab Invest 29:577, 1973
84. Shelley WB: Herpes simplex virus as a cause of erythema multiforme. JAMA 201:153, 1967
85. Shirai T, Mellors RC: Natural thymocytotoxic autoantibody and reactive antigen in New Zealand black and other mice. Proc Natl Acad Sci USA 68:1412, 1972
86. Short CL, Bauer W, Reynolds WE: Rheumatoid Arthritis. Cambridge, Mass, Harvard University Press, 1957

87. Siegel M, Lee SL, Peress NS: The epidemiology of drug-induced systemic lupus erythematosus. Arthritis Rheum 10:407, 1967
88. Steblay RW, Rudofsky V: Autoimmune glomerulonephritis induced in sheep by injections of human lung and Freund's adjuvant. Science 160:204, 1968
89. Stutman O: Lymphocyte subpopulations in NZB mice: Deficit of thymus dependent lymphocytes. J Immunol 109:602, 1972
90. Sugai S, Pillarisetty R, Talal N: Monoclonal macroglobulinemia in NZB/NZW F₁ mice. J Exp Med 138:989, 1973
91. Symposium on immunologic aspects of rheumatoid arthritis and systemic lupus erythematosus. Arthritis Rheum 6:402, 1963
92. Talal N: Immunologic and viral factors in the pathogenesis of systemic lupus erythematosis. Arthritis Rheum 13:887, 1970
93. Talal N, Steinberg AD, Jacobs ME, Chused TM, Gazdar AF: Immune cell cooperation, viruses and antibodies to nucleic acids in New Zealand mice. J Exp Med 134:525, 1971
94. Tan EM, Northway JD, Pinnas JL: The clinical significance of antinuclear antibodies. Postgrad Med 54:143, 1973
95. Thomas BA: The so-called Stevens-Johnson Syndrome. Br J Med 1:1393, 1950
96. Tonietti G, Oldstone MBA, Dixon FJ: The effect of induced chronic viral infection on the immunologic disease of New Zealand mice. J Exp Med 132:89, 1970
97. Tuffanelli DL, Winkelman RK: Systemic scleroderma: A clinical study of 727 cases. Arch Dermatol 84:359, 1961
98. Unanue ER, Dixon FS: Experimental glomerulonephritis: Immunological events and pathologic mechanisms. Adv Immunol 6:1, 1967
99. Vaughan JH: Rheumatologic disorders due to immune complexes. Postgrad Med 54:129, 1973
100. Vazquez JJ, Dixon FJ: Immunohistochemical analysis of amyloid by fluorescence technique. J Exp Med 104:727, 1956
101. Vernier RL: Clinical aspects of glomerulonephritis. In Immunological Diseases. Sampter M (ed). 2nd ed. Boston, Little, Brown and Co, 1971, p 1134
102. Verroust PJ, Wison CB, Cooper NR, Edgington TS, Dixon FJ: Glomerular complement components in human glomerulonephritis. J Clin Invest 53:77, 1974
103. Viets HR: Myasthenia gravis. N Engl J Med 251:97, 141, 1954
104. von Pirquet CF, Schick B: Serum Sickness, 1905, Schick B trans. Baltimore, Williams and Wilkins, 1951
105. Waksman BH, Raff MC, East J: T and B lymphocytes in New Zealand Black Mice. An analysis of the theta, TL and MBLA markers. Clin Exp Immunol 11:1, 1972
106. Weigle WO: Fate and biological action of antigen-antibody complexes. Adv Immunol 1:283, 1961
107. Westberg NG, Naff GB, Boyer JT, Michael AF: Glomerular deposition of properdin in acute and chronic glomerulonephritis with hypocomplementemia. J Clin Invest 50:642, 1971
108. Willerson JT, Asofsky R, Barth WF: Experimental murine amyloid. IV. Amyloidosis and immunoglobulin. J Immunol 103:741, 1969
109. Williams GM, Lee HM, Weymouth RF, Harlan WR Jr, Holden KR, Stanley CM, Millington GA, Hume DM: Studies in hyperacute and chronic renal homograft rejection in man. Surgery 62:204, 1967
110. Winkelman RK (ed): Symposium on Sclerodema. Mayo Clin Proc 46:83, 1971
111. Zabriskie JB: Mimetic relationships between group A streptococci and mammalian tissues. Adv Immunol 7:147, 1967
112. Zabriskie JB: The role of streptococci in human glomerulonephritis. J Exp Med 134:180, 1971
113. Zvaifler NJ: Further speculation on the pathogenesis of joint inflammation in rheumatoid arthritis. Arthritis Rheum 13:895, 1970
114. Zvaifler NJ: Immunoreactants in rheumatoid synovial fluid. J Exp Med 134:2765, 1971
115. Zvaifler NJ: Rheumatoid synovitis. An extravascular immune complex disease. Arthritis Rheum 17:297, 1974

14

Delayed Hypersensitivity (Tuberculin-Type, Cellular) Reactions

Delayed hypersensitivity (Fig. 14-1) is initiated by the reaction of *specifically modified lymphocytes* containing a receptor or mechanism capable of responding specifically to antigens deposited at a local site (8,63,109,188). The exact mechanism of this type of reaction is still uncertain. The reaction is manifested by the infiltration of cells, beginning with a perivascular accumulation of lymphocytes and monocytes at the site where antigen is located (199). Evidence obtained using labeled specifically sensitized cells transferred to normal donors indicates that only a few of the infiltrating cells are specifically sensitized. In some manner the reaction of these few sensitized cells with the antigen in the tissue causes large numbers of unlabeled cells to infiltrate the area, with subsequent tissue destruction. Specifically sensitized cells, upon reaction with antigen, may release mediators (109) capable of influencing the behavior of other non-sensitized mononuclear cells or of directly affecting the tissue cells in the area of the reaction (see below).

The term delayed is applied because the time course is measured in days or even weeks, in contrast to the anaphylactic reactions which reach their peak in a few minutes and the Arthus reaction which occurs in hours. The term tuberculin-type hypersensitivity is used because for many years the study of delayed hypersensitivity was essentially the study of the basic response to tuberculin and injection with tubercle bacilli. It is now known that delayed hypersensitivity also takes part in homograft rejection and autoallergic diseases and can be induced by purified protein antigens. It differs from the allergic reactions mentioned above in that 1) no humoral antibody is involved and reactivity cannot be transferred by serum, but

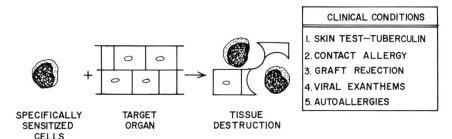

Fig. 14–1. Delayed hypersensitivity (cellular) reactions. Specifically modified lymphocytes containing substance or mechanism capable of recognizing antigen are the initiators, resulting in the release of factors affecting other mononuclear cells. Thus, most cells found in delayed hypersensitivity reactions are not specifically sensitized but are called into action by reaction of a few sensitized cells with antigen. Tissue damage occurs as direct reaction of sensitized cells to tissue cells containing antigen (as in graft rejection) or as a result of reaction of sensitized cells to antigen deposited in tissue (as in tuberculin skin reaction). Mechanism by which these cellular infiltrates destroy tissue cells is unknown, but death of tissue cells in affected areas occurs when these cells are separated and isolated from adjacent tissue cells by infiltrating inflammatory cells. Cellular hypersensitivity may provide protection from such events as viral infection, but as a result of reaction of sensitized cells with viral antigens, host's own tissue cells are destroyed (innocent bystander reactions). Clinical features of cellular hypersensitivity depend upon location of antigen (skin in contact dermatitis, thyroid in thyroiditis, kidney in renal allograft rejection).

only by cells or, in man, subcellular fractions; 2) the time course of the development of the lesion is much prolonged; and 3) the gross and microscopic appearance is different (Table 9–1).

CELL-MEDIATED IMMUNITY

The mechanism whereby sensitized lymphocytes kill target cells is unknown but considerable insight into this phenomenon is now being obtained by study of the killing effect of lymphocytes upon target cells in vitro. The term cell-mediated immunity has come to be applied to the destruction of target cells by lymphocytes in vitro (37,140). The target cell is either destroyed or inhibited in function so that the effect can be measured by 1) visual observation to determine the number of target cells remaining (51,156,211), 2) visual estimation of the number of cells killed by counting dead target cells that take up vital stains (126,181), 3) inhibition of cell metabolism such as a reduction of DNA, RNA or protein synthesis by target cells (71,210), 4) reduction of a biologic function, or inhibition of production of a biologically active product of the target cell (60), 5) reduction in the number of colonies found after transfer of a given number of target cells to tissue culture plates [colony inhibition (83,179)], 6) reduction in cell growth or function following transfer of treated target cells to living recipients [passive transfer (103,124)], or 7) release of intracellular components [lymphocyte-mediated cytolysis (31,33,86)].

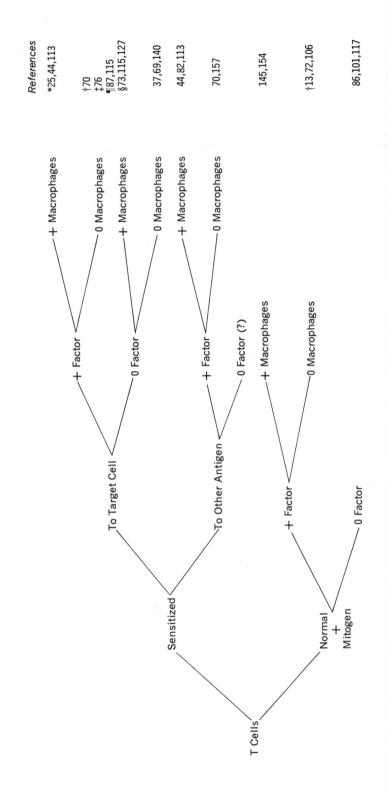

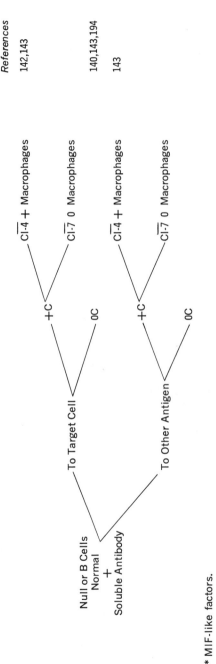

References

142,143

140,143,194

143

Cl-4 + Macrophages

Cl-7 0 Macrophages

Cl-4 + Macrophages

Cl-7 0 Macrophages

+C

0C

+C

0C

To Target Cell

To Other Antigen

Null or B Cells
Normal
+
Soluble Antibody

* MIF-like factors.
† Cytotoxic factor.
‡ Proliferation inhibitory factor.
§ Activated macrophages
‖ Cloning Inhibitory Factor

Fig. 14–2. Possible mechanisms of lymphoid cell-mediated cytotoxicity. T cells may kill target cells after specific sensitization or following mitogen activation. Cell killing may be mediated by direct contact, by release of cytoxic factors or by recruitment of macrophages. Antibody-dependent, cell-mediated cytolysis is accomplished by null (K) cells or B cells in the presence of soluble antibody and may be mediated by complement and macrophage activation. Since antibody may kill target cells in the absence of effector lymphocytes and antibody–antigen complexes may be cytotoxic to target cells (141), the role of lymphoid cells in antibody-dependent cytotoxicity may be difficult to identify. *Note:* Since antibody alone with C may be effective in vitro it is difficult to identify these mechanisms.

LYMPHOCYTE-MEDIATED CYTOLYSIS

Lymphocyte-mediated cytolysis has become the most frequently used assay for cell-mediated immunity. Intracellular components of target cells may be labeled by addition of isotopes such as ^{51}Cr (20,31,33,86), ^{86}Rb (205) or ^{99m}Tc (65), and cytolysis determined by the release of the label from the target cell. The way in which these isotopes label the target cells is not well understood. ^{51}Cr is presented to the target cells in the form of $Na_2^{51}CrO_4$ with the ^{51}Cr probably binding to intracellular protein (20). Upon addition of killer cells, the target cell is destroyed and the intracellular ^{51}Cr released. Cytolysis is then expressed as either the percent of ^{51}Cr released (20) or as the percent of specific cytolysis by subtracting the amount of ^{51}Cr released from target cells not treated with killer cells (control) from the experimental ^{51}Cr release (20,33).

TYPES OF CELL-MEDIATED IMMUNITY

Cell-mediated immunity may be demonstrated under three general circumstances: 1) the destruction of target cells by lymphocytes specifically sensitized to the target cell, 2) the production of killer cells or cell products by normal unsensitized lymphocyte populations following treatment with nonspecific lymphocyte stimulants, or 3) target cell killing by normal unsensitized lymphocytes in the presence of humoral antibody directed against the target cell or toward another antigen (antibody-dependent, cell-mediated lymphocytolysis). These various situations are adumbrated in Fig. 14-2. Direct target cell killing by specifically sensitized killer cells and mitogen-stimulated killer cells or cell products (lymphotoxins) are the result of T cell activation (37,140). Antibody-dependent, cell-mediated lymphocytolysis requires null cells* (lymphoid cells without T or B cell markers) or B cells as effectors [killer cells] (59,143). Sensitization of T cells (conversion to killer cells) may be induced in vitro (20,38,198). Macrophages are required for optimal sensitization of T cells but macrophages do not take part in the killer cell effector stage of the reaction (198). On the other hand, macrophages may acquire the capacity to kill target cells by reaction with a product made by specifically sensitized T cells on reaction with the target cells (25,44,113,115,116). Thus macrophages may become killer cells due to effects of activated T cell products and amplify cell-mediated immunity (see Immune Phagocytosis, page 273).

MECHANISMS OF CELL KILLING BY SENSITIZED LYMPHOCYTES

The direct destruction of target cells by specifically sensitized lymphocytes is the mechanism most likely operative in vivo (37,85,140), although the interaction of several different mechanisms may occur (see below). Agents that inhibit direct lymphocyte-mediated cytolysis have been used to study the mechanism of killing of target cells by specifically sensitized lymphocytes. Target cell killing may be divided into three phases: 1) initial recognition of target cell antigens by sensitized T cells, 2) increased protein synthesis by the killer cells, and 3) a secretory phase during which products

---

* Null killer cells are termed K cells.

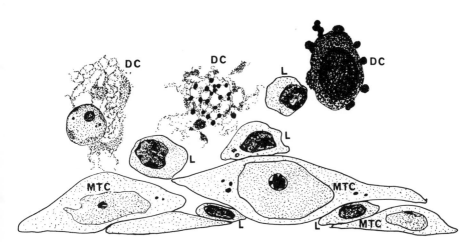

Fig. 14–3. Reaction of sensitized lymphocytes with target cells in vitro. Lymphocytes from sensitized donor infiltrate and surround monolayer target cells, seemingly without effect on viability or morphologic appearance of target cells. As a result of this infiltration, monolayer cells become separated from each other and from culture surface. Monolayer cells that retain contact with monolayer remain viable, but when isolated from other monolayer cells, morphologic changes consistent with cell death occur. These alterations do not occur in tissue culture cells that become separated from monolayer in presence of normal lymphocytes. Attempts to start monolayer cultures with fluids and washings taken from monolayers treated with sensitized lymphocytes have not been successful. DC, dead or dying cells separated from monolayers; L, lymphocytes; MTC, monolayer target cells. Contact between living sensitized lymphocytes and target cells in vitro is not absolutely required for destruction of the target cells, as extracts from sensitized cells cultured with antigens will also produce death of target cells. (Modified from Biberfield P, Holm G, Perlmann P. Exp Cell Res 52:672, 1968. Copyright © Academic Press)

of the T cell responsible for destruction of the target cell are released (85). However, because of difficulty in demonstrating lymphotoxins in the supernates of sensitized lymphocyte culture treated with antigen, the involvement of soluble mediators in direct lymphocyte-mediated cytolysis has been seriously doubted (36). A direct transfer of killer cell products to target cells is quite possible (85). Intimate contact of killer T cells with target cells is required for cell killing and toxic products may be passed from killer to target cell without significant release into supernates. On the other hand, lymphotoxins may be released into culture supernates as a result of antigen or mitogen stimulation of T cells in vitro (13,44,70,72,76, 87,106,113,115,145,154).

The interaction of sensitized lymphocytes and target cells may be studied morphologically by observing the effect of sensitized lymphocytes on target cells growing in monolayers (22,140). Plaques or holes occur in the monolayer when sensitized lymphocytes are added. Sensitized lymphocytes surround the target cells and eventually cause their detachment from the monolayer. Fig. 14–3 shows the destruction of monolayer target cells. As long as the target cell remains attached to the monolayer, it appears to be viable; however, upon separation from the monolayer, the target cell undergoes morphologic alterations indicative of cell death. These alterations include vacuolization and disintegration of the cytoplasm and condensation of nucleus and cytoplasm. Although close contact between the sensitized lymphocytes and target cells occurs, the exact mechanism of target cell death remains an enigma. An identical type of interaction between lymphocytes and target cells occurs in tissue reactions mediated by lymphocytes. Fig. 14–4 shows the pathologic changes occurring during the development of experimental allergic thyroiditis (57). As in the target cell monolayer system, lymphocytes pass between the thyoid follicular cells causing them to separate from each other and from the basement membrane, with eventual destruction of the thyroid cells. The basement membrane appears intact during the development of the lesion. Infiltration of mononuclear cells, with separation, isolation and destruction of target cells, may be observed in contact dermatitis, classic graft rejection and many autoallergic diseases believed to be mediated by specifically sensitized cells (e.g., destruction of myelin in experimental allergic encephalomyelitis, destruction of thyroid follicular lining cells in experimental allergic thyroiditis, and destruction of germinal epithelium in experimental allergic orchitis).

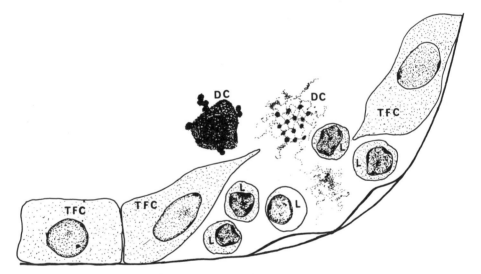

Fig. 14–4. Reaction of sensitized lymphocytes with target cells in vivo. (Morphologic changes in experimental allergic thyroiditis.) Changes similar to those illustrated in Fig. 14–3, for reaction of sensitized lymphocytes with tissue culture monolayers occurs with thyroid follicle-lining cells in allergic thyroiditis. Mononuclear cells appear first in perivenular areas and then invade stroma of thyroid. Invasion of follicles follows. Lymphocytes appear to pass through basement membrane of thyroid follicle, separating thyroid follicle-lining cells from basement membrane and from other follicular cells. Death of lining cells occurs when these cells are isolated from basement membrane and from other follicular cells. Essentially identical morphologic changes are seen in contact dermatitis, renal allograft rejection, and in epidermis of skin allograft rejection. Similar process is believed to occur in destruction of myelin observed in experimental allergic encephalomyelitis. **DC,** dead or dying cells; **L,** lymphocytes; **TFC,** thyroid follicle-lining cells (Modified from Flax MH: Lab Invest 12:199, 1963. Copyright © 1963, International Academy of Pathology)

LYMPHOCYTE MEDIATORS (LYMPHOKINES)

Lymphocyte mediators identified by their biologic activity, are substances that are released or can be extracted from sensitized lymphocytes after exposure to the specific antigen to which they are sensitized (109). The properties of these factors, determined by the system used to identify them, are poorly characterized. The following factors have been described:

1. Migratory-inhibitory factor (25) is extractable from lymphocytes and suppresses the in vitro migration of normal macrophages. It has a molecular weight of ~10,000 and is synthesized by sensitive lymphocytes upon contact with antigen.

2. Skin-reactive factor (19) is obtained the same way as migratory-inhibitory factor. When the factor is injected into the skin of a normal guinea pig, an inflammatory reaction ensues. Skin-reactive factor may serve to hold macrophages at the site of antigen injection and is believed to play a similar role in other reactions induced by specific antigen reacting with sensitized cells. Skin-reactive and migratory-inhibitory factors may be the same substance.

3. Transfer factor (110) is a material of relatively low molecular weight (~10,000), extractable from sensitized lymphoid cells, that induces a state of delayed sensitivity upon injection into a normal animal. Since transfer factor has been convincingly demonstrated only in man, complete characterization is difficult. Reports of transfer factor activity in other species have not been reproducible.

4. Cytotoxic factor (70) released by sensitized lymphocytes upon contact with antigen, causes destruction of target cells in vitro. This material is protein-like, has a molecular weight of ~85,000, is released from lymphoid cells of most mammalian species and causes the destruction of a wide variety of dissimilar cells.

5. Three macrophage-specific chemotactic factors have been identified (206). One of these is produced by sensitized lymphocytes upon contact with antigen; one is present in lysates of polymorphonuclear leukocytes, and the third is generated from serum by antigen–antibody complexes. Macrophage-specific chemotactic factor produced by reaction of sensitized lymphocytes with antigen appears to be different from migratory-inhibitory factor. These factors attract macrophages, which migrate toward areas containing chemotactic factors (206).

6. Lymphocyte-stimulating factor (172) is released from sensitized lymphocytes upon contact with antigen and causes normal lymphocytes in vitro to undergo blast transformation and subsequent mitosis. This material has not been found in all lymphocyte culture systems.

7. Lymphocyte-permeability factor (187) can be extracted from both sensitized and nonsensitized lymph node cells from various species and is capable of increasing vascular permeability. This factor can be detected in skin sites undergoing delayed hypersensitivity reactions. Antisera prepared to this factor cause a depression of delayed skin reactions.

8. Aggregation factor produces adherence of lymphocytes to macrophages. The presence of antigen in cultures containing lymphocytes

from sensitized animals and macrophages from normal animals causes not only an inhibition of migration of the macrophages, but also an adherence or aggregation of macrophages to macrophages (68) or lymphocytes to macrophages (161). This aggregation does not occur when migratory-inhibitory factor is added to normal mixed lymphocyte-macrophage cultures.

9. Proliferative-inhibitory factor (170) found in the supernatant from antigen-stimulated lymphocyte cultures, inhibits the growth of non-lymphoid cells in vitro, but does not kill them. It does not seem to affect other lymphoid cells.

10. Macrophage-activation factor (201) stimulates macrophage in vitro to assume a more active morphologic appearance and to adhere more firmly to plastic surfaces (128,133).

11. Interferon is a nonimmune factor that inhibits the growth of viruses (75).

12. Cytophilic antibody (81) may be produced by antibody-forming cells and become attached to macrophages, converting them into antigen-reactive cells.

The role of lymphocyte mediators in delayed hypersensitivity reactions remains obscure, but an interplay of such factors is possible. For instance, upon contact with antigen, lymphocytes release migratory-inhibitory, skin-reactive, macrophage-specific chemotactic and macrophage-activation factors; all of which serve to attract and hold macrophages in the reaction site. The number of specifically sensitized cells may be increased by transfer factor or cytophilic antibody (which confers upon previously neutral cells the capacity to recognize the antigen), and by lymphocyte-stimulating factor, which induces proliferation of lymphocytes. Cytotoxic factor may cause death of tissue cells in the reactive area, proliferative-inhibitory factor may inhibit nonlymphoid cell growth, and lymphocyte-permeability factor may increase the magnitude of the inflammatory reaction by causing more cells to accumulate. However, no direct role of any of these mediators has been convincingly demonstrated in delayed hypersensitivity in vivo.

DELAYED SKIN REACTION

The classic delayed type tuberculin skin reaction is elicited in sensitive individuals by intradermal injection of tuberculoprotein antigens [PPD, OT*] (8,109,188). Following injection of antigen into the skin of an individual sensitive in a delayed manner, there is little or no reaction until after 4–6 hours. The grossly visible induration and swelling usually reach a maximum at 24–48 hours. Histologically there is accumulation of mononuclear cells with proliferation around small veins. Later, mononuclear cells may be seen throughout the area of the reaction with massive infiltration in the dermis. Polymorphonuclear cells constitute less than one-third of the cells at any time, and very few are present at 24 hours or later unless the reaction is severe enough to cause necrosis.

* PPD, purified protein derivative; OT, old tuberculin. These materials are extracts from cultures of tubercle bacilli and contain tubercular antigens.

The evolution of the delayed skin reaction is presented in Fig. 14–5. This description incorporates the function of the lymphocyte mediators listed above. A simplified concept is that the lymphocyte initiates the reaction and the macrophage cleans it up.

CUTANEOUS BASOPHIL HYPERSENSITIVITY (CBH)

The term cutaneous basophil hypersensitivity (CBH) is used to denote a group of lymphocyte-mediated, basophilic reactions that differ histologically from classic delayed type (DH) reactions (155). Basophils are infrequent or rare in DH, but are numerous in the 24–48 hour delayed skin reaction to soluble protein antigens elicited after immunization of animals with those antigens in complete Freund's adjuvant which appears transiently prior to antibody formation (164). Basophils make up almost half of the inflammatory cells present in these reactions. Degranulation of these basophils is not a prominent feature during the reaction; these cells are not the same as mast cells involved in anaphylactic reactions. Basophils may also be found in other situations involving expression of cellular immunity including skin graft rejection, tumor rejection, viral immunity and contact allergy (48). CBH reactions require specifically sensitized lymphocytes. In contact dermatitis (see below) infiltration of lymphocytes precedes basophils by at least 12 hours, probably releasing a lymphokine responsible for attracting basophils (47). The function of the basophilic infiltrate is not known but might serve as an effective phagocytic cell which supplements the macrophage.

The term "Jones-Mote reaction" originally referred to the reappearance of a delayed type of sensitivity to serum proteins after the development and regression of an Arthus reaction, noted originally in humans by Jones and Mote (94,131). This term was extended to cover the transient form of delayed skin reaction to protein antigens occurring prior to antibody production in experimental animals (150,164), a finding also previously observed in humans (94,167). With a better appreciation of the basophilic nature of these reactions, the term cutaneous basophil hypersensitivity has been applied. As an immunologic reaction, the significance of CBH-type reactions remains unclear.

CONTACT ALLERGY

Contact allergy (contact eczema, dermatitis venenata) is represented by the common allergic reaction to poison ivy (52,104). It also occurs as an allergic response to a wide variety of simple chemicals in ointments, clothing, cosmetics, dyes, adhesive tape, etc. in any adequately exposed individual. The antigens are all highly reactive chemical compounds capable of combining with proteins; they are also lipid-soluble and so can penetrate the epidermis. The antigen is an incomplete antigen which combines with some constituent of the epidermis to form a complete antigen (antigen acts as hapten) (62). Sensitization occurs by exposure of the skin once or repeatedly to sufficiently high concentrations. All individuals are susceptible if exposed to the antigen in sufficient amounts. A greater amount of

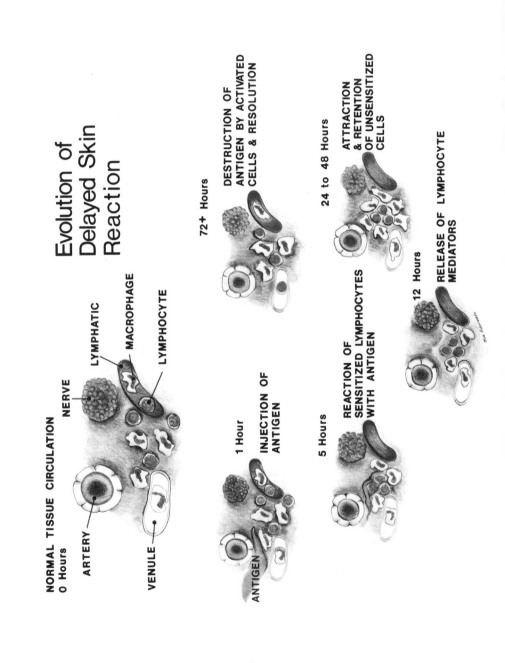

Evolution of Delayed Skin Reaction

NORMAL TISSUE CIRCULATION
0 Hours

NERVE

LYMPHATIC

MACROPHAGE

LYMPHOCYTE

ARTERY

VENULE

ANTIGEN

1 Hour
INJECTION OF ANTIGEN

5 Hours
REACTION OF SENSITIZED LYMPHOCYTES WITH ANTIGEN

12 Hours
RELEASE OF LYMPHOCYTE MEDIATORS

24 to 48 Hours
ATTRACTION & RETENTION OF UNSENSITIZED CELLS

72+ Hours
DESTRUCTION OF ANTIGEN BY ACTIVATED CELLS & RESOLUTION

antigen is needed for sensitization than for elicitation of skin reaction in an already sensitive individual. When United States soldiers moved into Japan after World War II, the military medical dispensaries noticed the widespread occurrence of a skin rash having the appearance of contact dermatitis. It was the distribution of the rash that was most unusual: It occurred on the elbows and buttocks. After diligent sleuthing, it was discovered that the bars and toilet seats of certain Japanese public establishments were coated with a laquer made from the sap of a tree that contained small amounts of a substance closely related to the poison ivy antigen. The amounts of this related antigen were not great enough to sensitize the native Japanese, but were sufficient to elicit the characteristic dermatitis in previously sensitized individuals. The American soldiers were sensitive owing to previous exposure to poison ivy.

The characteristic skin reaction is elicited in sensitized individuals by exposing the skin to the antigen (natural exposure, patch tests) (52,104). The reaction is a sharply delineated, superficial skin inflammation, beginning as early as 24 hours after exposure and reaching a maximum at 48–96 hours (Fig. 14–6). It is characterized by redness, induration and vesiculation. The reaction may take longer to reach a maximum than the tuberculin skin test because of the longer time required for the incomplete antigen to penetrate the epidermis. Histologically the dermis shows perivenous accumulation of lymphocytes and histocytes and some edema. The epidermis is invaded by these cells and shows intraepidermal edema (spongiosis), which progresses to vesiculation and death of epidermal cells. It was once assumed that the lesion was due to sensitization of the epidermal cells themselves. However, no reaction occurs when the local vascular supply is interrupted, and careful histologic study shows that infiltration of the epidermis with mononuclear cells precedes the epidermal cell damage. Since antibody is not involved, it is clear that hematogenous cells are the carriers of sensitivity, and epidermal death is comparable to the destruction of parenchyma (i.e., of the cells bearing the antigen) in homograft rejection and the autoallergies. In addition, sensitivity can be passively transferred with lymphocytes, and suppression of the circulating lymphocytes by radiation or by specific antiserum to lymphocytes suppresses the contact reactivity. Because the antigen is mainly present in the epidermis, it takes about 2 days for the reacting mononuclear cells (lymphocytes

Fig. 14–5. Evolution of the delayed skin reaction. In normal skin, lymphocytes pass from venules through the dermis to lymphatics which return these cells to the circulation. Production of delayed skin reaction involves recognition of antigen by sensitized lymphocytes (T cells), immobilization of lymphocytes at the site, production and release of lymphocyte mediators and accumulation of macrophages with eventual destruction of antigen and resolution of the reaction. This results in an accumulation of cells seen at 24–48 hours after antigen injection. Macrophages degrade the antigen. When the antigen is destroyed, the reactive cells are either disintegrated or return via the lymphatic to the bloodstream or draining lymph nodes. In this way specifically sensitized lymphocytes may be distributed throughout the lymphoid system following local stimulation with antigen.

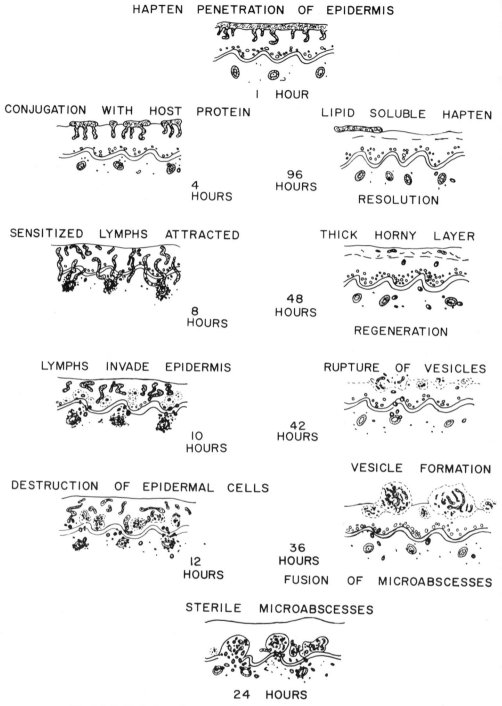

HAPTEN PENETRATION OF EPIDERMIS

1 HOUR

CONJUGATION WITH HOST PROTEIN

4 HOURS

SENSITIZED LYMPHS ATTRACTED

8 HOURS

LYMPHS INVADE EPIDERMIS

10 HOURS

DESTRUCTION OF EPIDERMAL CELLS

12 HOURS

STERILE MICROABSCESSES

24 HOURS

LIPID SOLUBLE HAPTEN

96 HOURS

RESOLUTION

THICK HORNY LAYER

48 HOURS

REGENERATION

RUPTURE OF VESICLES

42 HOURS

VESICLE FORMATION

36 HOURS

FUSION OF MICROABSCESSES

Fig. 14–6. Evolution of contact dermatitis reaction. A contact sensitizing hapten such as dintrophenol in a lipid solvent or poison ivy allergen needs to be in either a lipid solvent or lipid soluble in order to penetrate the epidermis. In so doing the contact sensitizing hapten joins to host proteins to become a complete antigen. In a sensitive individual, penetration of the epidermis brings the antigen into contact with specifically sensitized cells which react with the antigen and initiate a delayed hypersensitivity reaction.

and macrophages) to invade and react with all the antigen. As a result of this invasion and reaction epidermal cells are destroyed and small foci (sterile micoabcesses) are formed, eventually leading to vesicle formation which can be seen on the skin as small fluid filled blebs. Since all of the hapten may not be degraded in the vesicles, rupture of the vesicles by scratching may spread the antigen to uninvolved areas of the skin and provoke new reactions. Proliferation of the epidermal cells results in eventual sloughing of the affected epidermal cells. This process may take up to a week to 10 days depending on the amount of antigen present and the degree of sensitization of the individual.

GRAFT REJECTION

If solid tissue from one individual of a species is transplanted to a second, genetically different individual of the same species, a characteristic reaction termed allograft (homograft) rejection is observed (23,90,123,158). If transplantation occurs from one part of the body to another in the same individual (autograft) or between two genetically identical individuals (synograft) such as monozygotic twins, this reaction does not take place. If transplantation is made between individuals of different species (xenograft), a more brisk and intense rejection may result. The genetic control of transplantation antigens as demonstrated by the behavior of skin grafts among inbred strains of mice and their hybrid offspring is illustrated in Fig. 14–7. Transplantation antigens are usually inherited according to co-dominant Mendelian rules. Grafts between the parental strains are rapidly rejected. Since the F1 contains both specificities of each parental strain, F1 hybrids will accept grafts from each parental strain, but grafts from F1 mice will be rejected by each parental strain. F2 population, resulting from matings of F1 parents, will produce offspring half of which are similar to the F1 (heterozygous) and half of which are homozygous. The homozygous mice will be distributed equally between the genotype of the two parental strains. The results of grafting to and from the F2 mice to the F1 and to one of the parental strains can be predicted as indicated in Fig. 14–7. The results of a parental-F1 backcross (mating of F1 mice to one of the parental strains) is indicated at the bottom of Fig. 14–7. Half these offspring will be identical to the parental strain and half identical to the F1, and thus transplants to and from these mice will behave accordingly. Through the thorough study of the behavior of grafts among different strains of mice and their offspring and the correlation of this with the serologically identifiable lymphocyte antigens, the transplantation genetics and histocompatability loci of the mouse have been identified (see below).

The rejection reaction is perhaps best illustrated by the rejection of two skin grafts from the same donor to the same recipient, with the second graft placed about 1 month after the first graft (Fig. 14–8). During the second or third day following the first grafting procedure, revascularization begins and is complete by the sixth or seventh day. A similar response is observed for autografts, synografts, allografts, or xenografts, in that each type of graft becomes vascularized. However, at about 1 week the first signs of rejection appear in the deep layers of the allograft

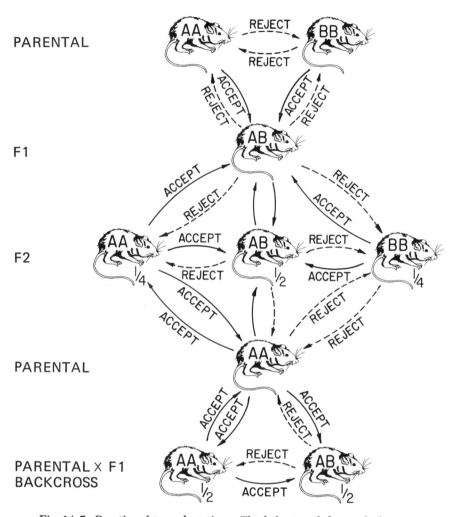

Fig. 14–7. **Genetics of transplantation.** The behavior of skin grafts between two inbred strains differing at a major histocompatibility locus (H2) and the behavior of grafts to and from various hybrids and backcrosses to one of the parental strains. Arrows indicate a graft from a given donor to a given recipient. Rejection occurs when the donor contains a specificity not present in the recipient. Capital letters indicate specificities present in inbred parental strains and designated progeny. Fractions indicate expected frequency of each genotype in the F2 and parental-F1 backcross populations. Dotted lines, rejection of graft; solid lines, acceptance.

or xenograft. A perivascular (perivenular) accumulation of mononuclear cells occurs similar to that seen in the early stages of a tuberculin skin reaction. The infiltration steadily intensifies, and edema is grossly visible. At about 9–10 days thrombosis of the involved vessels occurs, with necrosis and sloughing of the graft. This entire process usually requires 11–14 days and is called a first-set rejection. The synograft or autograft does not

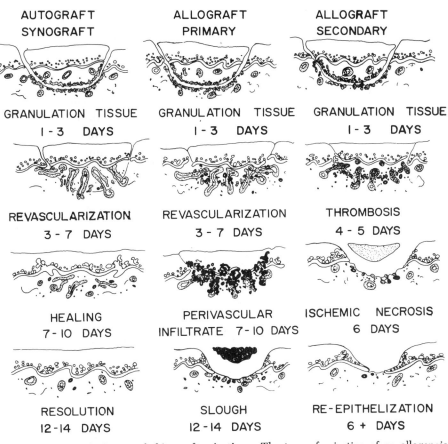

AUTOGRAFT   ALLOGRAFT   ALLOGRAFT
SYNOGRAFT   PRIMARY   SECONDARY

GRANULATION TISSUE   GRANULATION TISSUE   GRANULATION TISSUE
I - 3 DAYS   I - 3 DAYS   I - 3 DAYS

REVASCULARIZATION   REVASCULARIZATION   THROMBOSIS
3 - 7 DAYS   3 - 7 DAYS   4 - 5 DAYS

HEALING   PERIVASCULAR   ISCHEMIC NECROSIS
7 - I0 DAYS   INFILTRATE 7 - I0 DAYS   6 DAYS

RESOLUTION   SLOUGH   RE - EPITHELIZATION
12 - 14 DAYS   12 - 14 DAYS   6 + DAYS

Fig. 14–8. **Stages of skin graft rejection.**   The type of rejection of an allogeneic skin graft depends upon the degree of immune reactivity. An autograft or synograft will "take," i.e., survive and heal into the grafted site. An allograft to an unsensitized individual will be rejected after a stage of vascularization by a mononuclear cell infiltrate. An allograft to a sensitized recipient will not become vascularized and will be rejected by ischemic necroses within a few days after transplantation. (For details see text)

undergo this process, but remains viable with little or no inflammatory reaction. When a second graft is transplanted from the same genetically unrelated donor who provided the rejected first graft, a more rapid and more vigorous rejection occurs (second-set rejection). For the first 3 days after transplant the second-set graft is handled essentially the same as the first graft. However, vascularization is abruptly halted at 4–5 days, with a sudden onset of ischemic necrosis. Because the graft never becomes vascularized and the blood supply is cut off by the second-set rejection, there is little chance for cellular infiltration to occur. The primary target for the second-set rejection appears to be the capillaries taking part in revascularization. Essentially the same events follow grafting of other solid organs, such as kidney or heart.

ROLE OF DELAYED HYPERSENSITIVITY IN GRAFT REJECTION

Experimental evidence strongly indicates that graft injection is mediated by the cellular type of allergic reaction. This evidence can be summarized as follows: 1) the ability to reject a solid graft with a second-set reaction may be transferred from a sensitized individual to an unsensitized individual with cells, but not with serum, except under unusual circumstances (see below); 2) extracts of donor tissue injected into the skin of a sensitive recipient induce a delayed skin reaction; 3) individuals with depressed cellular reactivity but apparently normal ability to produce antibody (Hodgkin's disease) have prolonged homograft survival; 4) antilymphocyte serum (see Chapter 19) or other agents that affect delayed sensitivity more than humoral antibody are effective in prolonging the survival of homografts.

ROLE OF HUMORAL ANTIBODY IN GRAFT REJECTION

Humoral antibody may contribute to rejection of a tissue allograft or it may interfere with (block) the action of sensitized cells in rejection. Perhaps the first evidence that circulating antibody does play a role in graft rejection was that provided by Stetson (173), who demonstrated an acute necrotic rejection of skin allograft when specific antiserum to the graft was injected directly into the site of the skin graft. The failure of any circulation to be established resulted in complete ischemic necrosis–the white graft reaction.

GRAFT FACILITATION

Humoral antibody may also prolong graft survival. This paradoxical situation was first recognized in the 1930s when it was noted that prior immunization to tumor tissue might increase the incidence and growth of tumors in allogeneic systems (34). This phenomena was termed tumor enhancement (34,97) (see Chapter 20). Later it was noted that grafts of normal tissues would survive longer 1) if the animal was preimmunized in such a way as to produce circulating humoral antibody to allograft antigens rather than delayed hypersensitivity (24), or 2) if humoral antibody was passively transferred to the recipient (135). This effect was termed graft facilitation (196). The enhancement-facilitation effect may suppress other effects of delayed hypersensitivity, such as graft vs host reactions, rejection of fetal tissues by the mother, autoallergic diseases and tumor immunity (55,196) (see below).

The enhancement-facilitation effect of antibody interferes with a potential rejection reaction mediated by sensitized cells. The rejection reaction may be divided into three phases: afferent, central and efferent. Afferent refers to the delivery of antigen to the cells recognizing it; central refers to events following recognition, culminating in production of specifically sensitized cells; efferent refers to the delivery of the sensitized cells to the target tissue, the reaction of those cells with target cell antigens and destruction of the target cell by the sensitized killer cell. The theoretic sites of action of blocking (enhancing-facilitating) antibody are illustrated in Fig. 14–9. At present it is impossible to select one mechanism as the most important;

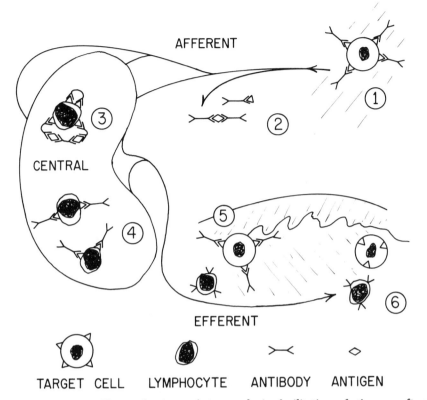

AFFERENT

CENTRAL

EFFERENT

TARGET CELL   LYMPHOCYTE   ANTIBODY   ANTIGEN

Fig. 14–9. Possible mechanisms of immunologic facilitation of tissue grafts. Blocking antibody may interfere with cellular reactions at one of the three stages of induction and expression of delayed hypersensitivity.

A. **Afferent.** Delivery of antigen to potentially responsive immunocompetent cells may be blocked by reaction of humoral antibody with antigen so that 1) the sites are masked and not recognizable or 2) the antigen is catabolized in such a manner as to avoid contact with potentially reactive cells.

B. **Central.** Antibody or antibody–antigen complexes may directly block surface receptors of reactive cells and 3) prevent antigen recognition, or 4) cellular interactions required for the induction of delayed hypersensitivity (67).

C. **Efferent.** Antibody-coated target cells may be 5) protected from attack by sensitized killer cells, or 6) antibody may induce disappearance of target cell surface antigens [modulation] (136).

it is likely that more than one mechanism is operative in a given situation. In particular, blocking antibodies may mask antigenic sites so that they are not available to recognition cells (afferent effect) or to killer cells (efferent effect). Interference with killer cells by masking of target cell antigens is supported by the finding that humoral antibody to a target cell may block immune attack by killer cells in vitro (27). In addition blocking antibodies, or complexes of blocking antibodies and antigen, may react directly with reacting or sensitized cells to block either the induction or expression of delayed hypersensitivity (196).

MORPHOLOGY OF REJECTION IN RENAL TRANSPLANTS

Further insight into the role different hypersensitivity mechanisms may play in graft rejection can be obtained from the morphologic changes observed in rejected renal allografts. Extensive morphologic studies on both dogs and humans are now available. The morphology of first-set rejections in untreated recipients is entirely consistent with cellular mechanisms. The main feature is the accumulation of mononuclear cell infiltrate. Within a few hours small lymphocytes collect around small venules; later many more mononuclear cells appear in the stroma. After a few days these mononuclear cells are much more varied in structure, with many small and large lymphocytes, immature blast cells and more typical mature plasma cells. Invasion of the renal tubular cells occurs, with isolation, separation, and death of these cells occurring in a way very similar if not identical to that described in Figs. 14–3 and 14–4 for tissue culture monolayers and thyroid follicular cells. The interstitial tissue of the rejecting kidney accumulates large quantities of fluid (edema). Finally the afferent arterioles and small arteries become swollen and occluded by fibrin–white cell thrombi. Occasionally these vessels show fibrinoid necrosis and contain immunoglobulins and complement consistent with deposition of antibody–antigen complexes. Therefore the first-set renal allograft rejection by an untreated recipient appears to occur primarily via cellular mechanisms, although there is evidence that humoral antibody may play a role.

A second renal allotransplant from the same donor who provided the first graft is rejected much more rapidly (within 1–3 days). There is little mononuclear cell infiltrate, presumably because adequate circulation necessary for the accumulation of blood mononuclear cells is never established. Morphologically the main features are destruction of peritubular capillaries and fibrinoid necrosis of the walls of the small arteries and arterioles. The glomeruli may contain intercapillary deposition of fibrin clots similar to those observed in the systemic Shwartzman reaction (see Chapter 21). By 24 hours there is widespread tubular necrosis, and the kidney never assumes any functional activity. Perfusion of a renal homotransplant with plasma from an animal hyperimmunized against the donor of the kidney produces a similar reaction. Therefore, the acute second-set rejection of renal allograft appears to be mediated by preformed circulating antibodies. This type of acute rejection of a renal allograft has been observed in humans when grafting was attempted across ABO blood group types. A renal allograft from a B or A donor to an O recipient resulted in a complete failure of circulation in the graft, with distention and thrombosis of afferent arterioles and glomerular capillaries with sludged red cells, presumably owing to the action of cytotoxic anti-blood-group antibodies upon blood group antigens located in the vasculature of the grafted kidney.

LATE REJECTION

Immunosuppressive therapy (see Chapter 19) is widely used to postpone allograft .rejection, and the use of immunosuppressive agents has resulted in a prolonged survival of human renal allografts (23). Such therapy appears to be effective in suppressing the development of rejection but does not prevent later rejection. Some patients with renal allografts have now survived for several years; however, rejection may still occur. Morphologically the major finding in such late rejection kidneys is a marked intimal proliferation and scarring of the walls of medium-sized arteries. The appearance is much like that of healed or late-stage polyarteritis nodosa. Unless proof otherwise is obtained, it must be concluded that such late rejections are the result of the antibody-mediated toxic complex reaction. The same humoral antibodies that block delayed hypersensitivity and facilitate graft survival may eventually cause the late rejection of the kidney due to a different effect (toxic complex reaction).

ORIGINAL DISEASE FACTORS IN RENAL TRANSPLANTS

An important factor in the survival of a renal transplant is the original disease which caused renal failure. Those recipients whose renal failure resulted from glomerulonephritis tend to develop glomerulonephritis in the transplanted kidney as well. This glomerulonephritis in the transplanted kidney appears due to the continued presence of circulating antibody in the blood of the recipient that reacts with glomerular antigens. This supports the concept that some cases of poststreptococcal glomerulonephritis are caused by production of antibodies that react directly with glomerular antigens, not with streptococcal antigen deposited on the membranes (see page 184).

DONOR-RECIPIENT MATCHING IN TRANSPLANTATION

Although immunosuppression has prolonged human graft survival, the results are not, as yet, satisfactory. Tissue matching of recipient and donor combined with less vigorous immunosuppression may be the most advantageous approach (182,195).

Histocompatibility antigens are those cellular determinants specific for each individual of a species that are recognized by genetically different individuals of the same species when attempts are made to transfer or transplant cellular material from one individual to another (2,3). Identical twins are the only known human individuals who share all histocompatibility antigens. Perhaps the best studied example of histocompatibility antigens is the ABO blood group system. The A and B antigens are found not only on erythrocytes but also on other tissue cells. Therefore, no attempt to transfer solid organs from one individual to another should be made across a known AB blood group difference. However, other histocompatibility antigens are obviously important, as matching of the ABO or other erythrocyte antigen systems between donor and recipient is not enough to provide a compatible relation.

During the 1960s many attempts were made to develop tests for histocompatibility antigens and matching tests for potential donors and recipients (2). Tests that have been used to select organ donors include in vivo tests: the third man test and normal lymphocyte transfer test, and in vitro: the mixed lymphocyte culture reaction (MLR) and the analysis and matching of histocompatibility antigens by serologic tests. The in vitro systems are not only useful for matching donors and recipients of grafts but provide a means of evaluating immunologic recognition and its significance.

Third-Man Test

This test (212) depends upon the rate of rejection of skin grafts from a series of skin donors by an unrelated individual who has been sensitized to the histocompatibility antigens of a prospective graft recipient. If the prospective recipient and one of the skin graft donors share antigens, the "third man" rejects the skin graft of the donor in a second-set rejection. However, the third man recognizes only antigens in common, not antigens that are different, between donor and recipient. The third man can be used to test compatibility for only one recipient; he cannot be used more than once because he becomes sensitized to antigens of each of the skin graft donors. These and ethical considerations make the third-man test unsuitable for any use.

Normal Lymphocyte Transfer Test

This test (74) depends upon the intensity of a skin inflammatory reaction occurring within 2 days of injection of washed peripheral blood lymphocytes from a prospective recipient into the skin of a prospective donor. The reaction presumably measures a graft-versus-host reaction (see below) in which the injected lymphocytes recognize histocompatibility antigens. Therefore, a minimal or negative reaction indicates a good histocompatibility match between donor and recipient. However, this test is not feasible on practical and ethical grounds. First, some reaction of the prospective donor against the lymphocytes of the prospective recipient appears to occur (a host-versus-graft reaction), and second, the transfer of cellular material from one individual to another may permit the transfer of viral hepatitis. The above in vivo tests are not used routinely for histocompatibility matching due to difficulties in interpretation, possible clinical complications and inconvenience in performing the test. The in vitro tests not only offer distinct advantages in methodology and interpretation but have permitted more detailed analysis of the major histocompatibility locus of man.

LYMPHOCYTE-DEFINED HISTOCOMPATIBILITY ANTIGENS

The mixed-lymphocyte reaction test [MLR] (11) is based on the observation that cultures of mixtures of lymphocytes from two genetically different individuals produce transformed immature blast cells that synthesize DNA. The degree of stimulation can generally be correlated with the degree of histocompatibility difference between the lymphocyte donors while the lymphocytes of both are still alive. This is a two-way test (a cross-match test) because the lymphocytes interact with each other. The test can be made one-way by killing the lymphocytes of one of the donors by radiation or by preventing the response of one set of lymphocytes by treatment with an antimetabolite, mitomycin C. In this way an estimation of a potential recipient (living cells) to a potential donor (treated cells) can be made. Although it was first suspected that MLR reactions depended upon the antigens defined by humoral antibodies (see HL-A Antigens below), it is now known that initiation of a mixed lymphocyte culture reaction is not dependent upon HL-A differences but other nonserologically defined structures that are more important (12,185). The genetic control of these MLR "antigens" is closely linked to control of the HL-A antigens (see below). These "antigens" have been termed lymphocyte-defined antigens because reaction of cellular antigens with living lymphocytes is required for identification. The cell that responds in the MLR is a T cell, therefore the recognition of MLR antigens requires T cell receptors of some kind (185). The stimulator cell, containing the antigen to which the responding T cell reacts, is a B cell. There is some, although not yet satisfactory, correlation between the degree of stimulation in mixed lymphocyte cultures and survival and function of solid tissue grafts.

SEROLOGICALLY DEFINED HISTOCOMPATIBILITY ANTIGENS

These antigens (2,3,204) are serologically defined cell membrane components which are recognized during allograft rejection and are directly related to the rejection reaction. The identification of histocompatibility antigens in the laboratory depends upon the serologic recognition of histocompatibility antigens on lymphocytes. Most tissue antigens appear to be shared by lymphocytes and solid tissue. The identification of a given antigen on a lymphocyte can be determined by the ability of an antiserum to react with the antigen, causing agglutination of lymphocytes containing the antigen or, in the presence of complement, causing the death of the lymphocytes. Lymphocytotoxicity is the method of choice (2,195).

Antihistocompatibility antisera that reacted with lymphocytes were recognized as long as 50 years ago, but the significance of such antibodies in regard to histocompatibility was not apparent until recently. Antibodies in human sera to human lymphocytes are found in patients with certain diseases (see Chapter 11), in multiparous women and in patients receiving multiple blood transfusions. These latter situations suggest genetically controlled differences in antigenic specificities among human individuals (allotypy). In the 1950s the reaction patterns of such antisera with lymphocytes from a number of different individuals were revealed. For instance, some antisera reacted with lymphocytes from essentially the same donors in a panel (e.g., 20 of 50 donors) while other antisera reacted with the lymphocytes of 20 different donors. The reaction patterns observed were extremely complicated and, it seemed, unresolvable. However, in the early 1960s Van Rood introduced computer analysis of the reaction patterns (195), a method that was soon adopted by others. This resulted in resolution of the reaction patterns of many different antisera. In the mid-1960s a number of individuals who had been testing such antisera held a series of conferences at which many of the problems involving detection techniques and reaction patterns were compared. The result was an example of the contribution that can be made to scientific understanding by unselfish cooperation of different investigators.

GENETICS OF HISTOCOMPATIBILITY ANTIGENS

It is now generally accepted that human histocompatibility antigens, comprising approximately 40 different specificities, are controlled by an allelic pair of autosomal cistrons termed the HL-A system (2,3,195,204).

The term cistron, a linear array of codons required for the synthesis of a single polypeptide chain, is used even though it is not yet clear whether the specificities under consideration are in one or more polypeptide chains (see below). Each cistron contains the information for two HL-A antigens, so that within a given family a given pair of specificities is inherited en bloc (3,195,204). The array of 42 specificities has been divided into a first and second segregant series [Table 14–1] (3,130,195,204). A third locus (Aj) may also be present (185). Each cistron contains information for one specificity in each series. A given individual can express a maximum of two specificities in each segregant series. For example, an individual may have one cistron coding for 2 and 5 and an allelic cistron coding for 1 and 7; 1 is the allelic specificity of 2, and 7 is the allelic specificity of 5. The situation is similar to the Gm specificities, Gm 1 and Gm 17 (see Genetics Analysis of Human Gm Allotypes, Chapter 5. The term *haplotype* has been applied to the pair of specificities controlled by one cistron of the HL-A system (2). Some of the specificities previously thought to be entities can be subdivided into two or more specificities. For example, in HL-A9, W23 and W24 are the narrowest specificities detected serologically but are part of larger genetic unit specificity HL-A9. The narrow specificities are termed *private* while the *broader* specificities are termed *public* (35,130). The private specificities are

TABLE 14–1
Two Segregant Series of HL-A Antigens and
Estimated Frequency in Caucasoid Populations

First (LA)		Second (four)	
HL-A1	0.16	HL-A5	0.04
HL-A2	0.34	HL-A7	0.16
HL-A3	0.17	HL-A8	0.13
HL-A9	0.10	HL-A12	0.16
W23 (HL-A 9.1)		HL-A13	0.01
W24 (HL-A 9.2)		HL-A14	0.01
HL-A10	0.10	HL-A17	0.03
W25 (HL-A 10.1)		HL-A27	0.05
W26 (HL-A 10.2)		W5	0.07
HL-A11	0.05	W10	0.11
HL-A28	0.05	W15	0.10
W19	0.07	W16	0.01
W29 (W 19.1)	0.04	W18	0.02
W30 (W 19.3)		W21	0.02
W31 (W 19.4)	0.03	W22	0.02
W32 (W 19.5)		407	0.01
		TT	0.01
		Sabell	0.01
		JA(KSO)	0.01
Blank	0.03*	Blank	0.03*

For details see reference 185.
  * Frequency of undetected HL-A specificities. Any given chromosome contains information for one specificity in column 1 and one specificity in column 2. A given individual may have from 2–4 HL-A specificities, although most individuals have 4.

probably controlled by single cistrons and present on single HL-A molecules, while public specificities may be controlled by linked cistrons essentially always inherited as a unit and shared by several HL-A molecules.

The number of possible HL-A genotypes possible in a total population may be calculated from the formula

$$\frac{n(n+1)}{2}$$

when n is the number of possible haplotypes. As shown in Table 14–1, there are 13 private determinants in the first series and 19 in the second. Allowing for one blank allele at each locus, 14×20, or 280 different haplotypes are possible. With $n = 280$, the number of genotypes for the two segregant series is 39,340. In addition, if a possible third segregant series contains 5 possible alleles, then 980,700 different genotypes are possible (185). Thus the chances of completely matching two unrelated individuals is about one in a million. However, some alleles occur more frequently in some populations: HL-A1 and HL-A8 in Caucasoid populations, W21 in American Indians and HL-A13 and W22 in Oceanic populations (185).

The distribution of cistrons within a family dictates that only four combinations of HL-A antigens occur among siblings (2). Each parent has an allelic pair of cistrons controlling a haplotype made up of two HL-A antigens, one from each series. If the cistrons are designated AB for one parent and CD for the other parent, the four possible cistron combinations in their children are AC, AD, BC, and BD. Thus, in a family of five children of the same parents at least two children must have identical HL-A cistrons.

HISTOCOMPATIBILITY TESTING USING SEROLOGICALLY DEFINED (HL-A) ANTIGEN AND LYMPHOCYTE-DEFINED (MLR) ANTIGENS

It was once hoped that the HL-A antigens could provide a means of identifying individuals who had similar or identical tissue antigens and who would not reject tissue grafts. Using skin grafts, it was observed that grafts between identical twins would survive indefinitely, grafts between unrelated HL-A nonidentical individuals being rejected at about 10 days. Grafts between HL-A identical unrelated individuals lasted only slightly longer than those between HL-A nonidentical unrelated individuals, while grafts between HL-A identical siblings survived 20–40 days. Clearly more than HL-A antigen matching is required to select a histocompatable donor (3). At least three other factors must be considered: 1) other HL-A loci, 2) minor histocompatibility loci (non-HL-A antigens), and 3) the lymphocyte-defined antigens responsible for the mixed lymphocyte reaction in vitro.

The existence of serologically detectable HL-A antigens in a third segregant series is likely (3,204). The presence of a third HL-A locus adds an additional multiple to the problem of tissue matching (see above). Since standard tissue typing (see below) has not taken into account this possibility, matches presently classified as identical indicate only identity at the first two HL-A loci, so that nonidentity at the third locus might explain some of the lack of correlation of matching to graft survival (185).

Transplantation studies in mice (171) have resulted in the concept of strong and weak histocompatibility antigens. At least 11 histocompatibility systems have been identified in the mouse. One of these, the H-2 system, appears to be analogous to the HL-A system of man. It is termed the strong histocompatibility system because organ grafts between individual mice differing in antigenic specificities controlled by the H-2 systems evoke strong rejection reactions. If organ donor and recipient are matched for the H-2 system, but differ in one of the other systems, rejection is not as rapid or severe. Therefore, these histocompatibility antigen systems are called weak. It is apparent that weak histocompatibility systems are also present in man, but remain to be defined. The evidence regarding weak histocompatibility antigens indicates that differences in these systems can be more readily overcome by immunosuppressive therapy than can differences in strong histocompatibility antigens.

The lymphocyte-defined MLR "antigens" described above also play an important role in matching. In HL-A identical siblings, it is likely that MLR antigens are also matched, because the MLR cistron is closely linked to the serologically defined HL-A cistron. The degree of reactivity in MLRs is usually closely related to the degree of HL-A disparity and were once thought to be measuring the same genetic difference (4). However, the MLRs of most HL-A identical, unrelated individuals give significant stimulation, although to a lesser extent than HL-A nonidentical control cells. In addition, stimulation of MLRs have been observed with HL-A identical siblings at a frequency of about 1%. The most likely explanation is that MLRs are controlled by a separate genetic locus closely linked to the HL-A loci. In fact, studies of families where recombination between HL-A1 and HL-A2 have occurred indicate that the MLR cistron is located between HL-A1 and HL-A2 (185). Therefore, matching in the human major histocompatibility locus requires HL-A identity as well as negative mixed lymphocyte cultures, a situation that occurs very rarely in unrelated individuals. This explains the observation that grafts between HL-A identical siblings (presumably also MLR negative) survive much better than grafts between HL-A identical unrelated individuals.

The clinical experience in regard to HL-A matching and renal graft survival is disappointing (130). A widely used system of grading a histocompatibility match between donor and recipient is that of Terasaki (2,182),

TABLE 14-2
Grading System for Tissue Matching

Grade	Description
A	Identical antigens
B	No antigens in donor that are not found in recipient
C	Donor has one antigen not found in recipient
D	Donor has more than one antigen not found in recipient*
E	Donor and recipient have a mismatch in both alleles of the HL-A cistron*
F	Positive cross-match between donor and recipient†

* Donor and recipient could have two HL-A antigen differences at the same allele, yet have one shared allele.
† Recipient contains antibody-to-donor erythrocytes.

presented in Table 14–2. The results of studies of related (particularly sibling), and unrelated donors indicate that survival of allografts from related donors is significantly better; grafts from sibling donors who are HL-A grade A (identical) do exceptionally well (2). However, close correlation of the Terasaki grade and survival of unrelated donor organs has not been found in most studies. There are a number of theoretical and technical reasons for this (129). The theoretical reasons have been described above, i.e., nontyped HL-A antigens, MLR antigens and minor histocompatibility antigens. The major technical problem is that HL-A typing of lymphocytes from cadaver donors is difficult and many errors may result. In centers where lymphocyte typing is carefully done, kidneys from matched donors function better, provoke fewer episodes of acute rejection, and survive longer than grafts from poorly matched donors (2).

Typing antisera are now compared at various lymphocyte-typing centers and the specificity of reactions verified. A reference bank of living donors of lymphocytes for a typing panel is required. Reference antisera can be obtained from the Collaborative Program in Transplantation and Immunology, National Institutes of Health, Bethesda, Maryland.

ISOLATION AND CHARACTERIZATION OF HL-A ANTIGENS

The nature of HL-A antigens is under intense study (152). In particular many attempts have been and are being made to extract antigen-containing molecules from lymphocytes and other cells and to characterize those molecules (134). Various methods, including the use of proteolytic enzymes, have resulted in the extraction of a polypeptide material with a molecular weight of 30,000 to 50,000. There is little doubt that HL-A antigens are polypeptide in nature. Small substitutions in the primary amino acid sequence could account for the different HL-A specificities as is the case for Ig allotypes (153). Progress in clearly defining the chemical nature of HL-A antigens has been slow due in part to the lack of selective procedures that will dissolve the antigenic molecules but not contaminating substances, and, in part, to the lack of specific in vitro assays for HL-A activity (152). Soluble extracts of donor tissue will induce delayed type skin reactions in sensitized recipients and block HL-A lymphocytotoxic test specifically (95). It is not clear if one (or more than one) polypeptide chain is present. Isolation and characterization of HL-A antigen would not only aid our understanding of the biology and genetics of transplantation, but also permit experimental manipulation, such as an attempt to induce tolerance to graft antigens.

MODULATION OF HL-A ANTIGENS

The effect of anti-HL-A sera upon the location of surface HL-A determinants demonstrates that HL-A determinants are mobile and that the specificities present are different molecules. Redistribution and capping of HL-A determinants on human lymphocytes occurs as a result of reactions with anti-HL-A sera. This modulation of HL-A occurs independently; anti-HL-A1 will cause redistribution of HL-A1 but will not affect HL-A8 or other HL-A determinants present on the cell surface.

HL-A AND B2 MICROGLOBULIN

The genetic control of immunoglobulin structure is not linked to the major histocompatibility system but a peculiar protein with properties similar to immunoglobulin, $\beta2$ microglobulin, may be closely associated with HL-A molecules. $\beta2$ microglobulin, a single polypeptide chain of about 100 amino acids, is present on the surface of human lymphocytes (77,144). Antisera to $\beta2$ microglobulin produces redistribution and capping of the latter on the lymphocyte surface. This treatment also removes all of the HL-A antigens on the cell surface (185). The loss of all HL-A antigens induced by anti-$\beta2$-microglobulin sera suggests that $\beta2$ microglobulin is bound in the cell membrane to the polypeptide molecules of each of the HL-A specificities. The role of $\beta2$ microglobulin as a receptor and the relationship of the structure cistrons of this protein to those of the HL-A proteins remains to be determined. (See page 40).

ANTI-HL-A AND THE MLR

Antisera to HL-A determinants will inhibit mixed lymphocyte reactions, suggesting that serologically defined (SD) determinants may play a role in lymphocyte-defined (LD) reactions. There are three possible explanations: 1) SD determinants are located close to LD determinants and the antiserum blocks by steric effects, 2) LD and SD determinants are on the same molecule and LD determinants are directly blocked or modulated by antisera to SD determinants or 3) the antisera used while only detecting SD determinants in the in vitro tests actually have in addition separate antibody activity to lymphocyte-defined determinants. Since SD determinants are individually modulated if LD determinants are associated with the SD determinants, antisera that react with only one HL-A specificity should not modulate those LDA-associated with other HL-As. Although poorly defined, antisera that may recognize LD determinants have been reported (185).

HL-A ANTIGENS AND DISEASE ASSOCIATION

Certain HL-A phenotypes are found associated with some human diseases (130). A counterpart of the HL-A system of man is the H2 system of the mouse, which is linked to the ability of some mouse strains to respond to certain antigens, i.e., the immune response (Ir) gene (see page 53). The relationship of HL-A phenotypes with human diseases suggests that similar Ir-type genes are linked to the HL-A system. A few scattered reports suggested a higher frequency of certain HL-A specificities in patients with leukemia or lymphoma, but further studies have failed to confirm the earlier observations. Therefore, it is not possible to state that there is a definite association of certain HL-A types with these diseases (130). More convincing data indicates higher frequencies of certain HL-A types with immunopathologic diseases. For instance, HL-A8 and HL-A15 may be increased in systemic lupus erythematosis; HL-A1 and HL-A8 with active hepatitis, myasthenia gravis and adult coeliac disease; and there is a very high incidence of W27 in patients with ankylosing spondylitis (28,163), Reiter's disease (30), acute anterior uvitis (29) and juvenile rheumatoid arthritis (149). The W27 specificity may be linked to an immune response cistron that influences a response to an infectious agent or to self antigens. An association between the haplotype HL-A2-12 and atopic sensitization to ragweed antigen was found in a large family; study of three generations provided a genetic map order of HL-A first locus, HL-A second locus and IrE (immune response to ragweed antigen E), so that IrE is considered as part of the major histocompatibility locus (26). An increased prevalence of HL-A13 and W17 is associated with psoriasis; and W5 with retinoblastoma (185). Associations of HL-A specificities with other forms of cancer are not consistently found (185). Further studies will most likely clarify an association of the serologically defined HL-A antigens and the lymphocyte-defined MLR antigens to different normal and abnormal immune responses in man as has been defined in the mouse (see page 53) and should result in a more complete genetic map for the major histocompatibility system of man.

BIOLOGIC SIGNIFICANCE OF THE MAJOR HISTOCOMPATIBILITY SYSTEM OF MAN

The major histocompatibility system of man must provide some type of surveillance or regulatory function. It is impossible to eliminate all histocompatibility antigens from the cell surface and maintain survival (102). Jerne postulated that lymphocytes have receptors that are directed against all histocompatibility antigens of other individuals within his species as well as receptors for his own (self) antigens. The self receptors are important in ontogeny to permit normal embryogenesis but are eliminated as immunologically functional so that the individual is tolerant to self antigens. On the other hand, cells with receptors for nonself antigens are stimulated to proliferate during ontogeny. Mutations of the cistrons controlling these receptors occur during this proliferation, leading to the production of millions of lymphocytes with receptors for different antigenic specificities (93). However, since no linkage between HL-A and immunoglobulin structural genes exists, it is difficult to explain how mutations in the major histocompatibility system could affect recognition by antibody. Thus Jerne's theory might explain generation of diversity of T cells but not B cells.

Burnet suggests that the major histocompatibility system prevents an individual from being invaded by cells from another individual (32). For example, cancer cells of one individual cannot survive in another individual because of histocompatibility differences. In addition, histocompatibility differences may prevent the mother from being invaded by fetal tissues and the fetus from being invaded by maternal cells (see below). Histocompatibility similarities may be required for cellular cooperation in induction of the immune response (see page 48) and somehow provide a mechanism to insure that T cells and B cells of a given individual can recognize each other for cooperation, yet bear receptors that recognize foreign structure at the same time.

PRESENT STATUS OF TRANSPLANTATION IN MAN

The initial success of solid tissue grafts indicates that the surgical techniques required for such procedures are well in hand. Most experience in human allografting has involved the kidney, and the results are now good enough to indicate that allografting is the treatment of choice for many types of renal failure (16). Clearly the use of sibling or parent donors is far superior for graft survival. However, most kidneys come from cadaver donors. Although the survival rate for recipients of unrelated cadaver donors is not as good as that of related donors, cadaver donors are much easier to obtain. It is also questionable whether a living relative should be asked to donate one of his kidneys. Fortunately for the recipient, a willing and related living donor is often available. For renal transplants done in 1968, 60% of sibling donor kidneys, 50% of parent and 30% of cadaver kidneys remained functional after five years (16). It is to be anticipated that better matching of cadaver kidneys and recipients will improve the survival rates of cadaver renal grafts.

Transplantation of other solid organs, i.e., heart, lung, liver and pancreas have received great publicity but the long-term results are not encouraging (5). The number of heart transplants has fallen from a peak notoriety of 101 in 1968 to 17 in 1972 (5,80). Clearly transplantation of the heart is not acceptable therapy at the present time and is restricted to a few experimental centers. The transplantation of solid organs other than the kidney has failed as much from physiologic and surgical difficulties as from immunologic rejection. The kidney is a simple organ to transplant, has considerable reserve in that, if damaged, a portion of the organ will maintain function, and patients with temporary renal failure or rejection reaction can be maintained on dialysis until measures can be taken to reverse rejection. The transplantation of bone marrow will be discussed below.

Because of the nature of the data and the presence of multiple uncontrolled variables, many of the results reported on human organ transplantation are uninterpretable. However, one thing appears clear: The survival of the recipient is dependent less upon exact tissue matching, organ source, choice of immunosuppressive treatment, or even surgical skill than upon careful pretransplant work-up and conditioning, and thorough and painstaking posttransplant follow-up of the patient by his physicians.

GRAFT-VERSUS-HOST REACTIONS

Graft-vs-host reactions result when immunologically competent cells from an allogeneic or xenogeneic donor are transferred to a recipient whose own immune responsiveness has been destroyed (irradiation) or is immature [newborn] (168). The transferred lymphoid cells colonize, recognize and react to the histocompatibility antigenic differences in the recipient. This reaction results in a characteristic runt syndrome or wasting disease. Graft-vs-host reactions become important clinically when grafts of lymphoid tissue, such as bone marrow or thymus, which contain immunologically reactive cells, are made.

Bone Marrow Transplantation

Bone marrow grafts have been used to treat patients with aplastic anemia (failure of blood cell production), in immune deficiencies and in patients with leukemia treated with irradiation (162). The use of bone marrow in immune deficiency diseases is discussed on page 309. With careful matching and follow-up, good results are obtained in about half the cases of aplastic anemia, if an HL-A identical sibling donor is used (174). Irradiation leads to failure of blood cell production and reduction in immune function (111). The degree and type of immune deficiency depends upon the dose of radiation given (180). Experiments on animals demonstrate that although doses sufficient to cause significant reduction in leukemia cell mass frequently result in death by infection, this can be circumvented by transfer of bone marrow from a healthy donor (40). However, unless a syngeneic donor is used, a fatal graft-versus-host reaction is the usual result. In some situations a fatal outcome can be avoided; the graft surviving, with the recipient eventually having both donor and host lymphoid cells (radiation chimera).

Clinically, bone marrow transplantation following radiation treatment of leukemia and aplastic anemia has had a limited success (39,174). Unless an identical twin is available, some degree of graft-versus-host reactivity seems inevitable (162,174). Efforts in improving bone marrow transplantation have centered on efforts to reduce the severity of the graft-versus-host reaction, yet provide sufficient bone marrow stem cells to reconstitute the irradiated recipient. Techniques used have included HL-A matching (39,120,162,184), particularly using HL-A-matched siblings (184), the use of mixtures of cells from a number of related donors with the hope that the most compatible donor cells will survive (120), the administration of immunosuppressive agents such as cyclophosphamide (169) or antilymphocyte serum (64,192), the fractionation of cells in an attempt to eliminate the immunologically reactive cells that would produce the graft-versus-host reaction (193), or the use of preserved autologous bone marrow obtained during a remission (121). None of these procedures can be considered satisfactory as yet, although some long-term remissions have been obtained (39,120,162,184). In most remissions a transient graft-versus-host-reaction occurs and the treated individual demonstrates both host and donor cells after the reaction, establishing radiation chimerism (120,184). A particularly interesting and perplexing observation has been that in a few cases of leukemia treated by whole body irradiation and bone marrow from an HL-A-matched sibling of the opposite sex, the donor's blood cells became established but developed leukemia (183). This could be due to 1; excessive antigenic stimulation of donor cells in a foreign environment, 2) and abnormal homeostatic mechanism in the recipient that also applies to donor cells, 3) fusion of donor and recipient cells resulting in transfer of donor chromosome markers to recipient leukemic cells or 4) transmission of an agent (oncogenic virus) from host to donor cells (56). Clearly use of bone marrow transplantation is clinically still an experimental procedure but preliminary results indicate that careful control of this procedure may result in a satisfactory therapy for leukemia.

GRAFT-HOST RELATIONS IN PREGNANCY

Except for matings within inbred strains of animals, a fetus in utero is a graft of tissue containing transplantation antigens to which the mother can react. Since half of the fetal genetic endowment is contributed by the father, the fetus is a hemiallogeneic graft. Paternal histocompatibility antigens are present on spermatozoa and are represented in fetal tissue (50). In spite of this potential for immune rejection as an allograft, the fetus is rarely affected (17). The fetus survives a longer time in the uterus than other foreign tissue grafts, and gestation is terminated by nonimmune events. The means by which the fetus avoids immune rejection is not fully understood. The following mechanisms have been proposed (17,18):

Paternal antigens are not present on embryonal or fetal tissues. This is certainly not true. Although histocompatibility antigens are present on postnatal cells in higher amounts than on fetal cells, tissue antigens have been demonstrated on embryonal and fetal cells at essentially all stages of development (50) and are present in sufficient amounts to be killed by sensitized lymphocytes in vitro (84) and in vivo (17).

The fetus is not rejected because half of its histocompatibility antigens are common with those of the mother. This is also an untrue statement, as a mother will reject skin grafts of fetal skin and surrogate mothers will support ova from unrelated parents when transplanted in utero.

The mother is tolerant of fetal tissues. While it is true that pregnancy does not induce transplantation immunity in that skin grafts of the paternal strain are not rejected with a second set reaction after delivery of F1 offspring, it is unlikely that the mother is rendered tolerant of fetal antigens during pregnancy. Fetal or paternal skin grafts will be rejected normally even though transplanted at the time of a normal pregnancy. Other evidence (see below) indicates that the mother does mount an immune response to fetal antigens.

The uterus is an immunologically privileged site. Skin grafts from F1 or paternal strains will be rejected if placed in the uterus of an histoincompatible female even if the recipient is hormonally prepared and the uterus has undergone a decidual reaction (i.e., the uterus is hormonally prepared for acceptance of a fertilized ovum). In addition, delayed hypersensitivity reactions can be elicited in the uterus by injection of antigen into the uterus of a sensitized animal.

The mother does not become immunized to fetal tissues during pregnancy. This also is unlikely as mothers will develop antibodies to fetal antigens; one of the common sources of HL-A typing sera is multiparous women. In addition, a significant hypertrophy of the draining lymph nodes occurs during pregnancy. Furthermore, protection is afforded to the fetus even if the mother is preimmunized to fetal tissues by injection of paternal antigens or rejection of paternal skin graft prior to pregnancy.

The placenta serves as a barrier to immunization and to maternal immune cells. The fetus is contained in a fluid-filled cyst of fetal origin, the amniotic sac, which separates the mother from the fetus except at the attachment of the placenta. At this point fetal tissue, the trophoblast, actually invades the endometrial wall of the uterus and comes into direct contact with the maternal circulation. Trophoblastic tissue, although containing histocompatibility antigens in low amounts (50), is not rejected if transplanted into sites outside the placenta. In fact the developing fetus may actually be maintained in the abdominal cavity outside of the uterus until nonimmune complications develop (ectopic pregnancy). Trophoblastic cells do not contain H, A or B blood group antigens; the endothelium of the vessels of the placenta and umbilical cord have only the basic H structure (177,178). In contrast, the endothelial cells of the fetus have a high amount of these antigens (178). The lack of ABH antigens in trophoblast prevents attack by maternal AB isoantibodies. The trophoblastic cells contain a large amount of glycocalyx, a cell coating of carbohydrate that masks transplantation antigens and repels lymphocytes (50). However, small numbers of maternal lymphocytes do cross the placenta, but evidently not in sufficient numbers to effect rejection of the fetus. That the placenta may contain lymphocytes that might attack the fetus is supported by the finding that placental size is increased in proportion to the degree of immunity of the mother to the fetus. It is possible that the placental tissue may contain histocompatibility antigens distributed in such a way that specifically sensitized lymphocytes react with placental tissue with minimal affect on placental function, but are prevented from passing into the fetal circulation. Maternal lymphocytes that do cross the placenta may not be reactive to fetal tissue antigens.

The production of blocking antibody prevents cellular reactivity to fetal antigens (196). It is well known that mothers will produce normal antibody to fetal antigens during pregnancy. While in general it has been impossible to induce a graft-vs-host reaction by immunization of the mother to fetal antigens, such runting can be observed under special circumstances. Fisher females who rejected DA skin grafts produced runted (graft-vs-host disease) offspring if mating to DA fathers took place at the time of rejection of the graft. If rejection of the graft took place two weeks prior to mating, runting was not observed. The runting is believed to be due to the presence of large numbers of lymphoid cells sensitized to fetal antigens at a time when no humoral antibody is present and the fetus is particularly susceptible to a graft-vs-host reaction; rejection of a graft two weeks prior to mating permits cellular sensitivity to decline and blocking antibody to rise so that the fetus is protected (55). Blocking factors have been described in mouse pregnancy sera which protect embryonal cells in vitro against the action of cytotoxic lymphocytes (84).

The early development of immune competence by the fetus in utero may provide a protective response for the immune elimination of the small number of maternal lymphocytes that get across the placenta. Under carefully defined conditions the passive transfer of cells from unrelated strains of mice immunized against the parental strain will produce runting of the offspring while no graft-vs-host reaction occurs in the mother. It is suggested that the passively transferred cells crossed the placenta and produced a graft-vs-host reaction in the fetuses that were not yet sufficiently immunologically competent to reject the specifically sensitized transferred cells; but the mother, who was immunologically mature did reject the transferred cells. In the human most instances of neonatal graft-vs-host disease are associated with an immune deficiency of the fetus. In fact there is speculation that the high incidence of lymphomas in children may be related to production of subclinical runt disease due to maternal lymphocytes that infiltrated the fetus during pregnancy and were not eliminated by an immune response of the fetus. The high incidence of "autoallergic" reactions found in patients with lymphomas and leukemias (42,43) suggests that the individual's lymphoid system may be responding to self antigens; perhaps this represents stimulation of maternally derived sequestered lymphocytes and is a graft-vs-host reaction.

A simple explanation of the mechanism of survival of the fetus under conditions which should provoke a rejection reaction (host-vs-graft) remains unestablished. Mothers do make an immune response to their unborn offspring and products of the immune response do cross the placenta to the fetus. Under certain conditions, this may cause extensive tissue damage and death. However, under normal circumstances adverse effects are rarely observed. The uterus is not a privileged site and the maternal immune system is not significantly abnormal during pregnancy. A combination of factors including the amount of histocompatibility antigens on fetal cells, the properties of the placenta, the effect of blocking (facilitating) antibody and the immune rejection response of the fetus to maternal lymphocytes must provide the fetus with the means of avoiding immune attack by its mother.

DELAYED HYPERSENSITIVITY AND VIRAL INFECTIONS

Delayed hypersensitivity reactions to viral antigens may be either protective by limiting viral infections or destructive by destroying functioning host cells that are expressing viral antigens.

VIRAL EXANTHEMS

It is now generally accepted that delayed hypersensitivity to virus is responsible for the lesions of the viral exanthems. von Pirquet in 1907 observed that the local lesion following smallpox vaccination (vaccinia) consisted of a two-stage reaction (197). Early (first 8 days), there is a papular vesicular lesion due to the growth of the inoculated virus; later (8–14 days) an indurated erythematous reaction (take) follows. The take reaction corresponds to the development of delayed hypersensitivity, since similar lesions appear at the same time on different parts of the body even though the different areas are inoculated with the virus at different times. The development of delayed hypersensitivity is advantageous, as animal experiments have shown that protection against the virus is associated with delayed hypersensitivity, not with circulating antibody, and that the infective virus disappears from the local lesion when the delayed reaction is maximal (21,78). The same concept was considered valid by von Pirquet for other viral exanthems (measles, varicella) in which multiple, disseminated lesions occur as a result of delayed reaction to viruses located at the sites of lesions. There is a suggestion that some of the lesions of the viral exanthems may be caused or contributed to by humoral antibody reacting with viral antigens to produce an Arthus-like reaction in the skin, however delayed hypersensitivity is the major mechanism in most instances.

LYMPHOCYTIC CHORIOMENINGITIS (LCM)

The role of delayed hypersensitivity in producing the lesions of some infectious diseases is exemplified by the viral disease of mice and men, lymphocytic choriomeningitis (89). The introduction of the specific virus in mice uniformly results in a fatal brain infection. Certain features of the experimental disease suggest that the brain lesions are due, not to the presence of the virus itself, but to a delayed hypersensitivity reaction to the viral antigens located in the brain. Intracranial injection of the virus results in much more severe disease than does intracutaneous injection. If a sublethal intracutaneous injection is followed by a lethal intracranial injection, the eventual outcome depends upon the interval between the cutaneous and cranial injections. If the cranial injection follows the cutaneous injection by less than 4 days, the outcome is invariably fatal, and the course of the disease is more rapid than when the virus is given only intracranially. If 7 days intervene between the cranial and cutaneous injections, the animals survive. The interpretation is that the sublethal cutaneous injection produces an immune response to the virus. If immunity is developed (7-day interval) when the cranial injection is administered, a specific delayed-type reaction prevents dissemination and growth of virus. However, if the virus is already distributed before the delayed reaction develops, the reaction of the specifically sensitized cells with the localized virus products the lesions. In the 4-day interval situation, the cutaneous injection initiates the development of delayed sensitivity so that it is partially developed, but not active (in the latent period) when the cranial injection is given. Since the induction of the delayed reactivity is already partially developed, the onset of symptoms occurs earlier than when the induction of the delayed reaction and the cranial injection of the virus occur at the same time. Further evidence that hypersensitivity is the mechanism responsible for the actual production of lesions is that procedures that suppress delayed hypersensitivity (administration of drugs such as amethopterin, x-irradiation, thymectomy at birth, or administration of antilymphocyte serum) markedly suppress the development of the symptoms of lymphocytic choriomeningitis. Some of the mice so treated may remain completely asymptomatic even though viable virus can be isolated from brain tissue. However, these mice may develop immune complex-mediated disease due to the production of humoral antibody to LCM virus and the formation of circulating antibody–antigen complexes.

CANINE DISTEMPER

The relationship of an inadequate or inappropriate immune response to a virus-induced disease is exemplified in a naturally occurring infectious disease of dogs, canine distemper (7). The canine distemper paramyxovirus is closely related to human measles virus and produces a disease in dogs similar to human measles and the related neurologic diseases–acute encephalitis, post infectious encephalitis and subacute sclerosing panencephalitis (SSPE). Canine distemper produces an acute systemic disease from which most animals recover. Following this a certain proportion of the affected animals go on to develop a demyelinating post infectious encephalomyelitis, the pathology of which is similar to experimental allergic encephalomyelitis (see below). The chronic phase of distemper is called "old dog encephalitis" and bears similarities to human SSPE. The distemper virus enters the brain during the acute systemic viremia and viral inclusions can be found in brain cells called glial cells (151). The postinfectious disease develops suddenly after a latent period of several weeks even though it can be assumed that the virus particles are in the brain throughout the latent period (105). Although the role of immunopathologic mechanisms in the disease remains unclear, antibodies to viral antigens and to myelin appear in high titers in the sera of affected dogs. Since the virus does not appear to cause tissue destruction, it is likely that the demyelination is due to sensitized lymphocytes reacting either to viral antigens present in myelinated tissue or to myelin antigens rendered immunogenic from the viral infection. Humoral antibody may play a role in initiating vascular reactions or may actually be protective (i.e., blocking antibody).

VIRAL ENCEPHALITIDES OF MAN

The viral encephalitides of man occur in a variety of forms depending upon the nature of the infecting agent and the type and intensity of the immune response. The disorders are classified as acute, postinfectious, latent, chronic, and slow (138,159,207,213).

In the acute encephalitides (poliomyelitis, rabies, herpes simplex), the virus destroys nerve cells directly in a predictable fashion. The immune response is protective in the sense that it blocks the destructive aspects of the disease by elimination of the virus.

Postinfection encephalomyelitis follows a mild virus infection and is caused by an autoallergic reaction of sensitized cells with myelin, presumably due to the presence of altered host antigen or virus antigen–host myelin combinations (see Autoallergic Diseases, below). The virus alone does not produce significant destruction. Such reactions may follow infections such as mumps, measles, distemper, or vaccination with rabies or vaccinia virus.

Latent viral infections are caused by a change in the relation of the host's immune response to a virus infection that has not produced clinical manifestations, so that clinical symptoms become manifest. This may occur because of an increase or a decrease in the host's immune state. Progressive multifocal leukoencephalopathy occurs in patients whose immune state is lowered (leukemia, lymphoma; see Secondary Immune Deficiencies, Chapter 20). Destruction of brain cells occurs in the absence of significant inflammation. Cytomegalic inclusion disease, a systemic virus infection, also occurs in patients with depressed ability to mount an immune response, e.g., kidney transplant recipients undergoing immunosuppression with drugs. On the other hand, symptoms related to lymphocytic choriomeningitis may be produced in experimental animals with latent infections by increasing their immune response to lymphocytic choriomeningitis. The lesions contain significant inflammatory reaction. Because of an immune response to the virus, infected cells are also destroyed (innocent bystander reaction).

Chronic encephalomyelitis features an irregular protracted course with variation in immune reactivity and brain cell destruction by virus. The condition of subacute sclerosing panencephalitis is believed to be a late manifestation in adults following measles infection in childhood. Affected patients have brain cell inclusions and high antibody titers to measles virus. Some change in the relation between protective immunity and virus infection is believed to occur, but it is not clear whether the allergic reaction or the virus itself is the cause of the destruction. Multiple sclerosis may also be related to a preceding measles infection as MS patients also have abnormally high antibody titers to measles virus (1). However, MS is a chronic remitting disease with the occurrence of repeated attacks while subacute sclerosing panencephalitis (SSPE) is an unremitting progressive disease due to dissemination of a defective yet replicating virus. SSPE is probably due to an inadequate protective immune response to the virus while MS may be caused by a delayed hypersensitivity response to myelin (see below).

Slow virus infections, represented by kuru and Jakob-Creutzfeldt disease (61), have a regular protracted fatal course following a long latent period. These diseases are characterized by abnormal membrane accumulations. The responsible agents have not been characterized, but appear to consist of membrane material with no RNA or DNA component. No inflammatory response or immune reactivity of the host can be demonstrated, the course of the disease being determined by characteristics of the agent. Kuru occurs in certain native tribes of New Guineans. Its incidence has decreased sharply since the ritual cannibalism involving removal of the brain and widespread contamination with tissue containing millions of infective doses of kuru has been discontinued (61). Kuru is caused by the progressive proliferation and dissemination of an agent which provokes no immune response and is normally not infective but becomes so if large amounts of the agent are introduced through the skin.

VIRAL HEPATITIS

Viral hepatitis (inflammation of the liver) is caused by at least two viruses: hepatitis A virus (infectious hepatitis) and hepatitis B virus (serum hepatitis). Although the clinical course and method of transmission of infectious hepatitis is believed to be different from that of serum hepatitis, there is a considerable overlap. The association of a specific virus with hepatitis was made possible by the study of Australia antigen (Au1), now known as hepatitis B antigen (HB Ag) (176). This antigen is detected in the serum of hepatitis patients or antigen carriers by double diffusion-in-agar or other immune reactions. The association with hepatitis was first made when a patient, previously found to be lacking the HB Ag antigen, was found to possess the antigen at the time of development of hepatitis. A systemic survey then demonstrated a high incidence of HB Ag antigen among patients with acute viral hepatitis and disappearance of the antigen upon their clinical recovery. The detection of HB Ag antigen is now being used to confirm the clinical diagnosis of hepatitis. The HB Ag specificity was found to reside in virus-like particles which can be isolated from the serum of hepatitis patients by differential centrifugation. Recently it has been reported that passage of the virus-like particles has resulted in viremia in experimental primates, raising the possibility that antigenic material may be obtainable for active immunization. The passage of viral hepatitis by transfusion (serum hepatitis) may be significantly reduced by screening blood donors for HB Ag (165).

Delayed hypersensitivity reactions to viral antigens expressed on the surface of infected liver cells or to liver cell antigens rendered immunogenic by association with viral particles may be the primary mechanism of liver cell destruction leading to elimination of virus infected cells and survival, or fatal destruction of liver cells (160). The viral antigen may be identified within the liver cells of infected individuals using immunofluorescence (49,91) and viral particles may be obtained from the blood of some patients during active stages of the disease (146,176). The blood bore particles consist mainly of viral coat particles whereas whole viral particles (coat and nucleoprotein core) are rarely found. In the infected cells the capsular antigen is found in the cytoplasm and the core antigen in the nucleus. The major lesion is a destruction of hepatocytes (liver cell necrosis) and a marked infiltration of mononuclear cells. The acute stage may be caused by virus-induced destruction of liver cells but many cells containing viral antigens are not destroyed unless there is an inflammatory cell infiltrate. Chronic active hepatitis may evolve from acute hepatitis or may arise without an acute phase. In particular, the form of chronic active hepatitis associated with Lupus Erythematosis has features consistent with an autoallergic disease (see below). The lesions of chronic active hepatitis are quite similar to those seen in livers undergoing graft rejection and experimental models of viral hepatitis implicate a delayed hypersensitivity mechanism (160).

Both humoral antibody and delayed hypersensitivity play a role in the disease. The liver destruction associated with mononuclear infiltrate is probably due to the action of specifically sensitized cells. Humoral antibody and HB Ag–antibody complexes are present in the sera of patients during or recovering from the disease (166). While humoral antibody may act to neutralize the virus, the presence of HB Ag-Ab complexes may lead to systemic toxic complex disease; polyarteritis has been found in patients with HB Ag-Ab complexes in their sera (66,148) [see page 191].

The passive transfer of antibody to HB Ag has been suggested as a possible therapy for patients with viral hepatitis (147) and a successful result in a pregnant patient with fulminant HB Ag positive hepatitis treated with plasmaphoresis and anti-HB Ag plasma has been reported (112). In summary, the destructive lesions of viral hepatitis are at least partially caused by a cellular reaction to the virus, while protection is effected by humoral antibody which probably acts to prevent spread of the infection from cell to cell. However, circulating HB Ag-Ab complexes may cause systemic immune complex disease.

AUTOALLERGIC DISEASES

The main criterion for classification of a disease process as autoallergic is the demonstration of a damaging effect of an *endogenous immune re-*

sponse to an endogenous antigen [Table 9–2] (15,45,63,200,202). Acquired hemolytic anemia (41), idiopathic thrombocytopenic purpura (14), experimental allergic glomerulonephritis (45,189), and lupus erythematosis are examples. However, most autoallergic diseases are the result of a delayed reaction. Experimentally, lesions are produced by immunizing an individual with constituents of his own tissues. When the hypersensitive state appears, reactions occur where antigen is situated in his tissues (203). So far, lesions have been produced by immunization of animals with lens, uvea, central nervous system myelin, peripheral nervous system myelin, thyroid, adrenal, testes, and (?) salivary gland (200). Antibody has been produced, but no lesions observed, with muscle (heart and skeletal), breast and pancreas. The lesions are irregularly distributed in regions of high antigen concentration (the white matter of the central nervous system in experimental allergic encephalomyelitis). Local inflammatory reactions occur around small veins and consist of lymphocytes, histiocytes, and other mononuclear cells (203). Necrosis, hemorrhage, and polymorphonuclear leptocyte infiltration occur only in very severe reactions and only in some species. Parenchymal destruction is coexistent with inflammation (i.e., demyelination, destruction of uvea pigment). Waksman has stressed that within the involved tissue the lesion distribution is determined by blood-tissue barriers (203). There is a good experimental correlation between the sites at which lesions appear preferentially and the passage of injected large colloids such as trypan blue from the blood into the tissues. Thus, in the testes, the most severe (though not the only) involvement is in the epididymis and the rete testes, both areas provided with numerous veins which permit passage of trypan blue. The experimental autoallergic diseases are of great interest since they provide good models for the human diseases of unknown etiology listed in Table 14–3. The animal diseases in general are chronic relapsing processes, since the antigen is consistently present in the tissues and the hypersensitive state may persist or be boosted from time to time by further immunization. The acute monocyclic disease may result from allergic reactions to viruses (92,98,122) or to combinations of bacterial products and tissues (?L-forms) (9,139). The morphologic similarity of these lesions to the autoallergies is indicated by the fact that the same hypersensitivity response is concerned in the production of lesions in both instances, even though antigens are different.

ENCEPHALOMYELITIS

Experimental allergic encephalomyelitis may be produced by the injection of central nervous system tissue incorporated into complete Freund's adjuvant (138,203). Hind leg paralysis occurs after 2–3 weeks and is associated with a disseminated focal perivascular accumulation of inflammatory cells involving small veins or venules (108). The inflammatory cells, which accumulate within the vessel wall and in the so-called perivascular space, are usually mononuclear, but polymorphonuclear leukocytes may be prominent in very acute reactions. Demyelination occurs in intimate association with the focal vasculitis and most likely is a result of the action of specifically sensitized cells (108); toxic complex activated polychemotaxis may be responsible for acute lesions. The antigen, encepholitogenic protein

TABLE 14–3
Relation of Experimental Autoallergic Diseases to Human Diseases

Experimental disease	Tissue involved	Histologically similar human disease	
		Acute monocyclic	Chronic relapsing
Allergic encephalo-myelitis	Myelin (CNS)	Postinfectious encephalomyelitis	Multiple sclerosis
Allergic neuritis	Myelin (PNS)	Guillain-Barré polyneuritis	
Phacoanaphylactic endophthalmitis	Lens		Phacoanaphylactic endophthalmitis
Allergic uveitis	Uvea	Postinfectious iridocyclitis	Sympathetic ophthalmia
Allergic orchitis	Germinal epithelium	Mumps orchitis	Nonendocrine chronic infertility
Allergic thyroiditis	Thyroglobulin	Mumps thyroiditis	Subacute and chronic thyroiditis
Allergic sialadenitis	Glandular epithelium	Mumps parotitis	Sjögren's syndrome
Allergic adrenalitis	Cortical cells		Cytotoxic contraction of adrenal
Allergic gastritis	Gastric mucosa		Atrophic gastritis
Experimental allergic nephritis	Glomerular membrane	Acute glomerulonephritis	Chronic glomerulonephritis

CNS, central nervous system; PNS, peripheral nervous system.
Modified from Waksman BH: Int Arch Allergy Appl Immunol 14 (Suppl.), 1959

(100), has been studied extensively and the amino acid sequence determined (53,209). The major encepholitogenic determinant is a nonapeptide with the amino acid sequence Phe-Ser-Trp-Ala-Glu-Gly-Gln-Lys, the important amino acids being Trp and Gln (209). The human disease takes three forms: acute hemorrhagic encephalomyelitis, acute disseminated encephalomyelitis, and multiple sclerosis (138).

Acute Hemorrhagic Encephalomyelitis

This is a rare disease which shows necrosis and fibrin deposits within the walls of venules, hemorrhages through the venule walls with intense polymorphonuclear infiltration, and demyelination in areas of the infiltration. This disease is similar to the acute forms of experimental allergic encephalomyelitis, and may be undetected by humoral antibody.

Acute Disseminated Encephalomyelitis

This takes two forms. The form that occurs following rabies antigen injection appears 4–15 days following injection of killed rabies virus and is histologically identical to experimental allergic encephalomyelitis. The lesion is caused by an allergic reaction to the brain tissue used to culture the virus used in the vaccine. This type of vaccine has been replaced by one prepared from duck embryos, and no proved case of postrabiesinoculation encephalomyelitis has been reported after introduction of the new vaccine. The second type of acute disseminated encephalomyelitis occurs after smallpox vaccination or infection with rubella, varicella, or variola. This rare disease is similar to experimental allergic and postrabies-injection encephalomyelitis. Individual cases suggest that acute hemorrhagic encephalomyelitis may progress to acute disseminated encephalomyelitis and then to multiple sclerosis.

Multiple Sclerosis

This may be the end stage or chronic form of the encephalitides. The lesions are multiple, sharply defined gray plaques, measuring up to several centimeters in diameter and composed of microglial cells, lymphocytes, and plasma cells usually located around small veins. At later stages scarring may obscure the small veins, and plaques may be found with no vascular component. Complement-fixing antibody is found in both the experimental and the human disease, but its titer is not related to the severity or course of the disease. A serum antibody capable of causing demyelination of myelin-containing cells in tissue culture has been reported. The titers of this antibody are not related to the titers of complement-fixing antibody in the same serum, and it is possible that the in vitro demyelinating antibody may play a role in demyelination in vivo, but this has not yet been established. There is some evidence to support the concept that the complement-fixing antibody may actually protect against development of the disease. Experimental allergic encephalomyelitis may be consistently transferred with cells but not with antiserum. The relationship of preceding viral infections to multiple sclerosis and other demyelinating diseases has been discussed above. Viral infections may produce an immunizing event leading to cellular sensitivity to myelin antigens.

NEURITIS

Experimental allergic neuritis is induced by the injection of peripheral nervous tissue in complete Freund's adjuvant (202). The lesions are limited to the peripheral nervous tissue; none are found in the central nervous system. The experimental disease is similar to a demyelinating syndrome that follows infection with certain microorganisms–the Guillain-Barré syndrome. An experimental allergic sympathetic neuritis may be induced by immunization with antigens obtained from sympathetic ganglia. The inflammatory lesions are limited to the sympathetic nervous system.

PHACOANAPHYLACTIC ENDOPHTHALMITIS

The lens was probably the first tissue to which an autoallergic reaction was recognized [1903] (203). Experimental lesions have been produced by scratching the lens of rabbits previously sensitized to lens material. The cornea becomes vascularized and infiltrated with histiocytes. Because the lens is not vascularized, specifically sensitized cells cannot come into contact with the antigen (lens) unless there is some release of the antigen into the anterior chamber of the eye or other tissue spaces. This is why

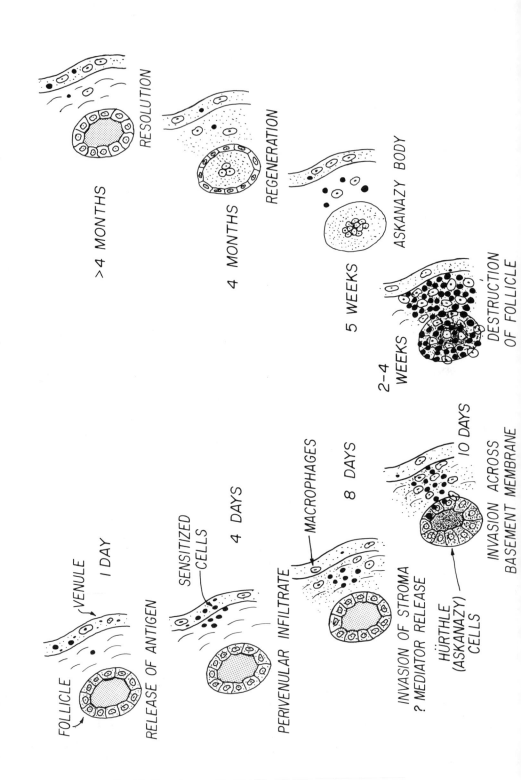

FOLLICLE
VENULE
1 DAY
RELEASE OF ANTIGEN

SENSITIZED
CELLS
4 DAYS

MACROPHAGES
PERIVENULAR INFILTRATE
8 DAYS

INVASION OF STROMA
? MEDIATOR RELEASE
HÜRTHLE
(ASKANAZY)
CELLS
10 DAYS
INVASION ACROSS
BASEMENT MEMBRANE

2-4
WEEKS
DESTRUCTION
OF FOLLICLE

5 WEEKS
ASKANAZY BODY

4 MONTHS
REGENERATION

>4 MONTHS
RESOLUTION

scratching the lens is necessary to induce the lesion. The disease is not related to circulating antibody, and no lesions are produced by washing the anterior chamber of the eye with large amounts of antibody. A not infrequent complication of cataract extraction is an intraocular inflammatory (presumably autoallergic) reaction. In some cases the inflammation may extend to involve the unoperated eye.

UVEITIS

Lesions similar to human disease can be produced in experimental animals by injection of uveal tissue in complete Freund's adjuvant (experimental allergic uveitis). The human condition, known as sympathetic ophthalmia, is an inflammatory lesion of the uveal tract that appears 2–6 weeks after a perforating wound of the eye and affects both the injured and normal eye. The early lesions are focal inflammatory infiltrations of lymphocytes in the choroid, usually related to small veins. As early as 1910, it was proposed that this disease represented an allergic response to uveal antigens (203). If an individual loses sight in one eye due to injury, the eye is usually removed as soon as possible because the incidence of inflammation occurring in the remaining eye is directly related to the length of time the damaged eye is allowed to remain in situ.

ORCHITIS

Focal perivenous accumulations of lymphocytes and histiocytes occur 8–14 days after sensitization of the animals with testes or spermatozoa in complete Freund's adjuvant (30a,186). The inflammatory infiltrate is found primarily in the vascular areas of the testes (epididymis) and causes progressive damage of germinal cells leading to aspermatogenesis. Complement-fixing, sperm-immobilizing, skin-sensitizing antibodies may be demonstrated. The destruction of seminiferous tubules is associated with a mononuclear infiltrate, while sperm passages have a polymorphonuclear reaction with IgG and C3 present. Therefore antibody and delayed hypersensitivity are both active in allergic aspermatogenesis. Mumps orchitis is a human disease that occurs approximately 14 days after mumps parotitis. The histologic picture is very similar to that of the experimental disease. It has not been possible to demonstrate viruses in the testes of patients with mumps orchitis.

Fig. 14–10. Evolution of experimental allergic thyroiditis. The lesions begin as perivascular infiltrates which extend through the interfollicular stroma to invade the follicular lining cells. Destruction of the lining cells occurs wherever mononuclear cells invade. Prior to destruction the lining cells may enlarge and become more densely stained in histologic sections (Hürthle or Askanazy cells). After the follicular lining cells are destroyed, the follicles may be filled with mononuclear cells (Askanazy body). In EAT the lesions always resolve, presumably due to regeneration of the follicular lining cells similar to that in epithelial cells after contact dermatitis (10,57).

THYROIDITIS

This is one of the most extensively studied experimental autoallergic diseases. It occurs 6–14 days following immunization of an experimental animal with thyroid extract or thyroglobulin in complete Freund's adjuvant (57,58). Evolution of the lesion is presented in Fig. 14–10. The lesion begins as a perivenous infiltration of lymphocytes and histiocytes, and destruction of the thyroid follicular epithelium is accomplished by the invasion of specifically sensitized cells similar to the lesion of contact dermatitis (57). The experimental disease almost always resolves, although some instances of a chronic lesion have been reported. The severity and course of the disease are not related to antibody titer, but do correlate with delayed hypersensitivity skin tests (58). Experimental thyroiditis may be transferred both with cells and with antiserum in rabbits (132). Antibody may play a role in initiation of lesions by increasing the permeability of venules to lymphocytes, permitting sensitized cells passage to contact with the target cells. In humans, a disease of unknown etiology, Hashimoto's disease, is characterized by intense lymphocytic infiltration and formation of lymphocytic follicles with prominent germinal centers. There are certain histologic similarities between Hashimoto's disease and experimental allergic thyroiditis, and there is a high incidence of antibodies in thyroglobulin and other thyroid antigens in patients with this disease. The role of humoral antibody in the pathogenesis of human thyroiditis remains unclear (see page 279), but electron dense deposits have been found in the follicular basement membrane of thyroids from patients with Hashimoto's disease which are similar to the deposits of toxic complex glomerulonephritis (96). In addition, patients with thyroiditis may have an increase (54) or a decrease (190) in circulating T cells. The significance of the difference in T cells as reported by the above groups is not clear at this time. Hashimoto's thyroiditis is often associated with other diseases of unknown etiology, such as Sjögren's syndrome, pernicious anemia, systemic lupus erythematosus, rheumatoid arthritis, and other diseases for which an autoallergic pathogenesis has been postulated (79).

Antibodies to different thyroid antigens have been found in patients with autoallergic thyroiditis (125).

1. *Antibody to thyroglobulin.* The original antibody discovered was to thyroglobulin. It can be demonstrated by many immunochemical techniques, including precipitation, passive hemogglutination, complement fixation, and binding of fluoresceine-labeled antibodies to thyroid colloid. The severity of the experimental disease does not correlate with the titer of this antibody, and the antibody is found in many other thyroid diseases as well as thyroiditis.

2. *Antibody to thyroid colloid antigen.* The immunoglobulins of some patients who give negative results with thyroglobulin antigen specifically bind to another antigen in the colloid of thyroid glands as demonstrated by the fluorescent antibody technique. The fluorescent staining pattern is different from that of antibody of thyroglobulin, indicating a different antigen specificity. The significance of this antibody is questionable. Its

correlation with the severity of the human disease is not good, but its correlation with the severity of the experimental disease is somewhat better.

3. *Antibody to microsomal antigen.* Antibodies with this specificity can be detected by complement fixation only when the antigen used is derived from hyperactive thyroid tissue (thyrotoxic glands). Fluorescent antibody binding, both in toxic glands and in normal glands, can be demonstrated to microsomes of thyroid cells but not to thyroid colloid.

4. *Cytotoxic antibody.* If antiserum from a patient with thyroiditis is placed on a monolayer of thyroid epithelial cells in tissue culture, death of the epithelial cells may occur. The specificity of this antibody appears to be different from those of antibodies mentioned above. Again, the significance of this antibody is questionable. It may be related to the microsomal antigen, as there is a correlation between the microsomal complement-fixation test and the in vitro cytotoxic antibody.

5. *Nuclear component.* Specific binding of fluorescein-labeled antibody to the nucleus of thyroid cells has been observed using the fluorescent technique with sera from some patients with thyroiditis. The binding is not specific for thyroid nuclei and occurs with nuclei of other tissue cells. This specificity may be related to that found in sera from patients with lupus erythematosus (see page 192).

The role of these antibodies in the pathogenesis of allergic thyroiditis remains obscure. There is some evidence that circulating antibody may actually suppress the development of experimental allergic thyroiditis. However, circulating thyroglobulin–antithyroglobulin complexes may cause a toxic complex glomerulonephritis.

SIALADENITIS

Mononuclear inflammatory lesions have been reported in experimental animals following the injection of salivary gland tissue in complete Freund's adjuvant. However, the validity of these observations is questionable, and the autoallergic nature of such lesions is not well established. It is convenient, however, to consider Sjögren's syndrome as an autoallergic disease. Thus human disorder, consisting of dryness of the eyes (keratoconjunctivitis sicca) and dryness of the mouth (xerostomia) is often associated with the connective tissue diseases (rheumatoid arthritis, systemic lupus erythematosus, scleroderma, polyarteritis nodosa). Clinically there is swelling of the salivary glands (if the parotid gland alone is involved the eponym Mikulicz's syndrome is used). Histologically there are lymphocyte and plasma cell infiltration of the salivary and lacrimal glands and fibrosis, acinar atrophy, and proliferation of the myoepithelial cells of the ducts with obstruction. Similar findings may be observed in the mucosal glands of the pharynx and larynx, and the submucosal glands of the esophagus, trachea, and bronchi. Precipitating and complement-fixing antibody to salivary gland tissue has been found associated with the disease, as have other serologic abnormalities such as lupus erythematosus factor, rheumatoid factor, and antibodies to thyroglobulin. The presence of antibodies to salivary ducts is associated with less cellular infiltrate in the salivary gland of patients with Sjögren's Syndrome when these lesions are compared to those of patients who lack this antibody (6). Thus, antibody to salivary gland may block cellular-mediated tissue destruction.

ADRENALITIS

Immunization of animals with adrenal tissue in complete Freund's adjuvant leads to mononuclear cell infiltration and necrosis of the adrenal cortex (203). Most cases of adrenal insufficiency in man (Addison's disease) are secondary to endocrine, infectious or neoplastic processes. However a type of adrenal insufficiency, primary cytotoxic contraction, is of unknown origin and may be a correlate of experimental autoallergic adrenalitis. Complement fixing antibodies have been found in some patients with Addison's disease caused by primary cytotoxic contraction of the adrenal.

ADJUVANT DISEASES

Following the injection of complete Freund's adjuvant alone, lesions may be found in joint synovia, colon, and skin that resemble human diseases of unknown, but suspected immune, origin (203). The joint lesions resemble, but are not identical with, those of rheumatoid arthritis. The lesion of rheumatoid arthritis in a villous or papillary thickening of synovial membrane and a vascular granulation tissue (pannus) which may erode the articular surface of the involved joint (see pages 197–199). Ulcerative colitis is a chronic disease of the colon. Its cause is unknown, and numerous attempts to isolate an infectious agent have been unsuccessful. Histologically, there are vascular congestion, edema, hemorrhage and superficial ulceration, with a mixed infiltration of polymorphonuclear leukocytes, lymphocytes, plasma cells and eosinophils. Associated with ulcerative colitis are hypergammaglobulinemia, a prevalence of atopic sensitivities, a prominent occurrence of other autoallergic diseases and antibodies to colonic tissue. Auer's colitis is a hemorrhagic necrotic lesion of the colon with a cellular infiltrate at the base of the crypts and perivascular polymorphonuclear leukocyte accumulation produced experimentally by the injection of antigen (egg albumen) into the colonic cavity of sensitized rabbits (Arthus reaction). Many skin diseases, such as psoriasis, scleroderma (progressive systemic sclerosis) and dermatomyositis, are suspected of having an allergic mechanism, but concrete evidence in favor of this view is not convincing (see Chapter 13).

LIVER DISEASE

Although direct evidence for the involvement of allergic mechanisms in the initiation or progression of human liver diseases is lacking, considerable circumstantial evidence (presumptive findings) is available to incriminate allergic mechanisms in chronic active hepatitis, primary biliary cirrhosis, some types of reactions to drugs causing jaundice and viral hepatitis (46,119,137) [see page 243]. These presumptive findings include diffuse (polyclonal) hypergammaglobulinemias, tissue lesions containing lymphocytes and plasma cells consistent with a cellular reaction, a depression of serum complement at some stages of the disease, a demonstration of immunoglobulin and complement in some early lesions, an association with other allergic diseases such as lupus erythematosus, a beneficial response to drugs that cause depressed immune response, and the presence of a variety of autoantibodies (118). These antibodies can be demonstrated by immunofluorescence to bind to the nuclei, ductular cells, and mitrochondria of the liver and to smooth muscle cells. Of particular interest is the automitochondrial antibody associated with primary biliary cirrhosis, chronic active hepatitis, and halothane hepatitis (drug-induced jaundice) but not in Laennec's cirrhosis, viral hepatitis, or extrahepatic biliary obstruction. Halothane is an anesthetic agent which has some very desirable properties but produces liver disease similar to viral hepatitis (175). This reaction rarely, if ever, occurs upon the first exposure to halothane but is induced only on subsequent exposures suggesting that a sensitization event occurs. The destructive lesions are associated with a mononuclear infiltrate similar to that seen in other delayed hypersensitivity reactions (191). It is possible that halothane acts like a hapten with affinity for a liver protein which leads to a contact dermatitis-like reaction in the liver. An animal model for autoallergic liver disease (experimental allergic hepatitis) has not been convincingly demonstrated through the induction of liver injury by immunization with liver extract, although mild inflammatory lesions may be observed in some immunized animals (137). An allergic role in alcoholic cirrhosis is unlikely.

PERIODONTAL DISEASE

Periodontal disease is a chronic inflammatory and proliferative reaction of the gums surrounding the teeth which may be at least partially caused by delayed hypersensitivity reactions. The disease begins as a marginal inflammation of the tissue surrounding the teeth (gingivitis) with a predominant lymphocytic infiltrate. The supporting collagen fibers of the gingiva are destroyed and an extensive reactive proliferation of the epithelial cells occurs. Subepithelial inflammation may extend into the marrow of the bone of the jaw leading to bony resorption and eventual loss of teeth in the involved zones. The role of allergic mechanisms in the production of periodontal disease has recently become of interest (114). While any of the allergically mediated inflammatory mechanisms may be responsible for tissue reactions in the oral cavity, the most likely cause of chronic periodontal disease is a delayed hypersensitivity reaction (88). The antigens responsible may be oral bacterial products, tissue breakdown products or dietary material. Periodontal disease is a result of poor dental hygiene and the best preventive action is keeping the oral cavity clean. The lesions of severe periodontal disease regress if the patient is treated with immunosuppressive therapy. This effect on periodontal disease has been noticed in patients with cancer or with a transplanted organ who have received immunosuppressive agents; gingival inflammation subsides while the patient is being treated.

AUTOANTIBODIES IN AUTOALLERGIC DISEASE

A number of antibodies to tissue or serum antigens have been observed in the sera of human patients with certain diseases. (Table 14-4)

TABLE 14-4
Some Human Diseases in Which Serum Antibodies to Serum or Tissue Antigens Have Been Found by Various Methods

Disease	Antigen	Method of anti-body detection
Addison's disease, idiopathic	Adrenal	CF,F
Dermatitis, chronic	Dermis	F,A
Glomerulonephritis, post-streptococcal	Kidney	CF,F,H,A
Other kidney diseases	Kidney	F,A
Viral hepatitis	Liver, spleen, smooth muscle	CF,F,H,A,P
Cirrhosis of liver	Liver, spleen, kidney	CF,F,H,A
Lung diseases (emphysema, asthma, tuberculosis)	Lung	CF, GC, P
Lupus erythematosus	Liver, spleen, kidney, muscle, platelets, blood cells, nucleoprotein, RNA, DNA, histone	CF,F,A
Multiple sclerosis	Brain or white matter	CF, tissue culture demyelination
Carcinomatous neuropathy	Neurons	F,CF (gray, white)
Other CNS diseases (cerebrovascular accident)	Brain	CF
Myasthenia gravis	Muscle, thymus, thyroid	CF,F,H,GC
Myocardial infarction	Heart	H,P
Orchitis, infertility	Sperm	A
Pancreatitis, chronic cystic fibrosis	Pancreas glandular epithelium	P,H
Pernicious anemia	Intrinsic factor, parietal cell microsomes	CF,F,inhibition
(Atrophic gastritis)	(Gastric mucosa)	
Rheumatic fever	Heart, muscle, joint	CF,F,H,GC
Rheumatoid arthritis	Heart, muscle, joint, subcutaneous nodules, denatured γ-globulin	P,H,A
Scleroderma, dermatomyositis	Kidney, muscle, joint, cell nuclei	F
Sjögren's syndrome	Salivary gland, liver, kidney, thyroid cell nuclei	CF,P,F,H
Syphilis	Wassermann antigen	CF,A
Thyroiditis, myxedema, thyrotoxicosis	Thyroglobulin, glandular epithelium, gastric mucosa cell nuclei	P,CF,H,F
Ulcerative colitis	Mucosal glands, mucus	CF,F,H,P
Uveal injury	Uveal pigment	CF

A, agglutination of other antigen-coated particles.
CF, complement fixation.
F, fluorescent antibody fixation.
GC, antiglobulin consumption.
H, hemagglutination, passive.
P, precipitation.
Modified from Waksman BH: Medicine 41:93, 1963. Copyright © 1962, Baltimore The Williams & Wilkins Co.

(45,63,107,125,200). While some of these autoantibodies have been recognized for some time (antibody to γ-globulin in rheumatoid arthritis, antibody to nucleoprotein in systemic lupus erythematosus, and the Wassermann antibody in syphilis), most are of recent discovery. Several are worth further consideration here.

Autoantibodies to cardiac muscle may be demonstrated in some patients following myocardial infarction (99). While the induction of these antibodies may be due to alteration of myocardial antigens secondary to necrosis, the antibodies found react (?cross-react) with normal myocardial antigens. It is inconceivable that these antibodies play a role in the original infarction, but they have been implicated by some in the postinfarction syndrome. Kaplan has shown that there are antigens of group A streptococci that cross-react with cardiac tissue (99). The occurrence of this type of antibody suggests that an appropriate streptococcal infection may break tolerance to normal cardiac tissue antigens, with the resulting autoallergic reaction and production of rheumatic fever. γ-Globulin may be revealed in the fibrinoid lesions of rheumatic carditis, but is not present in typical Aschoff bodies. Antibodies that bind with hapatocytic mitochondria may be detected by the fluorescent antibody technique in the sera of patients with biliary cirrhosis and hepatitis, but not in the sera of patients with other forms of cirrhosis or extrahepatic biliary obstruction (137). Autoantibodies are found associated with cytomegalic inclusion disease after cardiopulmonary bypass perfusion or massive blood transfusion (98).

The significance of most of these antibodies is unknown; in few cases has a pathogenic property been convincingly demonstrated. However antinuclear antibody in lupus erythematosis, rheumatoid factor in rheumatoid arthritis and antiheart antibody in rheumatic fever are almost certainly significant in the etiology of these autoallergic diseases. Until more evidence is obtained, one is left with the explanation that many other autoantibodies are more likely the result than the cause of tissue alteration or breakdown. It has been postulated that such antibodies actually function to clean up or clear the body fluids of the abnormal tissue components, since it is known that the presence of circulating antibody results in a rapid clearance of antigen from the blood stream. The relatives of individuals suffering from a disease associated with a circulating autoantibody have a higher incidence of autoantibodies than the general population.

ANTIGENS IN AUTOALLERGIC DISEASE

The specific antigens involved in autoallergic diseases have not been conclusively identified (200). The evidence suggests that the antigen may be thyroglobulin in thyroiditis, encephalitogenic peptide in experimental allergic encephalomyelitis (100), carbohydrate in orchitis, and protein in endophthalmitis. In each case, the antigen is a specific material belonging to a specialized tissue, and not shared with any other tissue. Some antigens, called tissue-specific, occur in the same tissue in different species; examples are central nervous system myelin and lens (203). This situation is exactly the opposite of what is found in allografts, where the antigen is material usually common to all the cells of one and only one individual. Nevertheless, the autoallergic lesion and the homograft reaction are allergic reactions of the same type (delayed), directed at antigens present in tissue.

GENERAL FEATURES OF AUTOALLERGIC DISEASES

The allergic response involved in most of the autoallergic diseases is the delayed type. The general characteristics can be summarized as follows:

1. The histologic picture is most consistent with a delayed reaction.
2. There is little or no correlation of disease with circulating antibody.
3. There is correlation between delayed skin or corneal reactions to tissue antigens and the disease process.
4. In general, production of the experimental lesion is possible only when mycobacterial adjuvant in combination with specific antigen is used or if repeated small doses of specific antigen are given—procedures that favor the production of delayed hypersensitivity.
5. Passive transfer of disease with serum is generally ineffective, while passive transfer with cells has been demonstrated for some of these diseases.
6. In some experimental situations (breast, muscle) good titers of circulating antibody may be produced, but no lesions are demonstrable. Antibody can cause damage only when antigens are readily available (vascular endothelium, circulating blood cells, glomerular basement membrane), but is unable to produce lesions in solid tissue. This is supported by tissue culture studies: Antibody is toxic for suspension or monolayer cultures, but solid cultures resist the action of antibody.
7. Direct destruction of organized tissue by sensitized cells occurs in other types of delayed reactions, such as homograft rejection and graft-vs-host reactions.

CRITERIA FOR IDENTIFICATION OF AUTOALLERGY

There are certain characteristics ideally identifiable in all immune responses which should be sought for in diseases of suspected autoallergic etiology. These include 1) a well-defined immunizing event (infection, immunization, vaccination; 2) a latent period (usually 6–14 days); 3) a secondary response (a more rapid and more intense reaction on second exposure to the antigen; 4) an ability to transfer the sensitive state with cells or serum from an affected individual to a normal individual; 5) a specific depression of the sensitive state by large amounts of antigen (desensitization); 6) identification and isolation of the antigen in a pure form and chemical characterization of the antigen. All, or even a few, of these criteria can rarely, if ever, be established for human diseases. The criteria are most closely approximated in certain blood dyscrasias and in acute disseminated encephalomyelitis.

Presumptive findings consistent with but not strong evidence for, an allergic mechanism in disease states include 1) a morphologic picture consistent with known allergic reactions; 2) the demonstration of antibody or a positive delayed skin reaction; 3) a depression of complement during some stage of the disease; 4) a beneficial effect of agents known to inhibit some portion of an allergic reaction (steroids, radiation, nitrogen mustard, aminopterin); 5) identification of a reasonable experimental model in animals that mimics the human disease; 6) an association with other possible autoallergic diseases; and 7) an increased familial susceptibility to the same disease or other autoallergic diseases.

THEORIES OF AUTOIMMUNIZATION

The explanation for autoimmunization is unknown and is the subject of much active research. Three major theoretic explanations have been suggested:

1. The tissues involved in autoallergic diseases are derived from ectoderm or endoderm and are regarded as foreign by the immune apparatus, which is mesodermal. These autoantigens are substances which are absent during the immune neutral period of development and, therefore, fail to induce tolerance like other body antigens. Blood-tissue barriers normally prevent these substances from ever reaching the circulation and the immune apparatus. When viral infection, injury, or other episodes cause breakdown of blood-tissue barriers, with release into circulation, allergic reaction may occur (9).

2. Viral infection or other events cause alteration of tissue substances not normally antigenic, so that they are recognized as antigen by the immune system. This hypothesis has received experimental support. Weigle (208) has been able to break tolerance using chemically modified antigens. By immunizing animals with aqueous homologous thyroglobulin to which arsanilic or sulfanilic acid had been coupled, he was able to induce experimental allergic thyroiditis; the supposition is that tolerance to autologous proteins can be broken by antigenically modified proteins of the same class.

3. According to the clonal selection theory of Burnet (see Chapter 7), an alteration, not in the tissue in which the lesion appears, but in the cells of the immune system, leads to autoallergy. Owing to an unknown mechanism some immunologically competent cells, which do not normally react against the tissues of the same animal, go out of control and recognize normal tissue substances as antigens.

4. The function of suppressor cells (see Suppressor T Cells, page 114) may be lost. Suppressor cells may prevent other immunologically competent cells from responding to self antigens. Presentation of the antigen in a particular manner may circumvent suppressor cell activity. Suppressor cells are short lived and may become less numerous with aging, permitting other cells to respond to self antigens. The incidence of autoallergic diseases and autoantibodies increases with age.

REFERENCES

1. Adams JM: Persistence of measles virus and demylinating disease. Hosp Pract 87:1970
2. Amos DB: Genetic and antigenetic aspects of human histocompatibility systems. Adv Immunol 10:251, 1969
3. Amos DB: Genetic aspects of human HL-A transplantation antigens. Fed Proc 29:2018, 1970

4. Amos DB, Bach FH: Phenotypic expressions of the major histocompatibility locus in man (HL-A): Leukocyte antigens and a mixed leukocyte culture reactivity. J Exp Med 128:623, 1968
5. Amos DB, Cooper T, DeBakey ME, Grondin P, Groth CC, Hanlon CR, Kayhoe DE, Murray JE, Najarian JS, Santos GW, Starzl TE: ACS/NIH Organ Transplant Registry. Third Scientific Report. JAMA 226:1211, 1973
6. Anderson LG, Tarpley TM, Talal N, Cummings NA, Wolf RO, Schall GL: Cellular-versus-humoral autoimmune responses to salivary gland in Sjögren's syndrome. Clin Exp Immunol 13:335, 1973
7. Appel MGJ, Gillespie JH: Canine distemper virus. Virology 11:1, 1972
8. Arnason BG, Waksman BH: Tuberculin sensitivity: Immunologic considerations. Adv Tuberc Res 13:1, 1964
9. Asherson GL: The role of microorganisms in autoimmune responses. Prog Allergy 12:192, 1968
10. Askanasy M. Pathologische-anatomische Beiträge zur Kenntnies des Morbus Basedouri, insbesondere über die dabie auftretende Muskelerkrankung. Dtsch Arch Klin Med 61:118–186, 1898
11. Bach FH: Transplantation: Pairing of donor and recipient. Science 168:1170, 1970
12. Bach FH (ed): The Histocompatibility Systems. Vol 4. Transplant Proc 1974
13. Badger AM, Cooperband SR, Green JA: Direct observations on the effect of proliferation inhibitory factor" on the clonal growth of target cells. J Immunol 107:1259, 1971
14. Baldini M: Idiopathic thrombocytopenic purpura. N Engl J Med 274:1245, 1302, 1360, 1966
15. Baldwin RW, Humphrey JH (eds): Autoimmunity. Philadelphia, Davis, 1965
16. Barnes BA, Bergan JJ, Braun WE, Fraumeni JF, Kountz SL, Mickey MR, Rubin AL, Simmons RL, Stevens LE, Wilson RE: The 11th report of the human renal transplant registry. JAMA 226:1197, 1973
17. Beer AE, Billingham RE: Immunobiology of mammalian reproduction. Adv Immunol 14:1, 1971
18. Beer AE, Billingham RE: The embryo as a transplant. Sci Am 230:36, 1974
19. Bennett B, Bloom BR: Reactions in vivo and in vitro produced by a soluble substance associated with delayed-type hypersensitivity. Proc Natl Acad Sci USA 59:756, 1968
20. Berke G, Amos GB: Mechanism of lymphocyte-mediated cytolysis: The LMC cycle and its role in transplantation immunity. Transplant Rev 17:71, 1973
21. Beveridge WIB: Acquired Immunity: Viral Infections. In Modern Trends in Immunology. Cruickshank R (ed). London, Whitefriars, 1963
22. Biberfield P, Holm G, Perlmann P: Morphologic observations on lymphocyte peripolesis and cytotoxic action in vitro. Exp Cell Res 52:672, 1968
23. Billingham RE: Tissue transplantation: Scope and prospect. Science 153:266, 1966
24. Billingham RE, Sparrow EM: The effect of prior intravenous injections of dissociated epidermal cells and blood on the survival of skin homografts in rabbits. J Embryol Exp Morphol 3:265, 1955
25. Bloom BR, Jimenez L: Migration inhibitory factor and the cellular basis of delayed hypersensitivity reactions. Am J Pathol 60:453, 1970
26. Blumenthal MM, Amos DB, Noreen H, Mendell NR, Yunis EJ: Genetic mapping of Ir locus in man: Linkage to second locus of HL-A. Science 184:1301, 1974
27. Bonavida B: Studies on the induction and expression of T cell-mediated immunity. II. Antiserum blocking of cell-mediated cytolysis. J Immunol 112:1308, 1974
28. Brewerton DA, Caffrey M, Hart FD, James DCO, Nichols A, Sturrock RD: Ankylosing spondylitis and HL-A27. Lancet 1:904, 1973
29. Brewerton DA, Caffrey M, Nichols A, Walter D, James DCO: Acute anterior uvitis and HL-A27. Lancet 2:994, 1973
30. Brewerton DA, Caffrey M, Nichols A, Walters D, Oates JK, James DCO: Reiter's disease and HL-A27. Lancet 2:996, 1973
30a. Brown PC, Glynn LE: The early lesion of experimental allergic orchitis in guinea pigs: An immunological correlation. J Pathol 98:277–282, 1969
31. Brunner KT, Mauel J, Rudolf H, Chapuis B: Studies of allograft immunity in mice. I. Induction, development and in vitro assay of cellular immunity. Immunology 18:501, 1970

32. Burnet FM: Multiple polymorphism in relation to histocompatibility antigens. Nature (Lond) 245:359, 1973
33. Canty TG, Wunderlich JR: Quantitative in vitro assay of cytotoxic cellular immunity. J Natl Cancer Inst 45:761, 1970
34. Casey AE: Experimental enhancement of malignancy in the Brown-Pearce rabbit tumor. Proc Soc Exp Biol Med 29:816, 1932
35. Ceppellini R: Old and new facts and speculations about transplantation antigens of man. Prog Immunol 1:973, 1971
36. Cerottini J-C: In Immunologic Intervention. Uhr JW, Landy M (eds). New York, Academic Press, 1971
37. Cerottini J-C, Brunner KT: Cell-mediated cytotoxicity, allograft rejection and tumor immunity. Adv Immunol 18:67–132, 1974
38. Cohen IR, Stavy L, Feldman M: Glucocorticoids and cellular immunity in vitro. Facilitation of the sensitization phase and inhibition of the effector phase of a lymphocyte with fibroblast reaction. J Exp Med 132:1055, 1970
39. Congdon CC: Comparative group on bone marrow transplantation in man. Exp Hematol 20:97, 1970
40. Congdon CC: Radiation injury: Bone marrow transplantation. Annu Rev Med 13:203, 1962
41. Dacie JV, Wolledge SM: Autoimmune hemolytic anemia. Prog Hematol 6:1, 1969
42. Dameshek W: Chronic lymphocytic leukemia–an accumulative disease of immunologically incompetent lymphocytes. Blood 29:566, 1967
43. Dameshek W, Schwartz RS: Leukemia and auto-immunization–some possible relationships. Blood 14:1151, 1959
44. David JR: Delayed hypersensitivity in vitro: Its mediation by cell free substances formed by lymphoid cell-antigen interaction. Proc Natl Acad Sci USA 56:72, 1966
45. Dixon FJ: Allergy and immunology: Autoimmunity in disease. Annu Rev Med 8:257, 1968
46. Doniach D: Autoimmune aspects of liver disease. Br Med Bull 28:145, 1972
47. Dvorak HF, Mihm MC Jr: Basophilic leukocytes in allergic contact dermatitis. J Exp Med 135:235, 1972
48. Dvorak HF, Dvorak AM: Basophilic leukocytes in delayed-type hypersensitivity reactions in animals and man. In Microenvironmental Aspects of Immunity. New York, Jankovic BD, Isakovic K (eds). Plenum Publishing Co., 1973, p 573
49. Edgington TS, Ritt DJ: Intrahepatic expression of serum hepatitis virus-associated antigens. J Exp Med 134:871, 1971
50. Edidin M: Histocompatibility genes, transplantation antigens and pregnancy. In Transplantation Antigens. New York, Academic Press, 1972, p 75
51. Ellison GW, Waksman BH, Ruddle NH: Experimental autoallergic encephalomyelitis and cellular hypersensitivity in vitro. Neurology 21:788–782, 1971
52. Epstein E, Clairborne ER: Racial and environmental factors in susceptibility to Rhus. Excerpta Med 12:357, 1958
53. Eylar EH: Amino acid sequence of the myelin basic protein. Proc Natl Acad Sci USA 67:1425, 1970
54. Farid NR, Munro RE, Row, VV, Volpe R: Peripheral thymus dependent (T) lymphocytes in Graves' disease and Hashimoto's thyroiditis. N Engl J Med 288:1313, 1973
55. Feldman JD: Immunological Enhancement: A Study of Blocking Antibodies. Adv Immunol 15:167, 1972
56. Fialkow PJ, Thomas ED, Bryant JI, Neiman PE: Leukemic transformation of engrafted human marrow cells in vivo. Lancet 1:251, 1971
57. Flax MH: Experimental allergic thyroiditis in the guinea pig. II. Morphologic studies on the development of the disease. Lab Invest 12:199, 1963
58. Flax MH, Jankovic DB, Sell S: Experimental allergic thyroiditis in the guinea pig. I. Relationship of delayed hypersensitivity and circulating antibody to the development of thyroiditis. Lab Invest 12:119, 1963
59. Forman J, Möller G: The effector cell in antibody-induced cell mediated immunity. Transplant Rev 17:108, 1973
60. Friedman H: Inhibition of antibody plaque formation by sensitized lymphoid cells: Rapid indicator of transplantation immunity. Science 145:607, 1964
61. Gajdusek DC: Kuru and Creutzfeldt-Jakob Disease. Experimental models of non-

inflammatory degenerative slow virus disease of the central nervous system. Ann Clin Res 5:254, 1973
62. Gell PGH, Benacerraf B: Delayed hypersensitivity to simple protein antigens. Adv Immunol 1:319, 1961
63. Gell PGH, Coombs RRA: Clinical Aspects of Immunology, 2nd ed. Oxford, Blackwell, 1968
64. Genogzian M, Edwards CL, Vodopick HA, Hubner KF: Bone marrow transplantation in a leukemic patient following immunosuppression with antithymocyte globulin and total body irradiation. Transplantation 15:446, 1972
65. Gillespie GY, Barth RF, Gobuty A: A new radioisotopic microassay of cell-mediated immunity utilizing technetium-99m labelled target cells. Proc Soc Exp Biol Med 142:378, 1973
66. Gocke DJ, Hsu K, Morgan C, Bombardieri S, Lockshin M, Christian CL: Association between polyarteritis and Australia antigen. Lancet 2:1149, 1970
67. Gorczynski R, Kontiainen S, Mitchison NA, Tigelar RE: Antigen–antibody complexes as blocking factors on the T lymphocyte surface. In Cellular Selection and the Immune Response. New York, Raven Press, 1974, p 143, Edelman CM (ed).
68. Gotoff SP, Vizral IF, Malecki TJ: Macrophage aggregation in vitro. Transplantation 10:443, 1970
69. Govaerts A: Cellular antibodies in kidney transplantation. J Immunol 85:516, 1960
70. Granger GA: Mechanisms of lymphocyte-induced cell and tissue destruction in vitro. Am J Pathol 59:469, 1970
71. Granger GA, Kolb WB: Lymphocyte in vitro cytotoxicity: Mechanisms of immune and non-immune small lymphocyte-mediated target L cell destruction. J Immunol 101:111, 1968
72. Granger GA, Laserna EC, Kolb WP, Chapman F: Human lymphotoxin: purification and some properties. Proc Natl Acad Sci USA, 70:27, 1973
73. Granger GA, Weiser RS: Homograft target cells: Contact destruction in vitro by immune macrophages. Science 56:97, 1966
74. Gray I, Russell PS: Donor selection in human organ transplantation. Lancet 2:863, 1963
75. Green JA, Cooperband SR, Kibrick S: Immune specific induction of interfereon production in cultures of human blood lymphocytes. Science 164:1415, 1969
76. Green JA, Cooperband SR, Rutstein JA, Kibrick S: Inhibition of target cell proliferation by supernatants from cultures of human peripheral blood lymphocytes. J Immunol 105:48, 1970
77. Grey HM, Kubo RT, Colon SM, Poulik MD, Cresswell P, Springer T, Turner M, Strominger JL: The small subunit of HL-A antigens is B2 macroglobulin. J Exp Med 138:1608, 1973
78. Hale JH: Duration of immunity in virus diseases. Adv Immunol 1:263, 1961
79. Hall R: Immunological aspects of thyroid function. N Engl J Med 266:1204, 1962
80. Haller JD, Cerruti MM: Heart transplantation in man: Compilation of cases. II. Am J Cardiol 24:554, 1969
81. Heise ER, Hans S, Weiser RS: In vitro studies on the mechanism of macrophage migration inhibitor in tuberculin sensitivity. J Immunol 101:1004, 1968
82. Heise ER, Weiser RS: Factors in delayed sensitivity: Lymphocyte and macrophage cytotoxins in the tuberculin reaction. J Immunol 103:570, 1969
83. Hellström KE, Hellström I: Lymphocyte-mediated cytotoxicity and blocking serum activity to tumor antigens. Adv Immunol 18:209, 1974
84. Hellström KE, Hellström I, Brawn J: Abrogation of cellular immunity to antigenically foreign mouse cells by a serum factor. Nature (Lond) 224:914, 1969
85. Henney CS: On the mechanism of T-cell mediated cytolysis. Transplant Rev 17:37, 1973
86. Holm G, Perlmann P: Quantitative studies on phytohaemagglutinin-induced cytotoxicity by human lymphocytes against homologous cells in tissue culture. Immunology 12:525, 1966
87. Holzman RS, Lebowitz AS, Valentine FT, Lawrence HS: Preparation and properties of cloning inhibitory factor. I. Inhibition of HeLa cell cultures by stimulated lymphocytes and their culture supernatants. Cell Immunol 8:249–258, 1973

88. Horton JE, Oppenheim JJ, Mergenhagen SE: A role for cell-mediated immunity in the pathogenesis of periodontal disease. J Periodontal 45:351, 1974
89. Hotchin JE: The Biology of Lymphocytic Choriomengitis Infection: Virus-induced Immune Disease. Cold Spring Harbor Symp Quant Biol 14:479, 1962
90. Howard JG, Michie JG: Transplantation Immunology. In Modern Trends in Immunology. Cruickshank R (ed). London, Whitefriars, 1963
91. Huang S-N, Millman I, O'Connell A, Aronoff A, Gault H, Blumberg GS: Virus-like particles in Australia antigen-associated hepatitis. Am J Pathol 67:453, 1972
92. Isacson EP: Myxoviruses and autoimmunity. Prog Allergy 10:256, 1967
93. Jerne NK: The somatic generation of immune recognition. Eur J Immunol 1:1, 1971
94. Jones TD, Mote JR: The phases of foreign sensitization in human beings. N Engl J Med 210:120, 1934
95. Kahan BD, Mittal KK, Reisfeld RA, Terasaki PI, Bergan JJ: The antigenic stimulus in human transplantation. Surgery 74:153, 1973
96. Kalderon AE, Bogaars HA, Diamond I: Ultrastructural alterations of follicular basement membrane in Hashimoto's thyroiditis. Am J Med 55:485, 1973
97. Kaliss N: Immunological enhancement of tumor homografts in mice. A review. Cancer Res 18:992, 1958
98. Kantor GL, Goldberg LS, Johnson L, Derechin MM, Barnett EV: Immunologic abnormalities induced by postperfusion cytomegalovirus infection. Ann Intern Med 73:553, 1970
99. Kaplan MH: Autoimmunity to heart and its relation to human disease. Prog Allergy 13:408, 1969
100. Kibler RF, Shapira R: Isolation and properties of an encephalitogenic protein from bovine, rabbit and human central nervous system tissue. J Biol Chem 243:281, 1968
101. Kirchner H, Blaese RM: Pokeweed mitogen-, concanavalin A-, and phytohemagglutinin-induced development of cytotoxic effector lymphocytes. An evaluation of the mechanisms of T cell-mediated cytotoxicity. J Exp Med 138:812, 1973
102. Klein E: Parental variants. Transplant Proc 3:1167, 1971
103. Klein G, Sjögren HO, Klein E, Hellström KE: Demonstration of resistance against methycholantherene-induced sarcomas in the primary autochthonous host. Cancer Res 20:1561, 1960
104. Kligman AM: Poison ivy (Rhus) dermatitis: Experimental study. Arch Dermatol 77:149, 1958
105. Koestmer A, McCullough B, Krakowka GS, Long JF, Olsen RG: Canine distemper: a virus-induced demyelinating encephalomyelitis. In Slow Virus Diseases. Zeman W, Lennette EH (eds). Baltimore, Williams and Wilkens, 1974, p 86
106. Kolb WP, Granger GA: Lymphocyte in vitro cytotoxicity. Characterization of human lymphotoxin. Proc Natl Acad Sci USA 61:1250, 1968
107. Kunkel HG, Tan EM: Autoantibodies and disease. Adv Immunol 4:231, 1964
108. Lampert PW: Mechanism of demyelination in experimental allergic neuritis: Electron microscopic studies. Lab Invest 20:127, 1969
109. Lawrence HS, Landy M (eds). Mediators of Cellular Immunity. New York, Academic Press, 1969
110. Lawrence HS, Valentine FT: Transfer factor and other mediators of cellular immunity. Am J Pathol 60:437, 1970
111. Leone CA (ed): Effects of Ionizing Radiations on Immune Processes. New York, Gordon and Breach, 1962
112. LePore MJ, McKenna PJ, Martinez DB, Stutman, LJ, Bonanno CA, Conklin EF, Robilotti JG Jr: Fulminant hepatitis with coma successfully treated by plasmapheresis and hyperimmune Australia-antibody-rich plasma. Am J Gastroenterol 58:381, 1972
113. Likhite V, Sehon A: Migration inhibition and cell-mediated immunity: A review. Rev Can Biol 30:135, 1971
114. Löe, M (ed): Possible Role of Immune Phenomena in Peridontal Tissue Destruction. J Periodontal 45:330, 1974
115. Lohmann-Matthes ML, Fischer H: T cell cytotoxicity and amplification of the cytotoxic reaction by macrophages. Transplant Rev 17:150, 1973

116. Lundgren G, Collste L, Möller G: Cytotoxicity of human lymphocytes: Antagonism between inducing processes. Nature 220:289, 1968
117. Lundgren G, Möller G: Non-specific induction of cytotoxicity in normal human lymphocytes in vitro: Studies of mechanism and specificity of the reaction. Clin Exp Immunol 4:435, 1969
118. Mackay IR: Lupoid hepatitis and primary biliary cirrhosis: Autoimmune diseases of the liver. Bull Rheum Dis 18:487, 1968
119. Mackay IR, Popper H: Immunopathogenesis of chronic hepatitis: A review. Aust NZ J Med 1:79, 1973
120. Mathe G, Schwarzenberg L, Amiel JL, Schneider M, Cattan A, Schlumberger JR, Tubiana M, Lalanne C: Immunogenetic and immunological problems of allogeneic haematopoietic radio-chimeras in man. Scand J Haematol 4:193, 1967
121. McGovern JJ Jr, Russell PS, Atkins L, Webster EW: Treatment of terminal leukemic relapse by total-body irradiation and intravenous infusion of stored autologous bone marrow obtained during remission. N Engl J Med 260:675, 1959
122. Mellors RC, Huang CY: Immunopathology of NZB/Bl mice. V. Virus-like (filtrable) agent separable from lymphoma cells and identifiable by electron microscopy. J Exp Med 124:1031, 1966
123. Merrill JP: Human tissue transplantation. Adv Immunol 7:276, 1967
124. Mikulska ZB, Smith C, Alexander P: Evidence for an immunologic reaction of the host directed against its own actively growing primary tumor. J Natl Cancer Inst 36:29, 1966
125. Milgrom F, Witebsky E: Autoantibodies and autoimmune diseases. JAMA 181:706, 1962
126. Möller E: Antagonistic effects of humoral isoantibodies on the in vitro cytotoxicity of immune lymphoid cells. J Exp Med 122:11, 1965
127. Möller E: Haemolytic activity of mouse peritoneal exudate cells in vitro. Immunology 16:609, 1969
128. Mooney JJ, Waksman BH: Activation of normal rabbit macrophage monolayers by supernatants of antigen stimulated macrophages. J Immunol 105:1138–1145, 1970
129. Morris PJ: Histocompatibility in organ transplantation in man. In Pathobiology Annal 1973. Ioachim HL (ed). New York, Appleton Century Crofts, 1973
130. Morris PJ: Histocompatibility systems, immune response and disease in man. In Contemporary Topics in Immunobiology. Cooper MD, Warner NL (eds). Vol 3. New York, Plenum Press, 1974, p 141
131. Mote, JR, Jones TD: The development of foreign protein sensitization in human beings. J Immunol 30:149, 1936
132. Nakamura RM, Weigle WO: Transfer of experimental thyroiditis by serum from thyroidectomized donors. J Exp Med 130:263, 1969
133. Nathan CF, Karnovsky ML, David JR: Alterations of macrophage functions by mediators from lymphocytes. J Exp Med 133:1356, 1971
134. Nathenson SG: Biochemical properties of histocompatibility antigens. Ann Rev Genet 4:69, 1970
135. Nelson DS: Immunological enhancement of skin homografts in guinea pigs. Br J Exp Pathol 43:1, 1962
136. Old LJ, Stockert E, Boyse EA, Kim JH: Antigenic modulation. Loss of TL antigen from cells exposed to TL antibody. Study of the phenomenon in vitro. J Exp Med 127:523, 1968
137. Paronetto F: Immunologic aspects of liver disease. Prog Liver Dis 3:299, 1970
138. Paterson PY: The demyelinating diseases: clinical and experimental correlates. In Immunological Diseases. Sampter M (ed). 2nd ed. Boston, Little, Brown, 1971, p 1269
139. Pease PE: L-Forms, Episomes, and Autoimmune Diseases. Edinburgh, Livingstone, 1965
140. Perlmann P, Holm G: Cytotoxic effects of lymphoid cells in vitro. Adv Immunol 11:117, 1970
141. Perlmann P, Perlmann H, Biberfeld P: Specifically cytotoxic lymphocytes produced by preincubation with antibody complexed target cells. J Immunol 108:558, 1972
142. Perlmann P, Perlmann H, Müller-Eberhard HJ, Manni JA: Cytotoxic effects of leukocytes triggered by complement bound to target cells. Science 163:937, 1969

143. Perlmann P, Perlmann H, Wigzell H: Lymphocyte-mediated cytotoxicity in vitro. Induction and inhibition by humoral antibody and nature of effector cells. Transplant Rev 13:91, 1972
144. Peterson PA, Rask L, Lindblom JB: Highly purified papain-solubilized HL-A antigens contain B-2-microglobulin. Proc Natl Acad Sci USA 71:35, 1974
145. Pick E, Brostoff J, Krejci J, Turk JL: Interaction between "sensitized lymphocytes" and antigen in vitro. II. Mitogen-induced release of skin reactive and macrophage migration inhibitory factors. Cell Immunol 1:92, 1970
146. Prier JE, Friedman H: Australia Antigen. Baltimore, University Park Press, 1973
147. Prince AM, Szmuness W, Woods KR, Grady GF: Antibody against serum-hepatitis antigen. Prevalence and potential use as immune serum globulin in prevention of serum hepatitis infections. N Engl J Med 285:933, 1971
148. Prince AM, Trepo C: Role of immune complexes involving SH antigen in pathogenesis of chronic active hepatitis and polyarteritis nodosa. Lancet 1:7713, 1971
149. Rachelefsky GS, Terasaki PI, Katz R, Steim ER: Increased prevalence of W27 in juvenile rheumatoid arthritis. N Engl J Med 290:892, 1974
150. Raffel J, Newel JM: The "delayed hypersensitivity" induced by antigen–antibody complexes. J Exp Med 108:823, 1958
151. Raine CS: Viral infections of nervous tissue and their relevance to multiple sclerosis. In Multiple Sclerosis. Wolfram F, Ellison GW, Stevens JG, Andrews JM (eds). New York, Academic Press, 1972, p 91
152. Reisfeld RA: Isolation and serological evaluation of HL-A antigens solubilized from cultured human lymphoid cells. In Methods in Membrane Biology. Korn ED (ed). New York, Plenum Press, 1974, p 143
153. Reisfeld RA, Pellegrino MA, Ferrone S, Kahan BD: Chemical and molecular nature of HL-A antigens. Transplant Proc 5:447, 1973
154. Remold HG, David RA, David JR: Characterization of migration inhibitory factor (MIF) from guinea pig lymphocytes stimulated with concanavalin A. J Immunol 109:578, 1972
155. Richerson HB, Dvorak HF, Leskowitz S: Cutaneous basophil hypersensitivity: A new interpretation of the Jones-Mote reaction. J Immunol 103:1431, 1969
156. Rosenau W, Moon HD: Lysis of homologous cells by sensitized lymphocytes in tissue culture. J Natl Cancer Inst 27:471, 1961
157. Ruddle NH, Waksman BH: Cytotoxicity mediated by soluble antigen and lymphocytes in delayed hypersensitivity. I. Characterization of the phenomenon. J Exp Med 128:1237, 1968
158. Russell PS, Monaco AP: The biology of tissue transplantation. N Engl J Med 271:502, 553, 610, 664, 718, 776, 1964
159. Russell WO: Viruses and autoimmune disease. Fifth annual ASCP Research symposium. Am J Clin Pathol 56:259, 1971
160. Sabesin SM, Koff RS: Pathogenesis of experimental viral hepatitis. N Engl J Med 290:944, 1974
161. Salvin SB, Nishio J: In vitro cell reactions in delayed hypersensitivity. J Immunol 103:138, 1969
162. Santos GW: Application of marrow grafts in human disease. Am J Pathol 65:653, 1971
163. Schlosstein L, Terasaki PI, Bluestone R, Pearson CM: High association of an HL-A antigen, W27, with ankylosing spondylitis. N Engl J Med 288:704, 1973
164. Sell S, Weigle WO: The relationship between delayed hypersensitivity and circulating antibody induced by protein antigens in guinea pigs. J Immunol 83:257, 1959
165. Senior JR, Sutnick AI, Goeser E, London WT, Dahlke MB, Blumberg BS: Reduction of post-transfusion hepatitis by exclusion of Ausralia antigen from donor blood in an urban public hospital. Am J Med Sci 267:171, 1974
166. Shulman NR, Barker LF: Virus-like antigen–antibody and antigen–antibody complexes in hepatitis measured by complement fixation. Science 165:304, 1969
167. Simon FA, Rackeman FF: The development of hypersensitiveness in man. I. Following intradermal injection of the antigen. J Allergy 5:439, 1934
168. Simonsen M: Graft-versus-host reactions: Their natural history and applicability as tools of research. Prog Allergy 6:349, 1962
169. Slavin RE, Santos GW: The graft versus host reaction in man after bone marrow

transplantation: Pathology, pathogenesis, clinical features and implication. Clin Immunol Immunopathol 1:472, 1973
170. Smith RT, Baucher JAC, Adler WH: Studies of an inhibitor of DNA synthesis and a nonspecific mitrogen elaborated by human lymphoblasts. Am J Pathol 60:495, 1970
171. Snell GD, Stimpfling JH: Genetics of Tissue Transplantation. In Biology of the Laboratory Mouse. Green EL (ed). 2nd ed. New York, McGraw-Hill, 1966
172. Spitler LE, Lawrence HS: Studies on lymphocyte culture: Products of sensitive lymphocyte-antigen interaction. J Immunol 103:1072, 1969
173. Stetson CA: The role of humoral antibody in the homograft rejection. Adv Immunol 3:97, 1963
174. Storb R, Thomas ED, Buckner CD, Clift RA, Johnson FL, Fefer A, Glucksberg H, Giblett ER, Lerner KG, Neiman P: Allogenic marrow grafting for treatment of aplastic anemia. Blood 43:157, 1974
175. Subcommittee on the National Halothane Study: Summary of the National Halothane Study: Possible Association between Halothane Anesthesia and Post-Operative Hepatic Necrosis. JAMA 197:775, 1966
176. Sutnick AI, Millman I, London WT, Blumberg BS: The role of Australia antigen in viral hepatitis and other diseases. Annu Rev Med 23:161, 1972
177. Szulman AE: The A, B and H blood-group antigens in the human placenta. N Engl J Med 286:1028, 1972
178. Szulman AE: The histologic distribution of the blood group substances in man as determined by immunofluorescence. III. The A, B and H antigens in embryos and fetuses from 18 mm in length. J Exp Med 119:503, 1964
179. Takasugi M, Klein E: A microassay for cell-mediated immunity. Transplantation 9:219, 1970
180. Taliaferro WH, Taliaferro LG, Jaroslow BN: Radiation and Immune Mechanisms. New York, Academic Press, 1964
181. Taylor HE, Culling CFA: Cytopathic effect in vitro of sensitized homologous and heterologous spleen cells on fibroblasts. Lab Invest 12:884–894, 1963
182. Terasaki PI, Mickey MR, Singal DP, Mittali KK, Patel R: Serotyping for transplantation. XX. Selection of recipients for cadaver donor transplants. N Engl J Med 279:1101, 1968
183. Thomas ED, Bryant JI, Buckner CD, Clift RA, Fefer A, Neiman P, Ramberg RE, Storb R: Leukemic transformation of engrafted bone marrow. Transplant Proc 4:567, 1972
184. Thomas ED, Buckner CD, Rudolph RH, Fefer A, Storb R, Neiman PE, Bryant JI, Chard RL, Clift RA, Epstein RB, Fialkow PJ, Funk DD, Giblett ER, Lerner KG, Reynolds FA, Slichter S: Allogeneic marrow grafting for hematologic malignancy using HL-A matched donor–recipient sibling pairs. J Hematol 38:267, 1971
185. Thorsby E: The human major histocompatibility system. Transplant Rev 18:51, 1974
186. Tung KSK, Unanue ER, Dixon FJ: The immunopathology of experimental allergic orchitis. Am J Pathol 60:313, 1970
187. Turk JL, Polak L: A comparison of the effect of anti-lymph-node serum and anti-granulocyte serum on local passive transfer of the tuberculin reaction and the normal lymphocyte transfer reaction. Int Arch Allergy Appl Immunol 34:105, 1968
188. Uhr JW: Delayed hypersensitivity. Physiol Rev 46:359, 1966
189. Unanue ER, Dixon FJ: Experimental glomerulonephritis: Immunological events and pathologic mechanisms. Adv Immunol 6:1, 1967
190. Urbaniak SJ, Penhale WJ, Irvine WJ: Circulating lymphocyte subpopulations in Hashimoto's thyroiditis. Clin Exp Immunol 15:345, 1973
191. Uzunalimoglu B, Yardley JH, Boitnott JK: The liver in mild halothane hepatitis. Light and electron microscopic findings with special reference to the mononuclear cell infiltrate. Am J Pathol 61:457, 1970
192. Van Bekkum DW: Mitigation of acute secondary disease by treatment of the recipient with anti-lymphocyte serum before grafting of allogeneic hemopoietic cells. Exp Hematol 20:3, 1970
193. Van Bekkum DW: Use and abuse of hemopoietic cell grafts in immune deficiency diseases. In Lymphoid Cell Replacement. Möller G (ed). Transplant Rev 9:3, 1972

194. Van Boxel JA, Paul WE, Green I, Frank M: Antibody-dependent lymphoid cell-mediated cytotoxicity: Role of complement. J Immunol 112:398, 1974
195. Van Rood JJ, Eernisse JG: The detection of transplantation antigens in leukocytes. Prog Surg 7:217, 1967
196. Voisin GA: Immunological facilitation, a broadening concept of the enhancement phenomenon. Prog Allergy 15:328, 1971
197. von Pirquet CF: Klinische Studien über Vakzination und Vakzinale Allergie. Leipzig, Deuticke, 1907
198. Wagner H, Röllinghoff M, Nossal GJV: T-cell-mediated immune responses induced in vitro: A probe for allograft and tumor immunity. Transplant Rev 17:3, 1973
199. Waksman BH: A Comparative Histopathological Study of Delayed Hypersensitivity Reactions. In Cellular Aspects of Immunity. Wolstenholme GEW, Connor CE (eds). Boston, Little, Brown, 1960
200. Waksman BH: Autoimmunization and the lesions of autoimmunity. Medicine 41:93, 1962
201. Waksman BH: Discussion of Biological Activities of Lymphocytic products. In Mediators of Cellular Immunity. Lawrence HS, Landy M (eds). New York, Academic Press, 1969, pp 278–283
202. Waksman BH: Experimental allergic encephalomyelitis and the "autoallergic" diseases. Int Arch Allergy Appl Immunol 14 (Suppl), 1959
203. Waksman BH: The distribution of experimental autoallergic lesions: Its relationship to the distribution of small veins. Am J Pathol 37:673, 1960
204. Walford RL, Waters H, Smith GS: Human transplantation antigens. Fed Proc 29:2011, 1970
205. Walker SM, Lucas ZJ: Cytotoxic activity of lymphocytes. I. Assay for cytotoxicity by rubidium exchange at isotopic equilibrium. J Immunol 109:1223, 1972
206. Ward PA, Remold HG, David JR: Leukotactic factor produced by sensitized lymphocytes. Science 163:1079, 1969
207. Webb HE, Gordonsmith CW: Relation of immune response to development of central nervous system lesions in virus infections of man. Br Med J 2:1179, 1966
208. Weigle WO: The induction of autoimmunity in rabbits following injection of heterologous or altered homologous thyroglobulin. J Exp Med 121:289, 1965
209. Westall FC, Robinson AB, Caccam J, Jackson J, Eylar EH: Essential chemical requirements for induction of allergic encephalomyelitis. Nature (Lond) 229:22, 1971
210. Williams TW, Granger GA: Lymphocyte in vitro cytotoxicity: Mechanisms of lymphotoxic-induced target cell destruction. J Immunol 102:911, 1969
211. Wilson DB: Quantitative studies on the behavior of sensitized lymphocytes in vitro. I. Relationship of the degree of destruction of homologous target cells to the number of lymphocytes and to the time of contact in culture and consideration of the effects of isoimmune serum. J Exp Med 122:143, 1965
212. Wilson RE, Henry L, Merrill JP: A model system for determining histocompatibility in man. J Clin Invest 52:1497, 1963
213. Zeman W, Lennette EN: Slow-Virus Diseases. Baltimore, Williams & Wilkens, 1974

15

Granulomatous Reactions

The reasons for considering granulomatous reactions separately from delayed hypersensitivity have been clarified by Epstein (6). Granulomatous reactions (Fig. 15-1) are identified by appearance of reticuloendothelial cells, including phagocytes, histiocytes, epithelioid cells and giant cells. The characteristic epithelioid cell has a prominent eosinophilic amorphous cytoplasm and a large, oval, pale-staining nucleus with a sharp, thin nuclear membrane and large nuclei. These cells have been called epithelioid because of their superficial resemblance to epithelial cells. They are arranged into tubercles or granulomas—the most characteristic feature of granulomatous hypersensitivity reactions. Although it is not always possible, these reactions should be differentiated from banal chronic inflammatory reactions in which mononuclear cells, plasma cells, and eosinophils accumulate. Epstein considers the granulomatous reaction an immune response to poorly soluble substances. It may be induced by foreign bodies or by a hypersensitivity reaction to insoluble antigens. Perhaps the most common granulomatous reaction may be found surrounding insoluble suture material.

The origin of the most characteristic cell of granulomatous hypersensitivity reaction—the epithelioid cell—remains uncertain (6). It has been generally thought that the epithelioid cell arises from a phagocyte that has ingested foreign material. However, this concept is difficult to reconcile with the observations that 1) epithelioid cells do not necessarily contain phagocytized material, 2) epithelioid cells arise in areas where mitosis of monocytes is much more frequently observed than phagocytosis, 3) many epithelioid cells may be found in areas where there appears to be little substance to be phagocytized, and 4) there is no evidence that epithelial cells are phagocytically active. In conclusion, it is likely that epithelioid cells differentiate from actually dividing mononuclear cells. In the lung, epithelioid cells and giant cells may arise from bronchial lining cells.

The relation of granulomatous hypersensitivity to delayed type reactions or other immune reactions is also unknown. Morphologically, granulomatous hypersensitivity reactions are clearly different from pure delayed reactions, although there are similarities (6). The onset of granulomatous hypersensi-

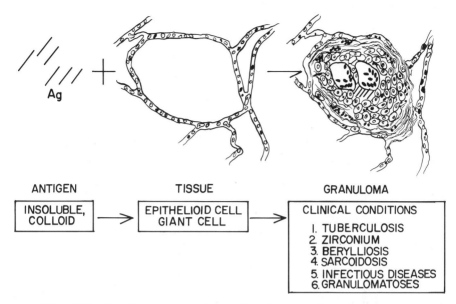

ANTIGEN	TISSUE	GRANULOMA
INSOLUBLE, COLLOID	EPITHELIOID CELL GIANT CELL	CLINICAL CONDITIONS 1. TUBERCULOSIS 2. ZIRCONIUM 3. BERYLLIOSIS 4. SARCOIDOSIS 5. INFECTIOUS DISEASES 6. GRANULOMATOSES

Fig. 15–1. Granulomatous reactions. Granulomatous hypersensitivity reactions may be identified morphologically by appearance of reticuloendothelial cells, including histiocytes, epithelioid cells, giant cells, and, in some instances, lymphocytes arranged in a characteristic round or oval laminated structure called a granuloma.

tivity reactions is much more delayed than that of delayed hypersensitivity, requiring weeks or even months to develop. Many diseases demonstrate both granulomatous reactions and vasculitis, varying from essentially pure granulomatous lesions to pure vasculitis (Fig. 15–2) and suggest a possible relationship between granulomatous reactions and toxic complex arteritis.

The diseases associated with granulomatous hypersensitivity include tuberculosis, zirconium granuloma, berylliosis, sarcoidosis, leprosy, parasitic infestations and other diseases in which epithelioid granulomas appear, but are not a primary feature.

TUBERCULOSIS

Tuberculosis is the classic example of a granulomatous diseases (3). Only tuberculosis in man is considered here, as infection of other species with tubercle bacilli results in a significantly different response from that of man (6). Infection with tubercle bacilli may result in different types of immune responses, including 1) circulating antibody, 2) classic delayed hypersensitivity, 3) immune phagocytosis, and 4) granulomatous hypersensitivity. That some type of immunity does occur is indicated by finding of a primary (Ghon) complex in many patients at autopsy, indicating that the patient resisted a previous tuberculosis infection by a granulomatous reaction, and by the failure of many patients with clinical symptoms of primary tuberculosis to develop significant further disease. This immunity

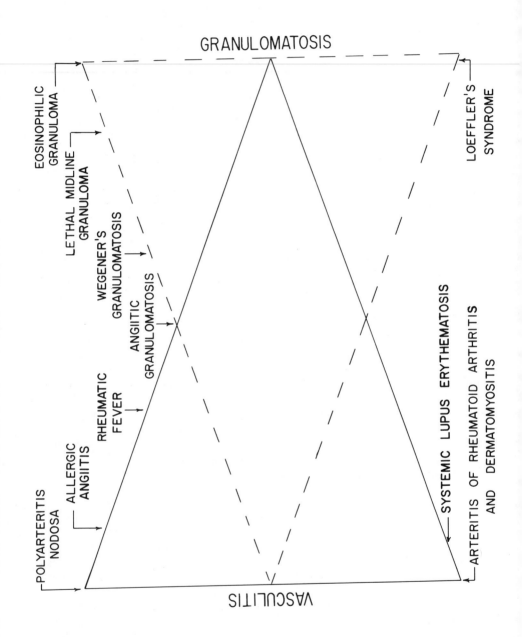

may be mediated through one or a combination of the above four mechanisms. Evidence that the granulomatous reaction is protective is not always clear. Epstein, in fact, states that the event which signals the breakdown of the immune defense against tuberculosis in the onset of granulomatous hypersensitivity (6). The granulomatous response may not destroy the bacillus, and may even protect it from the other defensive reactions of the host. However, it is more generally accepted that a granulomatous tubercle isolates the bacillus and limits dissemination. Clearly a granulomatous reaction represents a defensive reaction on the part of an infected individual; the fact that this reaction is not always successful in limiting the infection does not mean that is is not a potentially protective response.

ZIRCONIUM GRANULOMA

Some 6 months following the marketing of stick deodorants containing zirconium salts, individuals were observed with axillary granulomas. The injection of zirconium into the skin of such patients resulted in the delayed appearance of a typical epithelioid granuloma. Further studies have clearly implicated zirconium as the causative agent. Some type of hypersensitivity was suspected because only relatively few individuals who used such deodorants actually developed lesions.

BERYLLIOSIS

Chronic progressive pulmonary disease featuring multiple small non-caseating granulomas may be caused by the inhalation of beryllium salts (4,16). The conclusion that a type of hypersensitivity is involved is based on the observations that only a small number of the exposed individuals actually develop the disease and that there is a delay of months or years from the time of exposure to the development of berylliosis (9,16). The chronicity may also be due to the fact that beryllium tends to remain in the tissues indefinitely. It has been reported that patients with berylliosis give positive patch test reactions with the antigen, but the validity of this observation has been questioned. Further studies have shown that beryllium is an active inducer of contact (delayed-type) sensitivity, and a patch test probably does not measure granulomatous hypersensitivity but delayed hypersensitivity. A more valid test is the production of a granuloma upon intradermal application of beryllium in patients with berylliosis.

Fig. 15–2. Spectrum of association of granulomatous reactions and vasculitis. The lesions of Loeffler's syndrome and eosinophilic granuloma are essentially pure granulomas; those of the vasculitis found with polyarteritis nodosa and collagen diseases are almost pure arteritis. On the other hand, a number of diseases, such as rheumatic fever and Wegener's granulomatosis, demonstrate a mixture of granulomatous reactions and vasculitis (1).

The lymphocytes of patients with berylliosis will transform in vitro upon exposure to beryllium sulfate (5), further suggesting that cellular sensitization to beryllium occurs. Zirconium as well as beryllium may bind serum proteins and function as a hapten in the production of contact sensitivity. However, the relation of this mechanism to the development of granulomas remains obscure.

SARCOIDOSIS

Boeck's sarcoidosis is a systemic granulomatous process prominently involving the lymph nodes, lungs, eyes, and skin, with lesions that may be indistinguishable from those of tuberculosis, fungus infections or other granulomatous hypersensitivity reactions (6). It is remarkable for its geographic prevalence in the eastern United States and its rarity in the western United States. Most patients have a negative tuberculin reaction and generally suppressed delayed hypersensitivity. However, a cutaneous granulomatous reaction may be elicited 3–4 weeks after the subcutaneous injection of crude extracts of sarcoid lymph nodes (Kveim reaction). The specificity of this reaction and its use as a diagnostic test are questionable. The role of an infectious agent remains undefined. No infectious agent has been isolated.

LEPROSY

Leprosy occurs in three forms—tuberculoid, lepromatous and mixed. The tuberculoid type is characterized by an organized epithelioid granuloma, while in the lepromatous large foamy lepra cells filled with organisms are found. The tuberculoid form is the more benign. The induction of a granulomatous hypersensitivity response produces the tuberculoid form and provides protection against the spread of the infection (see page 290).

PARASITIC INFESTATIONS

Granulomatous reactions occur in response to parasitic infestations, particularly those due to certain helminths (worms; see also Chapter 18). Schistosomiasis and filariasis are worthy of further comment. In infestations with *Schistosoma mansoni* the eggs are released into the portal bloodstream and lodge in the portal veins of the liver. Here the eggs evoke a severe granulomatous inflammatory reaction that may gradually increase and lead to extensive fibrosis of the portal areas (pipestem fibrosis). If the liver involvement is severe, collateral circulation of the portal system develops as the portal radicals in the liver become obstructed. The eggs may then pass from the portal system through collateral channels to the pulmonary arteries resulting in multiple small granulomatous lesions resembling miliary tuberculosis (pseudotubercles). The eggs of other schistosomes (*S. haematobium* and *S. japonicum*) are deposited in large numbers in the subepithelial connective tissue of the urinary bladder. A severe granulomatous reaction may occur resulting in obstruction of urinary flow.

The adult worms of *Wuchereria bancrofti* (filaria) reside in the larger lymphocytic channels, particularly those of the extremities. In some individuals the presence of these worms evokes an extensive granulomatous inflammatory reaction that causes obstruction to lymphatic flow. This obstruction may lead to massive swelling (lymphedema) of the involved area (elephantiasis). Only a small number of individuals with filaria infestation develop this complication, and it is believed that those individuals who do not develop clinical manifestations do not have granulomatous sensitivity to the organism. Therefore, the granulomatous reaction, although it leads to death and isolation of the offending agent, is definitely deleterious to the host.

GRANULOMATOUS-LIKE DISEASES

Epithelioid granulomas occur in such diseases as tertiary syphilis, certain fungus infections and some foreign body reactions (e.g., around urate deposits in gout). Granulomas are also a prominent feature of silicosis, but the formation of silica granulomas is most likely due not to granulomatous hypersensitivity but to an effect on phagocytosis. Ingested silica is toxic for phagocytic cells. Cells that take up silica die, and the silica is rephagocytized by other cells.

WEGENER'S GRANULOMATOSIS

Wegener's granulomatosis is a triad of granulomatous arteritis, glomerulonephritis and sinusitis (7). The glomerulonephritis may or may not be present, and the granulomas may be disseminated but are usually prominent in the lungs, nasal and oral cavities, and spleen. The granulomatous lesions are destructive and contain fibroblastic proliferation, necrosis and prominent Langhans' giant cells. This disease may be related to polyarteritis nodosa (2), and some authors have called it polyarteritis of the lungs or a type of hypersensitivity angiitis. However, the lesions of Wegener's granulomatosis are distinctive enough to warrant a separate diagnosis, and polyarteritis nodosa does not usually involve the lung. The relation of Wegener's granulomatosis to other necrotizing granulomatous processes such as midline lethal granuloma of the face and Cogan's syndrome (a middle ear granuloma) is also unclear (2), and these appear to be clinically separate entities. No infectious agent has been consistently isolated from patients with any of these diseases.

EXTRINSIC ALLERGIC ALVEOLITIS

Allergic reactions to organic dusts, bacteria, or mold products in the lung are believed to be causative in certain types of interstitial pneumonitis, termed extrinsic allergic alveolitis by Pepys (14) [Table 15-1]. The primary allergic reaction appears to be granulomatous; however, the frequent coexistence of other types of reactions such as anaphylactic, toxic complex or

TABLE 15–1
Source and Type of Antigen-Producing Extrinsic Allergic Alveolitis

Disease	Source of antigen	Antigen against which precipitating antibody is present
Farmer's lung	Moldy hay	*Micropolyspora faeni, Thermoactinomyces vulgaris*
Bagassosis	Moldy bagasse*	*T. vulgaris*
Mushroom-worker's lung	Mushroom compost	*M. faeni, T. vulgaris*
Fog-fever in cattle	Moldy hay	*M. faeni*
Suberosis	Moldy oak bark, cork dust	Moldy cork dust
New Guinea lung	Moldy thatch dust	Thatch
Maple-bark pneumonitis	Moldy maple-bark	*Cryptostroma (Coniosporium) corticale*
Malt-worker's lung	Moldy barley, malt dust	*Aspergillus clavatus* *Aspergillus fumigatus*
Bird-fancier's lung	Pigeon/budgerigar/ parrot/hen droppings	Serum protein, droppings
Pituitary snuff-taker's lung	Heterologous pituitary powder	Serum protein, pituitary antigens
Wheat-weevil disease	Infested wheat flour	*Sitophilus granarius*
Sequoiosis	Moldy sawdust	*Graphium* *Aureobasidium pullulans (Pullularia)*
Cheese-washer's lung	Moldy cheese	*Penicillin* spp.

* Residue of sugar cane after extraction of syrup.
Modified from Pepys J: Hypersensitivity diseases of the lungs due to fungi and organic dusts. Monogr Allergy. Vol 4, Basel/New York, S. Karger, 1969.

delayed may produce a complex clinical and pathologic picture in a given patient. The pathologic reaction is mixed, but inflammation of the alveolar walls is the primary feature, usually consisting of epithelioid cell granulomas. Plasma and lymphoid cell infiltration may also be prominent, and granulomas are not always present. In fact, a variety of lymphoid cell infiltrates and inflammatory reactions may be found in the lung (10), suggesting that a mixture of different types of immune or allergic reactions may be manifested at any given time (12). In many cases, precipitating antibodies may be demonstrated to test antigens. However, vasculitis is not a prominent feature, although there are notable exceptions. Patients with these chronic pulmonary diseases often have acute attacks of asthma on exposure to the antigen, which may be caused by the existence of anaphylactic antibodies.

GRANULOMATOUS HEPATITIS

Circumscribed granulomas consisting of epithelioid cells surrounded by plasma cells and lymphocytes may be seen in the liver, and are associated with a variety of diseases including sarcoidosis, histoplasmosis, tuberculosis, cirrhosis, lymphomas, Wegener's granulomatosis, immune deficiency diseases and malignant tumors (8,13,15). However, in a substantial number of patients no specific disease association occurs (13,15). It is likely that the reaction represents an allergic reaction to a drug or response to an unidentified infectious agent.

GRANULOMATOUS DISEASE OF CHILDREN

Granulomatous disease of children consists of chronic pulmonary disease, recurrent suppurative lymphadenitis, and chronic dermatitis with scattered granulomas in many organs. This disease appears to be a specific deficiency in the cellular enzymes necessary to kill bacteria following phagocytosis which results in formation of nonallergic granulomas (See Chapter 19).

REGIONAL ENTERITIS

Regional enteritis is a peculiar chronic inflammatory lesion of unknown etiology. The primary feature is thickening and scarring of the intestinal wall which may occur at any level of the gastrointestinal tract, but usually involves the terminal ileum. Histologically, the inflammatory changes vary from those consistent with a delayed hypersensitivity reaction (dense infiltration of mononuclear lymphoid follicles containing germinal centers) to those of granulomatous hypersensitivity (typical epithelioid granulomas with prominent giant cells, essentially identical with the pulmonary lesions of sarcoidosis). These tissue reactions may be due to immune reactions to antigenic materials crossing the wall of the intestine, although no inciting antigenic material has yet been identified and direct demonstration of hypersensitivity has not been possible. The mononuclear inflammation of regional enteritis may be the result of the development of delayed hypersensitivity to soluble antigens in the diet, and the granulomatous inflammation may be due to the development of granulomatous hypersensitivity to insoluble antigens in the diet.

IMMUNE PHAGOCYTOSIS

Mackaness and Blanden (11) have recently reviewed the characteristics of a type of "cellular immunity" that is clearly different from the usual delayed type of hypersensitivity reactions. An acquired cellular resistance to microbial infection may be observed in an infected host whose mononuclear phagocytes have an increased capacity for destroying infected organisms. Once such an increased capacity has been established, it is active against infections caused by unrelated organisms. Macrophages that develop an increased functional capacity are termed activated. A number of agents have been found that cause activation of macrophages. These include Bacillus Calmette-Guérin (BCG), Listeria monocytogenes, toxoplasma, endotoxin and polynucleotides (Fig. 15–3). A considerable interest in the role of this phenomenon in enhancing tumor immunity has developed because of the possibility of effecting tumor growth with activated macrophages (see Chapter 20). Because of the nonspecific nature of this antimicrobial reaction, some alteration in the nonimmune metabolic activity of such phagocytes may have occurred. This type of cellular immunity

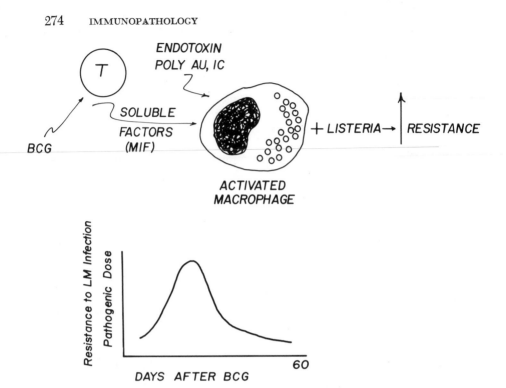

Fig. 15–3. **Nonspecific macrophage activation.**   Macrophages may acquire an increased capacity to destroy infective organisms or target cells after treatment with a variety of agents. BCG acts upon a T cell which produces a soluble factor that affects macrophages. Endotoxins and polynucleotides act directly on macrophages. The mechanism of action of these agents is not understood, but as a result of macrophage activation, an experimental animal will resist a normally infectious challenge dose of an infectious agent. The chart (**bottom**) indicates that the dose of *L. monocytogenes,* which is required to kill an experimental animal, is significantly higher after treatment of the animals with BCG.

is termed immune phagocytosis even though this "immunity" is nonspecific. The relation between immune phagocytosis and granulomatous hypersensitivity or other specific immune or hypersensitivity reactions is unclear.

REFERENCES

1. Alarcon-Segovia D, Brown AL: Classification and etiologic aspects of necrotizing angiitis. An analytic approach to a confused subject with a critical review of the evidence for hypersensitivity in polyarteritis nodosa. Mayo Clin Proc 39:205, 1964
2. Chrug J: Allergic granulomatosis and granulomatous vascular syndromes. Ann Allergy 21:619, 1963
3. Dannenburg AM: Cellular hypersensitivity and cellular immunity in the pathogenesis of tuberculosis specificity, systemic and local nature, and associated macrophage enzymes. Bacteriol Rev 32:85, 1968
4. Denardi JN, Van Ordstrand HS, Curtis GH, Zielinski J: Berylliosis. Arch Industr Hyg 8:1, 1953

5. Deodhar SD, Barna B, Van Ordstrand HS: A study of the immunologic aspects of chronic berylliosis. Chest 63:309, 1973
6. Epstein WL: Granulomatous hypersensitivity. Prog Allergy 11:36, 1967
7. Fahey JL, Leonard E, Chrug J: Wegener's granulomatosis. Am J Med 17:168, 1954
8. Gugkian JC, Perry JE: Granulomatous hepatitis of unknown etiology: An etiologic and functional evaluation. Am J Med 44:207, 1968
9. Kanarek DJ, Wainer RA, Chamberlin RI, Weber AL, Kazemi H: Respiratory illness in a population exposed to beryllium. Am Rev Resp Dis 108:1295, 1973
10. Liebow AA, Carrington CB: Hypersensitivity reactions involving the lungs. Trans Stud Coll Physicians Phila 34:47–70, 1966
11. Mackaness GB, Blanden RV: Cellular immunity. Prog Allergy 11:89, 1967
12. McCombs RP: Diseases due to immunologic reactions in the lungs. N Engl J Med 286:1186–1245, 1972
13. Mir-Madjlessi SH, Farmer RG, Hawk WA: Granulomatous hepatitis: A review of 50 cases. Am J Gastroenterol 60:122, 1973
14. Pepys J: Hypersensitivity Diseases of the Lungs Due to Fungi and Organic Dusts. In Monographs in Allergy. Vol. 4. Kallós P, Hašek M, Interbitzen TM, Miescher P, Waksman BH (eds). Basel, Karger, 1969
15. Simon HB, Wolff SM: Granulomatous hepatitis and prolonged fever of unknown origin: A study of 13 patients. Medicine 52:1, 1973
16. Tepper LB, Hardy HL, Chamberlin RI: Toxicity of Beryllium Compounds. Amsterdam, Elsevier, 1961

16

Comparison of Immunopathologic Mechanisms

ANTIBODY-MEDIATED DISEASE

Neutralization, cytotoxic, atopic, and toxic complex reactions result when circulating or humoral antibody combines in vivo with antigen. Considered as immune phenomena, these four types of reactions have the following properties in common:

1. The hypersensitive state is induced by previous exposure to antigen (or passive transfer of antibody).
2. There is a definite induction or latent period comparable to that of other immune responses (1–2 weeks).
3. The reaction occurs only on exposure to the specific antigen or to closely related chemical substances that cross react.
4. The reaction is determined mainly by the biologic properties of the antibody, or species of animal (i.e., details of anaphylaxis depend on distribution of smooth muscle). The type of tissue reaction or effect also depends upon the nature and location of the antigen.
5. The degree of hypersensitivity tends to diminish with time. Reexposure to antigen results in reappearance of hypersensitivity more rapidly and in more intense form than primary exposure (secondary or anamnestic response).
6. The hypersensitive state can be passively transferred with serum (antibody).
7. Administration of antigen with proper precautions to avoid anaphylactic death can result in temporary desensitization—loss of the ability to react due to saturation of antibody available at the given time.

276

CELL-MEDIATED DISEASE

Delayed Hypersensitivity

This is characterized by the reaction of specifically sensitized cells (lymphocytes) with antigen. As a result of such reactions, a number of mediators may be released which increase the intensity of the tissue response by the recruitment of other mononuclear cells. The major difference between this type of allergic response and those discussed above is that delayed hypersensitivity reactions cannot be transferred or initiated by circulating immunoglobulin antibody.

Granulomatous Hypersensitivity

This is characterized by the formation of organized collections of altered mononuclear cells called granulomas. The nature of antigen recognition in granulomatous hypersensitivity remains unknown, but this type of hypersensitivity may be due to delayed reactivity to insoluble antigens. The immune characteristics of granulomatous reactivity are not well documented.

INTERACTIVATIONS OF ALLERGIC MECHANISMS

The classification of allergic diseases presented herein has stressed the unique characteristics of each type of reaction. However, not only may more than one mechanism be active at a given time, but the activation of one mechanism may result in side effects due to interactivations of another allergic mechanism. Some possible interactivations of allergic mechanisms are illustrated in Fig. 16–1.

The central position of toxic complex reactions is emphasized in Fig. 16–1 because these reactions may be activated by each of the other allergic mechanisms, and toxic complex reactions may play a role in damage induced by each of the other mechanisms (1). Neutralization by reaction of antibodies with circulating antigen may result in the formation of soluble antibody–antigen complexes, in turn causing a toxic complex glomerulonephritis. In fact, neutralization reactions may be considered as a variation of toxic complex reactions. Anaphylactic reactions may be activated by mast cell lysis by release of enzymes from polymorphonuclear leukocytes due to toxic complex action. The release of anaphylactic mediators may contribute to the vascular lesions of toxic complex reactions. The reaction of immune complexes with platelets may induce serotonin release, which causes increased vascular permeability, toxic complex deposition, polymorphonuclear infiltrate and subsequent tissue damage. Anaphylactic mediators released from antigen-activated mast cells may cause separation of endothelial cells, exposing the basement membrane and thus forming foci where immune complexes can fix and stimulate basement membrane damage by an Arthus mechanism. Binding of antibody–antigen complexes to red cells may result in their destruction by activation of complement (the innocent

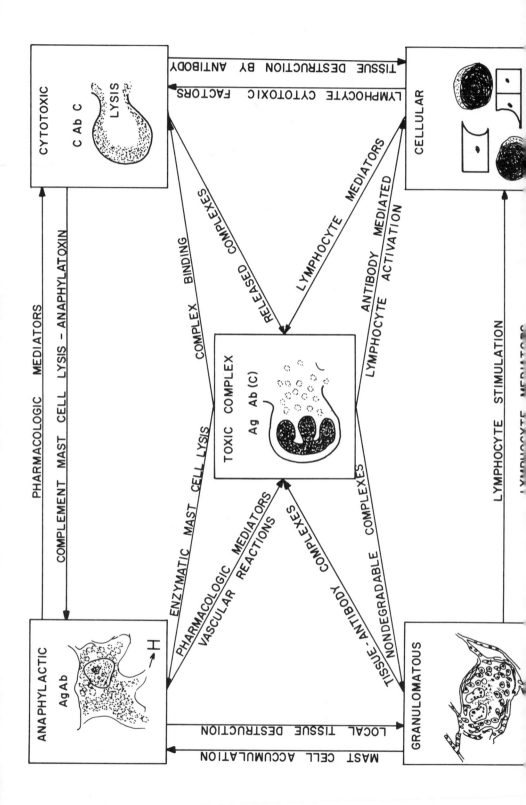

bystander reaction), and soluble complexes released by lysed cells may contribute to a toxic complex effect. Antibodies may cause destruction of tissue cells in graft rejection or autoallergic diseases mainly mediated by sensitized cells. Although sensitized cells reacting with lymphocytic choriomeningitis (LCM) virus antigens in host cells are thought to be responsible for most of the tissue destruction observed in LCM disease, antibody to LCM virus causes destruction of LCM-infected cells in vitro in the presence of complement. Immunoglobulin and complement can be identified early in the lesions of experimental allergic encephalomyelitis (7), although the role of toxic complexes in the production of the demyelination characteristic of the disease is not clear (5,8,11). Mediators released from sensitized lymphocytes upon contact with antigen may be chemotactic for polymorphonuclear leukocytes, thus producing a tissue reaction similar to that induced by toxic complex reactions. In general, circulating antibodies are effective in destroying cells either in suspension or in direct contact with the circulation, whereas sensitized cells effect the destruction of cells in solid tissue. Both immunoglobulin and antibody may play a role in the lesions seen in autoallergic disease such as thyroiditis, encephalomyelitis or orchitis (10). The formation of nondegradable antibody–antigen complexes may initiate granuloma formation, whereas tissue-antibody or breakdown products produced by granulomatous reactions may lead to toxic complex glomerulonephritis.

Other allergic mechanisms may also interreact. Complement-induced mast cell lysis (cytotoxic reaction) may cause anaphylactic symptoms, and pharmacologic mediators and vascular reactions may contribute to cytotoxic effects. Cytotoxic antibody may contribute to cell-mediated tissue destruction (e.g., aspermatogenesis); cytotoxic factors released by activated lymphocytes may produce lysis of cells. Lymphocyte mediators may contribute to the evolution of a granulomatous reaction by attracting and activating macrophages; release of lymphocyte-stimulating factors from granulomatous inflammatory sites may contribute to the cellular component of such reactions. Finally, although the mechanism is less clear, granulomatous lung diseases (such as farmer's lung) frequently have asthmatic (anaphylactic) components. Granulomatous inflammation may increase the number of mast cells present, and tissue destruction by anaphylactic mechanisms may contribute to granuloma formation. Interactivation of anaphylactic and cellular reactions, and of cytotoxic and granulomatous reactions, may also occur, although these are not indicated in Fig. 16–1.

The confusion that can arise when one immunopathologic mechanism is accepted over another on the basis of one set of observations is illustrated by thyroiditis in experimental animals. The onset and severity of experimental allergic thyroiditis in guinea pigs can be correlated with the intensity of delayed sensitivity and not with titers of circulating antibody (2). In addition, the disease may be transferred with lymph node cells from sensi-

Fig. 16–1. Possible interactivation of allergic mechanisms.   For description see text.

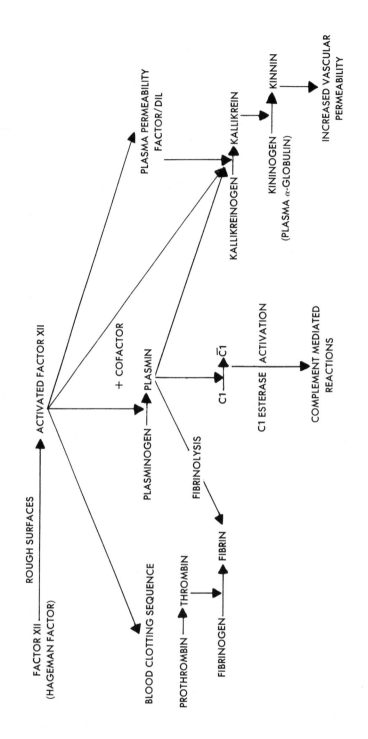

tized guinea pigs, but not with antiserum. On the other hand, thyroiditis has been transferred with antiserum in rabbits (6). Thymectomy of chickens, which suppresses delayed reactions, inhibits the induction of experimental allergic thyroiditis, but bursectomy, which suppresses antibody formation, does not affect the induction of thyroiditis (3). However, a naturally occurring thyroiditis in the obese strain of chickens (4) is suppressed by bursectomy and made worse by thymectomy (12). On the basis of these observations some workers concluded that thyroiditis is mediated only by sensitized cells while others considered that immunoglobulin antibody was necessary for the induction of thyroiditis. It is likely that both sensitized cells and immunoglobulin antibody play a role in allergic thyroiditis or that there may be species differences.

Other systems, such as the blood clotting and the kinin systems, may be activated during the evolution of an inflammatory reaction which also involves allergic reactions. For example, the role that Hageman factor (factor XII of the blood sequence) plays in involvement of other systems is illustrated in Fig. 16–2 (9). Conversion of plasmogen to plasmin produces activation of complement which may induce lytic or inflammatory reactions. Kinins increase vascular permeability and may expose basement membranes for toxic complex deposition. Complement may be activated by nonimmunologic mechanisms (see Alternate Pathway, Chapter 11). Interaction of these "nonimmune" inflammatory mechanisms with allergic (immune) mechanisms further complicates interpretation of a given inflammatory situation.

It is not difficult to imagine how confusing it may be to evaluate the inflammatory processes taking place in a given patient. One must try to determine the role played by allergic and nonallergic mechanisms. In addition, the contribution of each allergic mechanism must first be considered separately.

REFERENCES

1. Cochrane CG: Immunologic tissue injury mediated by neutrophilic leukocytes. Adv Immunol 9:97, 1968
2. Flax MH, Jankovic BD, Sell S: Experimental allergic thyroiditis in the guinea pig.

Fig. 16–2. Interrelations of inflammatory and clotting mechanisms. Activation of first component of blood clotting mechanisms (Hageman factor) also results in activation of other biologic reactions including plasmin, complement and kinin systems. Plasmin induces fibrinolysis; complement, local inflammation and cell lysis; kinin, a biologically active polypeptide fragment that is split off plasma α-globulin, enhances vascular permeability and causes dilatation of small vessels. Reaction of an individual to a variety of inciting events sets off an interrelated series of responses, both immune and nonimmune, leading to blood clotting, clot lysis, inflammation, and cell lysis. (Modified from Ratnoff OD: Interrelations of clotting and immunologic mechanisms. Hosp Pract 6:119, 1971)

I. Relationship of delayed hypersensitivity and circulating antibody to the development of thyroiditis. Lab Invest 12:119, 1963

3. Jankovic BD, Isvaneski M, Popeskovic L, Mitrovic K: Experimental allergic thyroiditis (and parathyroiditis) in neonatal thymectomized and bursectomized chickens. Int Arch Allergy Appl Immunol 26:18, 1965

4. Kite JH, Wick G, Twarog B, Witebsky E: Spontaneous thyroiditis in an obese strain of chickens. II. Investigations on the development of the disease. J. Immunol 103:1331, 1969

5. Lampert PW: Mechanism of demyelination in experimental allergic neuritis: Electron microscopic studies. Lab Invest 20:127, 1969

6. Nakamura RM, Weigle WO: Transfer of experimental thyroiditis by serum from thyroidectomized donors. J Exp Med 130:263, 1969

7. Oldstone MB, Dixon FJ: Immunohistochemical study of allergic encephalomyelitis. Am J Pathol 52:251, 1968

8. Paterson PY: Experimental allergic encephalomyelitis and autoimmune disease. Adv Immunol 5:131, 1966

9. Ratnoff O: The interrelationship of clotting factors and immunologic mechanisms. In Immunology. Good RA, Fisher DW (eds). Stanford, Conn, Sinaver Assoc, Inc, 1971, p 135

10. Tung KSK, Unanue ER, Dixon FJ: The immunopathology of experimental allergic orchitis. Am J Pathol 60:313, 1970

11. Waksman BH: The distribution of experimental autoallergic lesions: Its relationship to the distribution of small veins. Am J Pathol 37:673, 1960

12. Wick G, Kite JH, Witebsky E: Spontaneous thyroiditis in the obese strain of chickens. IV. The effect of thymectomy and thymobursectomy on the development of the disease. J Immunol 104:54, 1970

17

Drug Allergy

The untoward or undesirable effects of a drug may be due to: 1) overdosage, a normal reaction to too much of the drug; 2) intolerance, an increased sensitivity to the normal action of the drug; 3) idiosyncrasy, a qualitatively abnormal pharmacologic response to the drug; 4) side effect, a normal but not the desired effect of the drug; 5) secondary effect, a normal undesired effect of the drug occurring as a result of producing the desired effect; or 6) an allergic reaction to the drug (2). Drug allergy includes various immunologically mediated hypersensitivity reactions to drugs. These reactions may be classified, on the basis of the immune mechanism involved, as 1) neutralization or inactivation of biologically active molecules, 2) cytotoxic or cytolytic reactions, 3) atopic or anaphylactic reactions, 4) toxic complex (Arthus) reactions, 5) delayed hypersensitivity reactions, or 6) granulomatous reactions (see Chapters 10 through 15).

Allergic reactions to drugs, therefore, include one or more of the immune mechanisms listed above. A given patient may express drug resistance, anaphylactic shock, asthma, fever, thrombocytopenia, agranulocytosis, hemolytic anemia, serum sickness, a systemic delayed reaction or granulomatous hepatitis, or a mixture of one or more of the above (1). Perhaps the most common allergic drug reactions recognized are manifested in the skin and thus are easily seen. A wide variety of skin reactions may be associated with drug allergy, such as exanthematic rashes, urticaria, angioedema, serum sickness, serpiginous lesions, contact dermatitis, erythema multiforme, erythema nodosum, purpura and eczema. These most likely are due to some one or more allergic mechanisms.

DRUGS AS HAPTENS

Many drug allergies involve the in vivo combination of the drug (acting as a hapten, or incomplete antigen) with a body constituent, to produce a complete antigen. This is usually the mechanism in contact allergies and in atopic reactions to, for example, aspirin. It is also the mechanism in penicillin allergy. Levine (3) has shown that penicillin acts as a hapten that combines with serum or tissue proteins to form a complete antigen. Such combinations occur in three different chemical forms owing to the ability of benzyl penicillin (penicillin G) to rearrange in vivo and to bind to protein in different forms. The administration of the simple compound benzyl penicillin to experimental animals and to man may lead to the production of antibodies with at least three different antigenic specificities. This raises the possibility that an individual may produce reaginic (atopic) antibody to one haptogenic determinant and precipitating (Arthus) antibody to another, or may produce different types of antibodies to the same determinant, thus creating the potential for a bizarre clinical picture produced by a combination of different types of allergic reactions. In fact, penicillin has been incriminated as eliciting each type of allergic mechanism. Every individual for whom penicillin therapy is being considered must be carefully questioned to rule out a previous allergic response to the drug. In addition, every patient should be warned that an allergic reaction might occur and every physician must be prepared to counteract an allergic reaction.

CLINICAL TESTING OF PENICILLIN SENSITIVITY

Recently, testing to determine an individual's potential for manifesting a serious allergic reaction to penicillin has been attempted (4,5). Studies show that many people with a history of a reaction to penicillin are able to tolerate a therapeutic dose and that the presence of circulating antibodies is not always associated with allergic reactions to penicillin. However, a positive skin reaction to intradermal injection of penicllin is associated with a high incidence of allergic reactivity (4,5). Thus, when penicillin is the drug of choice, it can, with careful evaluation and supervised administration, be given to a patient with a history of allergic reaction to penicillin. However this procedure is not advisable for general use at the present time.

REFERENCES

1. Cluff LE, Johnson JE III: Drug fever. Prog Allerg 8:149, 1964
2. de Weck AL: Drug reactions. In Immunological Diseases. 2nd ed. Sampter M (ed). Boston, Little, Brown, 1971, p 415.
3. Levine BB: Immunochemical mechanisms involved in penicillin hypersensitivity in experimental animals and in human beings. Fed Proc 24:45, 1965
4. Levine BB, Zolov DM: Prediction of penicillin allergy by immunological tests. J Allergy 43:231, 1969
5. Voss HE, Redmond AP, Levine BB: Clinical detection of the potential allergic reactor to penicillin by immunologic tests. JAMA 196:679, 1966

III

Immunity

18

Immune
Resistance to
Infection

The same immune mechanisms that produce the immunopathologically mediated diseases discussed in the preceding section of this book are also responsible for specific resistance to infection (acquired immunity). These immune mechanisms most likely evolved, and were selected as a means of protecting the individual from the destructive effects of parasitic organisms and their products, or as a means of resisting the growth of neoplastic cells (see Chapter 20). However, under some circumstances, these protective immune reactions behave as pathogenic hypersensitivity reactions. The subject of this chapter is the role of immune mechanisms in resistance to infection.

REACTIONS TO INFECTIOUS AGENTS

Innate Immunity

The survival of an individual depends upon his ability to resist a wide variety of infections (viral, bacterial, fungal, etc.). The mechanisms of resistance include nonspecific innate characteristics and specific immune reactions (19). Each species has inherent resistance to many infectious agents by virtue of factors such as pH, temperature and metabolic products (6). These factors are immunologically nonspecific in that they operate upon antigenically unrelated agents. Other factors that inhibit growth of infectious agents may be released by certain cells after stimulation. Interferon is a soluble substance induced by a variety of stimulatory events that inhibits viral infections (13). In addition to this innate resistance which does not require previous contact with the specific infectious agent, there is an acquired immunity dependent upon immune mechanisms (19).

Acquired Immunity

A specific immunity usually follows recovery from an infectious disease. The primary infection results in a state of decreased susceptibility to a subsequent attack by the organism which was responsible. This is a naturally developing state of specific active immunity (acquired immunity). Resistance to an immunologically unrelated organism is not affected.

Natural Immunity

Antibodies to certain infectious agents appear in the sera of "normal" individuals who have had no known contact with the antigen. The formation of natural antibodies is most likely due to contact with cross-reacting antigens in intestinal flora, with killed organisms in food, or from subclinical infections (42). Such natural antibodies are usually of the IgM class of immunoglobulin and are often directed against organisms found in the gastrointestinal tract (enteric organisms).

SPECIFIC ACQUIRED ACTIVE IMMUNITY

Specific active immunity is mediated through specific immunoglobulin antibody or specific cellular sensitivity. The importance of these immune mechanisms in maintaining the integrity of the individual is best exemplified by those diseases in which immune reactions are depressed or absent (see Chapter 19). The type of immune reaction differs with different infectious agents and with different reacting individuals (Table 18–1). In general, the mechanisms mediated by humoral antibody (immunoglobulin) are effective against infectious agents that exist extracellularly while cellularly mediated reactions (delayed hypersensitivity and granulomatous reactions) are effective against intracellular parasites.

Bacterial Infections

Specific immunity to the destructive effects of bacterial or bacterial products is usually mediated by humoral antibody (1). The mechanisms of antibody-mediated protection against bacterial infections are illustrated in Fig. 18–1. Destruction of infecting organisms is accomplished by the

TABLE 18–1
Major Immune Defense Mechanisms for Infectious Diseases

Type of infection	Major immune defense mechanism(s)
Bacterial	Antibody
Viral	Delayed and antibody
Mycobacterial	Granulomatous (delayed)
Protozoal	Delayed and antibody
Worms	Anaphylactic and granulomatous
Fungal	Delayed (granulomatous)

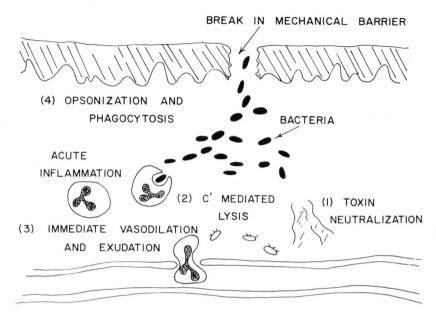

BREAK IN MECHANICAL BARRIER

(4) OPSONIZATION AND
PHAGOCYTOSIS

BACTERIA

ACUTE
INFLAMMATION

(2) C' MEDIATED
LYSIS

(1) TOXIN
NEUTRALIZATION

(3) IMMEDIATE VASODILATION
AND EXUDATION

**Fig. 18–1. Antibody-mediated mechanisms of protection against bacterial infec-
tions.** Bacterial infections may be resisted by each of the antibody-mediated
immune mechanisms including 1) neutralization of bacterial toxins, 2) cytotoxic
lysis by antibody and complement, 3) acute anaphylactic vascular events leading
to immediate exudate of inflammatory cells and fluids, and 4) acute polymorphonuclear infiltration (Arthus reaction) and opsonization of bacteria leading to increased phagocytosis.

activation of complement following the reaction of antibody with the organism, which leads to increased susceptibility of the organism to phagocytosis
(toxic complex reaction) or destruction by lysis (cytotoxic reaction). The
effectiveness of antibody-mediated protection depends upon the normal
function of the associated systems of complement and phagocytosis since
the killing effect of antibody upon an infectious organism in vivo depends
upon amplification by these systems. Enhanced states of phagocytosis (see
Immune Phagocytosis, page 273) may increase the effectiveness of antibody-mediated protection. Some bacteria produce disease not by direct
effects of the organism but by the release of products called toxins which
may have severe destructive effects distant from the site of infection. Destructive bacterial toxins are rendered harmless by reaction with antibody
(neutralization reaction).

Viral Infections

Immunologic resistance to viral infections is usually mediated by cellular sensitivity (32,48), but humoral antibody does play a role (Fig. 18–2).
Most viral agents live within the host's cells, and some viruses can spread
from cell to cell without contacting extracellular fluid. To be effective
in attacking intracellular organisms, an immune mechanism must have the

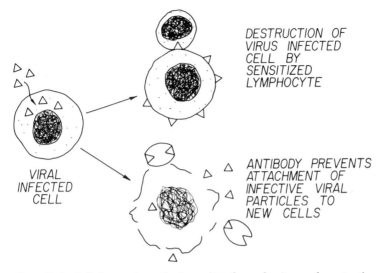

DESTRUCTION OF
VIRUS INFECTED
CELL BY
SENSITIZED
LYMPHOCYTE

VIRAL
INFECTED
CELL

ANTIBODY PREVENTS
ATTACHMENT OF
INFECTIVE VIRAL
PARTICLES TO
NEW CELLS

Fig. 18–2. Cellular and antibody-mediated mechanisms of protection against viral infections. Sensitized lymphocytes may destroy virus infected cells that express viral antigens on the surface while antibody can react with released viral particles and prevent their attachment to uninfected cells, thus inhibiting spread of the infection.

capacity to react with cells in tissue. This is property of cell-mediated reactions. Many cells infected with a virus will, at some stage of the infection, express viral antigens on the cell surface. It is at this stage that specifically sensitized cells can destroy the virus-infected cell (48). Adverse effects of this reaction occur if the cell expressing the viral antigens is important functionally, as is the case for certain viral infections of the central nervous system (see page 242). Humoral antibody can prevent the entry of virus particles into cells by interfering with the ability of the virus to attach to a host cell, and secretory immunoglobulin–antibody can prevent the establishment of viral infections in humans. However, once the virus is within cells, it is protected from the effects of antibody. The most convincing evidence that antibody is less important than cellular hypersensitivity in resistance to viral infections, is that patients with deficiencies in antibody production do not have serious viral infections but do tend to develop bacterial infections. Patients with defects in delayed hypersensitivity develop serious and sometimes fatal virus infections (see Chapter 19).

Mycobacterial Infections

Infections such as tuberculosis and leprosy are resisted by cellular mechanisms—including granulomatous hypersensitivity. At one time it was thought that the development of tuberculosis required the effect of delayed hypersensitivity (33), and in fact some of the lesions seen, i.e., granulomata, do depend upon immune mechanisms for their formation. However these lesions are not really the cause of the disease but an unfortunate untoward effect of the protective mechanisms. As may occur with delayed hypersensitivity to virus infections, the immunologic inflammatory reaction to the infective mycobacteria results in destruction of normal tissue. In the lung for instance extensive damage may be done by the formation of large granulomas in response to a tuberculosis infection, resulting in respiratory failure. In these cases it is the opinion of some that the immunologic reaction to eliminate the tuberculosis infection prior to dissemination causes the disease. The immunologic response produces the lesion, but the mycobacterium causes the disease.

The role of granulomatous reactions in protection is best exemplified in leprosy (46). If a granulomatous reaction develops, a limited form of the disease occurs (tuberculoid leprosy) but if the infected individual produces no granulomatous reaction the leprosy bacilli multiply and produce marked tissue destruction (lepromatous leprosy), see page 270. Therefore it is clear that the granulomatous reaction is a major protective response to mycobacterial infections. The role and relationship of delayed hypersensitivity to granulomatous reactions remains unestablished.

Protozoal Infections

The mechanism of protection to protozoal infections, like viral infections, depends upon the location of the agent in the host. Protozoa are unicellular organisms which may be located intracellularly, extracellularly in the blood, both intracellularly and in the blood, or primarily in the gastrointestinal tract. Intracellular protozoans such as Leishmania are resisted by delayed and granulomatous reactions similar to the response to leprosy (45,46). In certain types of leishmaniasis the organism is limited to focal inflamed areas of the skin which have histologic characteristics of a delayed hypersensitivity reaction (24). If this delayed hypersensitivity is lost, dissemination of the organisms may occur. Trypanosomiasis is an example of a blood-borne parasite which may also be found intracellularly, the major defense appears to be via humoral antibody, Malaria protozoa multiply intracellularly, but disseminate through release into the bloodstream. Malarial immunity is mediated by IgG antibody (7,22) which can effectively attack the blood-borne organism but is not effective against the intracellular stage (7). Therefore, humoral immunity is effective only during a short period of the malarial protozoal life cycle (7). Even highly immune infected persons may be unable to clear the parasites completely due to protection of the intracellular stages, but the number of organisms present in the body is controlled and the host lives in balance with his infection. Entamoeba histolytica is an intestinal protozoan infection of man. Although antibodies are produced, the protective effect of these antibodies remains to be demonstrated; immune protection for intestinal protozoa has not been established.

Helminth (Worm) Infections

The response to worm infections also depends upon the location of the infestation. Worms are located in the intestinal tract and/or tissues.

Tapeworms, which exist only in the intestinal lumen, promote no protective immunologic response. On the other hand, worms with larval forms which invade tissue do stimulate an immune response. The tissue reaction to Ascaris and Trichenella consists of an intense infiltrate of polymorphonuclear leukocytes featuring eosinophils. Anaphylactic antibodies (IgE) are also frequently associated with helminth infections, and intradermal injection of worm extracts elicits a wheal-and-flare reaction. Children infested with Ascaris lumbricoides have attacks of urticaria, asthma, and other anaphylactic or atopic types of reactions. An eosinophilic pulmonary infiltrate (pneumonia) may be found associated with migration of helminth larvae through the lung. The possible protective role of this anaphylactic sensitivity is not clear (40), but it has been suggested that expulsion of parasitic worms from the gastrointestinal tract occurs following the induction of peristalsis and diarrhea due to intestinal anaphylactic reactions to worms (34).

Schistosomes are examples of helminths that exist primarily in tissue, in which they elicit a striking granulomatous reaction (see page 270). While these granuloma do isolate the organisms, the surrounding tissue may be extensively disrupted, leading to secondary effects such as obstruction of lymphatics or destruction of liver (10,14,47). Humoral antibodies of both anaphylactic and other classes may be demonstrated to schistosomes, but their role in the disease is not known (9,47).

Fungal Infections

Cellular immunity appears to be the most important immunologic factor in resistance to fungal infections although humoral antibody certainly may play a role. The importance of cellular reactions is indicated, 1) by the intense mononuclear infiltrate and granulomatous reactions that occur in tissues infected with fungi, and 2) by the fact that fungal infections are most frequently associated with depressed immune reactivity of the delayed type (opportunistic infections) (29). Chronic mucocutaneous candidiasis refers to a heterogeneous group of fungus diseases characterized by persistent or recurrent infection by candida albicans of mucous membranes, nails and skin. Patients with this disease generally have a depression of cellular immune reactions (27,37).

Insect Stings

Immune reactions to insect stings are generally believed to be responsible for most of the irritating skin reactions (16,43). Individuals vary markedly in their immune reactions to insect stings (25). Clearly the reaction of a given individual to an insect sting depends upon the dominant type of immune response. Most people react to insect stings, including mosquito bites, by acute cutaneous anaphylactic reaction (25) and desensitization or hyposensitization can be achieved (16,43). Systemic shock and death from wasp or bee stings, while infrequent, may develop in hyperreactive individuals (38). In fact, insect stings are responsible for more deaths than snake bites (4). Stebbings (43) postulates two possible protective functions of anaphylactic reactions: 1) Immediate avoidance behavior by the recipient, which serves to reduce antigen contact, and 2) anaphylactic reactions preventing toxic complex reactions or delayed hypersensitivity reactions. Since potentially fatal anaphylactic reactions require much less antigen contact than other allergic reactions, the latter mechanism seems unlikely. In fact, hyposensitization via the production of blocking IgG antibodies is attempted clinically to reduce the possibility of anaphylactic reactions to insect bites (see page 168). An anaphylactic reaction to insect stings may be protective in producing avoidance behavior. However, in all likelihood, anaphylactic reactions to insect bites are not protective reactions but examples of potentially protective immune reactions being used inappropriately.

ROLE OF ALLERGIC REACTIONS IN IMMUNITY

From the preceding discussion it can be appreciated that each of the six types of allergic reactions responsible for immune disease also has important functions in resistance to infection.

1. Neutralization or inactivation of biologically active toxins by antibodies is highly desirable. This is precisely what is accomplished by immunization with diphtheria toxoid.
2. Cytotoxic or cytolytic reactions directly affect the infecting organisms, leading to their death or lysis.
3. The effect of histamine release (the anaphylactic mechanism) at the usual dose level results in slight vasodilation and increased capillary permeablity, both effects interpreted in classic pathology as aiding defense. Smooth muscle contraction and diarrhea induced by the anaphylactic mechanism may cause expulsion of intestinal parasites.
4. The inflammatory effect of antigen–antibody precipitate in the Arthus mechanism results in stickiness of leukocytes, platelets and endothelium, and increases permeability. These effects promote defense by localization and diapedesis of leukocytes. At the dose level of a usual infection, this effect is not harmful to the host. Precipitating antibody and complement, as means of enhancing phagocytosis (opsonization), are responsible for protection against many bacterial infections.
5. Delayed hypersensitivity at the dose level occurring in infection results in local mobilization of phagocytes and effective destruction of infecting agents.
6. Granulomatous hypersensitivity may serve to isolate or localize insoluble toxic materials or organisms.

CLINICAL IMMUNIZATION

Since it was first demonstrated that a previous natural exposure to an infectious agent or product thereof may produce a state of specific immune resistance to reinfection, many satisfactory procedures for intentionally inducing immunity have been developed. Immunization is the process of artifically inducing a state of specific immunity in an individual by transferring preformed antibody or sensitized cells (passive immunity), or by providing a direct stimulus for an immune response by contact with antigen (active immunity).

Passive Immunity

The transfer of immune products (humoral or cellular) from a sensitized individual to a nonimmunized individual may produce a state of immunity in the recipient. For humoral antibody this may be accomplished by injection of a serum containing antibody from immunized animals or by injection of pooled human immunoglobulin in which specific antibody is present (30). Horse antiserum has been used following exposure to toxins of botulism, diphtheria, gas gangrene, and tetanus. Although the horse antitoxin neutralizes the toxins, the administration of horse serum frequently leads to serum sickness as the host responds to the horse serum proteins by forming precipitating antibody (see Chapter 13). Therefore, horse serum should be used only in life-threatening circumstances and only after careful testing fails to detect a preexisting allergy to horse serum. Pooled human immunoglobulin is used after exposure to hepatitis or measles, or rubella (German measles) during the first trimester of pregnancy (30). Passive immunity occurs naturally in fetal life. Maternal antibodies cross the placenta and provide specific immunity for the newborn until about 3–4 months of age, when the infant begins to produce its own antibody.

The passive transfer of cellular immune reactions using living cells is generally not satisfactory due to immune rejection of the transferred cells (5). Passive transfer of cellular sensitivity may be accomplished if the recipient is unable to reject transferred living lymphoid cells or by using a product of sensitized cells known as transfer factor (28). The former is possible with transfers between identical twins. Cellular reactivity may also be transferred if lymphoid cells are given to a recipient who is incapable of reacting due to an immunologic deficiency (31). However, the transferred cells may react to the recipient's tissues (Graft-vs-Host reaction, see page 236). Successful cell transfer depends on histocompatibility matching of donor and recipient (18,31), with transfer factor used successfully in a limited number of human immunodeficiency diseases (37,41). [For a further discussion of the use of lymphoid cells or cell products as therapy for immune deficiencies, see Chapter 19.)

Active

Active immunity occurs upon recovery from a naturally acquired infection or by the process of artificially inducing immunity by inoculation, ingestion or inhalation of a modified form of an infectious organism or a product of an organism, so that the immunizing material retains the antigenicity of the intact organism but does not have the capacity to cause disease. The types of artificial immunogens that have been used include 1) low doses of a product of the organism, 2) altered products such as chemically modified toxins [toxoid] (20,21), 3) antibody-neutralized toxin, 4) killed organisms (8), 5) low doses of virulent organisms given by nonpathogenic or relatively innocuous routes (24), 6) living attenuated (avirulent) strains (12,35), and 7) organisms altered in such a way that they can infect but cannot complete a complex life cycle (e.g., immunization of cattle against lung worm). Attenuated strains are produced by culturing virulent organisms in vitro or in unnatural hosts so that the organisms are no longer pathogenic for the natural host but retain the antigenic specificity of the virulent strains (12).

Prophylactic Immunization

Some diseases for which active prophylactic immunization is available are listed in Table 18–2. Diseases for which immunization is widely employed include diphtheria, whooping cough (pertussis), tetanus, measles (rubeola), poliomyelitis, rubella and mumps (2,8,11,26,36,44). Vaccination against smallpox, although an effective procedure, produces a significant number of untoward reactions and has been discontinued in countries that do not have endemic disease. Immunizations in clinical practice are scheduled as a compromise between immunization efficiency and convenience of administration, i.e., to obtain safe, adequate protection with a minimum number of visits to the doctor. Most immunizations usually require two to three applications and occasional booster injections. Children are usually immunized with diphtheria toxoid, killed pertussis organisms, and tetanus toxoid by three injections of the combined antigens (DPT) between 2–6 months of age, with another booster at 18–24 months. Infants younger than 2 months of age give poor immune responses. One inoculation with attenuated measles and mumps virus and two or three oral doses of attentuated poliovirus are given between 7–11 months of age or along with DPT immunization. Vaccination for smallpox is accomplished between 1–2 years of age using a relatively avirulent related virus (cowpox, vaccinia).

The use of vaccinia inoculation for immunization against smallpox was reported by Edward Jenner in 1798 (23). The vaccinia virus has low pathogenicity for man and contains antigens that cross react with smallpox virus. Dermal inoculation induces delayed-type hypersensitivity which results in a typical delayed skin reaction at the site of inoculation approximately 8 days after application (32). This long-lasting cellular sensitivity protects the vaccinated individual against smallpox. The term vaccination, now used to cover all kinds of protective immunization, is derived from the vaccinia virus. Inoculation with normal strains of vaccinia virus leads to complications such as postvaccinial encephalitis or disseminated vaccinia in a small but significant number of vaccinated individuals. Preliminary studies of an attenuated strain of vaccinia virus indicate the induction of good protective immunity and an absence of significant complications, but these studies are not yet conclusive. In fact, there is some evidence that the vaccines now in use are really derived from an attenuated smallpox strain and not vaccinia virus.

Immunization for diseases such as cholera, typhoid, typhus and yellow fever is not done routinely, but is indicated for an individual traveling to areas where the disease is endemic. Work is now underway to produce and evaluate immunogens for meningococci, streptococci, pneumococci, atypical mycoplasma, viral hepatitis and other agents (2). Attempts have been made to immunize patients with treated organisms grown from cul-

TABLE 18-2
Prophylactic Immunization for Human Infectious Diseases

Disease	Antigen preparation	Indication	Immunization route	Result
		Toxoids		
Diphtheria	Formaldehyde-treated toxin	All children	Intramuscular	Satisfactory
Botulism	Formaldehyde-treated toxin	On exposure	Intramuscular	Needs improvement
Tetanus	Formaldehyde-treated toxin	All children	Intramuscular	Satisfactory
		Killed Organisms		
Pertussis	Thiomersalate-treated	All Children	Intramuscular	Needs improvement
Typhoid	Acetone-treated	Travelers†	Subcutaneous	Needs improvement
Cholera	Phenol-treated	Travelers†	Subcutaneous	Needs improvement
Plague	Formalin-killed	On exposure	Subcutaneous	Needs improvement
		Attenuated Organisms		
Poliomyelitis	Tissue culture	All children	Oral	Satisfactory
Measles	Tissue culture	All children	Subcutaneous	Satisfactory
Mumps	Tissue culture	All children	Subcutaneous	Satisfactory
Rubella	Tissue culture	All children	Subcutaneous	Satisfactory
Yellow fever	Tissue culture	Travelers†	Subcutaneous	Needs improvement
Influenza	Tissue culture (4 strains)	High-risk group	Subcutaneous	Needs improvement
Tuberculosis	Bacille Calmette-Guérin	High-risk group	Intradermal	Needs improvement
		Killed Partially Attenuated Organisms		
Typhus	Chick embryo culture	Travelers†	Subcutaneous	Satisfactory
Rabies	Duck embryo culture	On exposure	Multiple subcutaneous	Satisfactory
	Premylinated Mouse Brain			
		Avirulent Organisms		
Smallpox	Vaccinia (cow pox) virus*	All children	Intradermal or subcutaneous	Needs improvement
		Virulent Organisms		
Cutaneous Leishmaniasis	Controlled route and dose	Exposed children	Intradermal	Needs improvement

*Attenuated vaccinia virus may reduce complications.
† Travelers to areas where disease is endemic.

tures of the patient's own tissues [autogenous vaccines (39)] but such procedures have not been clinically rewarding. The sine qua non for production of a vaccine is the availability of an experimental animal host or in vitro culture to produce an attenuated strain, or enough of the agent for chemical modification. The breakthrough in the production of both attenuated and killed poliomyelitis vaccines was the development of in vitro conditions for culture of the virus (15). Regardless of the care taken to produce specific antigens for immunization it is virtually impossible to rule out dangerous contaminating materials. Although it was impossible to know at the time, the original Salk polio vaccine was contaminated with SV 40 virus which may be responsible for the production of a different disease (3).

Evaluation of Immunization

Evaluation of the effectiveness of a vaccine poses considerable problems. If an experimental animal is available, the vaccine can be tested for its ability to protect the infected animal. In many cases either an animal model is not available or the experimental disease is not like the human disease (17). The ability of the vaccine to induce antibody formation or active delayed hypersensitivity in humans can be tested, but the presence of antibody or cellular sensitivity may not necessarily be correlated with resistance to disease. The only valid method is to test the ability of the vaccine to reduce the incidence or severity of disease in human clinical trials. This requires painstaking planning and evaluation. Protection of the immunized individual may not be the sole criterion of effectiveness. For instance, in evaluation of immunization with formalin-killed poliomyelitis virus, factors in addition to protection of the immunized individual must be considered. Oral immunization by ingestion of attenuated virus may prevent passage of the virus through fecal contamination, while injection of killed virus is ineffective in this regard (35). Polio infections are contracted by swallowing of virus-contaminated materials. In an unprotected individual the virus passes into the blood stream leading to a systemic infection. Disease occurs when the virus attacks the anterior horn cells of the medulla and spinal cord. Antibody induced by injection protects by preventing the systemic spread of the virus, but the gastrointestinal phase may still occur. Oral immunization leads, in addition, to local immunity in the gastrointestinal tract presumably due to secretory antibody. This prevents the gastrointestinal phase and limits the spread of the virus. Individuals inoculated with the killed virus may be protected from disease but can still serve as carriers to disseminate the virus during an epidemic. If a substantial portion of a population has received the oral vaccine, even the unimmunized portion of the population will be protected from epidemic disease (35).

Immunity as a Relative Condition

Specific or nonspecific resistance to infection is a relative state. The effect of different doses of infectious agents or their products upon experimental animals clearly demonstrates that administration of sufficiently large numbers of organisms can overcome the resistance of a highly immune animal. In addition, doses of toxins can be given that cause the death of animals that have high titers of neutralizing antibody. Thus immunity to infection is not an absolute condition, but depends upon a large number of complex variables including not only the resistance of the host but also the dose, route of contact and virulence of the infecting agent.

DELETERIOUS EFFECTS OF PROTECTIVE REACTIONS (ALLERGY)

Immune mechanisms are believed to have been selected during evolution because of their protective activity. However, under some circumstances, these protective mechanisms may be responsible for tissue destruction or loss of normal function.

The use of abnormally high doses (as in laboratory or medical practice) and of unphysiologic (intravenous) routes of administration may produce deleterious reactions (anaphylaxis, tuberculin shock, serum sickness, transfusion reactions, graft rejection) which do not occur naturally. Frequent administration, ingestion, and contact with drugs and other chemicals produce unnatural diseases. However, there are naturally occurring hypersensitive diseases—some hemolytic anemias, leukopenias, purpuras, erythroblastosis fetalis, neonatal thrombocytopenic purpura, atopy, hay fever, anaphylaxis due to the sting of insects, polyarteritis nodosa (rare, many cases may be related to immune reactions to drugs), contact dermatitis (poison ivy), some autoallergic diseases, and granulomatous reactions to worm infestations. In these naturally occurring diseases infectious agents are not primarily pathogenic and it may properly be said that the immune apparatus is being used for the wrong purpose. In infection, the necrosis associated with granulomatous reactivity is clearly harmful to the host; yet prominent necrosis occurs in only a few infectious diseases (tuberculosis). In other diseases (most viral infections) immune reactions are a highly effective mechanism of defense.

Earlier thinking considered hypersensitivity quite separate from immunity to infectious diseases. Delayed hypersensitivity was considered different from other types of immunity, causing necrosis of sensitized tissues and having no protective effect (for a detailed discussion, see reference 33). This view was based on the killing of sensitive cells in tissue culture by antigen, and a number of experiments which suggested that delayed hypersensitivity was dissociated from immunity. This has been contradicted by other evidence. Therefore, it is incorrect to assume that hypersensitivity and immunity are two qualitatively distinct immune reactions.

REFERENCES

1. Austin KF, Cohn ZA: Contribution of serum and cellular factors in host defense reactions. N Engl J Med 268:933, 994, 1056, 1963
2. Artenstein MS: The current status of bacterial vaccines. Hosp Pract 8:49, 1973
3. Baguley DM, Glasgow GL: Subacute sclerosing panencephalitis and Salk Vaccine. Lancet 2:763, 1973

4. Barr SE: Allergy to hymenoptera stings. Review of the world literature: 1953–1970. Ann Allergy 29:49, 1971
5. Billingham R, Silvers W: The immunology of transplantation. Englewood Cliffs, NJ, Prentice-Hall, 1971
6. Braude AI: Resistance to infection. In Clinical Physiology. Grollman A (ed). New York, McGraw-Hill, 1957, p 773
7. Brown IN: Immunologic aspects of malaria infection. Adv Immunol 11:268, 1969
8. Cannon DA (ed). A Symposium on Immunization in Childhood Edinburgh, Livingstone, 1960
9. Capron A, Biguet J, Tran Van Ky P, Moschetto Y: Immunological studies in various types of schistosomiasis. NY Acad Sci 160:863, 1969
10. Cheever AW: A quantitative post-mortum study of schistosomiasis in man. Am J Trop Med Hyg 17:38, 1968
11. Cvjetanovic B: Immunization programmes. WHO Chron 27:66, 1973
12. D'Arcy Hart P: Efficacy and applicability of mass BCG vaccination in tuberculosis control. Br Med J 1:587, 1967
13. DeClerq E, Merigan TC: Current concepts of interferon and interferon induction. Ann Rev Med 21:17, 1970
14. Edington GM, Von Lichtenberg F, Nwaboebo I, Taylor JR, Smith JH: Pathologic effects of schistosomiasis in Ibadan, Western State of Nigeria. I. Incidence and intensity of infection, distribution and severity of lesions. Am J Trop Med Hyg 19:985, 1970
15. Enders JF, Weller TH, Robbins FC: Cultivation of the Lansing strain of poliomyelitis virus in cultures of various human embryonic tissue. Science 109:85, 1949
16. Frazier CA: Biting insect survey: A statistical report. Ann Allergy 32:200, 1974
17. Frenkel JK: Models for infectious disease. Fed Proc 28:179, 1969
18. Githens J: Hematopoietic and immunologic tissue grafting. Clin Peditr 10:138, 1971
19. Gladstone GP: Pathogenicity and Virulence of Micro-Organisms. In General Pathology. 4th ed. Florey HW (ed). Philadelphia, Saunders, 1970
20. Glenny AT, Hopkins BE: Diphtheria toxoid as an immunizing agent. Br J Exp Pathol 4:823, 1923
21. Holt LB: Developments in Diphtheria Prophylaxis. London, Heinemann, 1950
22. Immunology of malaria: Report of a WHO Expert Committee. WHO Tech Rep Ser 396, 1968
23. Jenner E: Inquiry into the Cause and Effects of the Variolae Vacciniae. Low, 1798; republished in 1896 by Cassell
24. Katzenellenbogen I: Vaccination against oriental sore: Reports of 555 inoculations. Arch Dermatol 50:239, 1944
25. Killby VA, Silverman PH: Hypersensitive reactions in man to specific mosquito bites. Am J Trop Med Hyg 16:374, 1967
26. Krugman S, Perkins FT: Vaccination against communicable diseases. Am J Dis Child 126:406, 1973
27. Landau JW: Chronic mucocutaneous candidiasis-associated immunologic abnormalities. Pediatrics 42:227, 1968
28. Lawrence HS: Transfer Factor. Adv Immunol 11:195, 1969
29. Lurie HI, Duma RJ: Opportunistic infections of the lungs. Hum Pathol 1:233, 1970
30. Merler E (ed): Immunoglobulins: Biological Aspects and Clinical Uses. Washington, DC, National Academy of Sciences, 1971
31. Moller G (ed): Lymphoid Cell Replacement. Transplant Rev 9, 1972
32. von Pirquet CF: Klinische Studien über Vakzination and Vakzinale Allergie. Leipzig, Deuticke, 1907
33. Rich AR: The Pathogenesis of Tuberculosis, 2nd ed. Springfield, Ill, Thomas, 1951
34. Robbins JB: In Immunologic Incompetence. Kagan BM, Stiem ER (eds). Year Book Med Pub, Chicago, 1971, p 357
35. Sabin AB: Present position of immunization against poliomyelitis virus with live virus vaccines. Br Med J 1:663, 1959
36. Schiff P: Modern trends in immunization. Med J Aust 1:551, 1973
37. Schulkind ML, Adler WH III, Altemeier WA, Ayoub EM: Transfer factor in the treatment of a case of chronic mucocutaneous candidiosis. Cell Immunol 3:606, 1972
38. Shulman S: Allergic responses to insects. Ann Rev Entomol 12:323, 1967

39. Smith DT: Autogenous vaccines in theory and practice. Arch Intern Med 125:344, 1970
40. Soulsby EJL: The Mechanism of Immunity to Gastro-Intestinal Nematodes. In Biology of Parasites. New York, Academic Press, 1966
41. Spitler LE, Levin AS, Stites DP, Fudenberg, HH, Pirofsky B, August CS, Stiehm ER, Hitzig WH, Gatti RA: The Wiscott-Aldrich syndrome. Results of transfer factor therapy. J Clin Invest 51:3216, 1972
42. Springer GF, Horton RE, Forbes M: Origin of anti-human blood group B agglutinins in white leghorn chicks. J Exp Med 110:221, 1959
43. Stebbings JH: Immediate hypersensitivity: A defense against arthropods. Perspect Biol Med 17:233, 1974
44. Stokes J Jr: Recent advances in immunization against viral diseases. Ann Intern Med 73:829, 1970
45. Taylor AER (ed): Immunity to Parasites. Oxford, Blackwell, 1968
46. Turk JL, Brvceson ADM: Immunological phenomena in leprosy and related diseases. Adv Immunol 13:209, 1971
47. Warren KS: The immunopathogenesis of schistosomiasis: a multidisciplinary approach. Trans Roy Soc Trop Med Hyg 66:417, 1972
48. Wheelock EF, Toy ST: Participation of lymphocytes in viral infections. Adv Immunol 16:123, 1973

FOR ADDITIONAL READING

Perkins FT (ed): International Symposium on Vaccination Against Communicable Diseases. Basel, S. Karger, 1973

19

Immune
Deficiency
Diseases

The occurrence of repeated infections in an individual almost certainly is due to a deficiency in his defense against infection. Such a deficiency must be especially considered if the infecting organism is one that is not usually responsible for human disease (48). The type of infection observed is determined by the kind of immune abnormality present. Immune deficiency diseases may be classified according to etiology into primary and secondary (27,72,75,76). Primary immune deficiencies result from genetic abnormalities in the development of immune maturity; secondary deficiencies result from diseases that interfere with the expression of a mature immune system.

Multiple levels of defensive reactions must be considered in evaluating resistance to infection. Infections may occur with increased frequency in elderly individuals, in debilitated patients, or when natural nonimmune barriers are affected. The depression of pulmonary clearing mechanisms due to the loss of the ciliary activity of bronchial lining cells found associated with exposure to cigaret smoke is an example. Because of the complexity of immune deficiencies and the manner of clinical presentation of deficiency, a careful systematic diagnostic work-up must be carried out in order to select appropriate therapy (7,57). This chapter will emphasize specific immunologic deficiencies in host defense.

DEVELOPMENT OF IMMUNE MATURITY

Good and his co-workers (28,29,63) have made an extremely useful attempt to correlate the role of different organs in the development of immune maturity in experimental animals with the various manifestations of immune deficiency diseases in man. The evidence to date indicates that there is a common ancestral cell for all white cells, including immunologi-

300

cally competent cells, arising from a bone marrow precursor. In order for potential immunologically competent cells to develop to maturity and obtain the capacity to recognize antigen, they must come in contact with, or be affected by, products of endodermal tissue. The embryonal "central" lymphoid tissue consists of the thymus, tonsils, appendix, liver, Peyer's patches, and in fowl, the bursa of Fabricius. The peripheral lymphoid tissue is the remaining lymphoid tissue, including lymph nodes and spleen (78).

ROLE OF THE THYMUS

The thymus appears to be necessary for the proper development of cellular (delayed-type) immune reactions mediated by lymphocytes (53,54). The thymus develops from the third and fourth pharyngeal pouches and the mature thymus contains remnants of epithelial tissue (Hassall's corpuscles) in the medulla (see page 25). Surgical extirpation of the thymus in newborn mice leads to failure of expression of delayed-type immune reactions. Neonatally thymectomized mice develop a characteristic wasting syndrome, most likely because of their inability to defend successfully against normally nonpathogenic organisms. This hypothesis is supported by the finding that wasting does not occur in neonatally thymectomized germ-free mice, even though such mice give evidence of impaired cellular reactions in that they do not reject skin allografts [homografts] (50). The serum immunoglobulin levels of neonatally thymectomized mice are usually normal, although selective deficiencies in the production of specific antibodies may be observed. The mechanism of thymus action is unknown. The presence of a humoral factor produced by the thymus and acting upon the peripheral lymphoid tissue of the body is supported by the ability of thymus grafts in millipore chambers to restore the immune capacity of neonatally thymectomized mice. For a further discussion of thymic humoral factors, see page 38.

ROLE OF THE GASTROINTESTINAL TRACT

Other areas of the embryonal gastrointestinal tract have been implicated as necessary for the development of humoral antibody-mediated immune capacity (63). Surgical or hormonal bursectomy (removal of the bursa of Fabricius) in chickens leads to deficiency in circulating immunoglobulins and antibody responses, while cellular reactions (allograft rejection) are not affected (17,35,91). In mammals, maturation of cells required for expression of humoral immunity may take in the liver, Peyer's patches or appendix (17a), which also arise from gastrointestinal anlage.

DUAL MECHANISM

Lymphoid tissue associated with the intestinal epithelium appears responsible for the development of humoral antibody formation, while the lymphoid tissue associated with the thymus is responsible for development of cellular reactions. The peripheral lymphoid tissue may then be subdivided into the thymus-dependent system (T cells) and the immunoglobulin-producing system (B cells).

Thymectomized animals have lymphopenia and aplastic zones in the lymph nodes (paracortical) and spleen (parafollicular) (41,62,87) that in the normal animal are associated with the development of cellular immunity. Bursectomized chickens have aplastic germinal centers and very few or absent plasma cells in lymphoid organs (17,35), structures that are associated with the synthesis of immunoglobulin antibody.

Although it is clearly not possible to be certain that this dual developmental mechanism is operative in the human, such a system does provide a convenient scheme for understanding the various immune deficiencies of man (63,75,76).

RESPONSE OF IMMATURE ANIMALS

Fetal and neonatal animals may be induced to form antibody or develop high levels of immunoglobulins if given strong antigenic stimuli. However, neonatal animals normally are protected by maternal antibody received by placental transfer or by absorption of colostral antibodies shortly after birth (63,67). The newborn animal begins to produce its own antibodies due to natural stimulation. The development of "normal" lymphoid tissue and "normal" immunoglobulin levels depends upon contact with antigen; germ-free animals that have a markedly reduced antigenic load maintain only very low levels of serum immunoglobulins and have undeveloped, immature lymphoid tissue, but will promptly respond if stimulated by antigen exposure.

INFANT HYPOGAMMAGLOBULINEMIA

A temporary delay in the production of immunoglobulins by a newborn may cause a transient hypogammaglobulinemia of infancy (67). Hypogammaglobulinemia occurs when the normal catabolism of placentally transferred maternal IgG commencing after birth is associated with an abnormal delay in the onset of the immunoglobulin synthetic capacity. This temporary immunoglobulin deficiency usually terminates between 9-18 months of age. Since it is only temporary, it is not considered a primary immune deficiency disease; if it continues, however, a true permanent immune deficiency disease must be considered.

PRIMARY IMMUNE DEFICIENCIES

Fundamental developmental abnormalities result in a permanent loss of some immune capacity. Such abnormalities may occur at one of the major sites of immune development mentioned above—the ancestral anlage the thymus-dependent system, or the immunoglobulin-producing system (63) (See Fig. 19-1). For specific references to each syndrome, see references 25, 75 and 76.

In the discussion below, the terminology given in parentheses refers to nomenclature recommended by a committee of the World Health Organization (24). In general, immune deficiencies may be cellular, humoral, or both (combined immune deficiency). The classification presented below refers to specific clinical syndromes. It may be extremely difficult to classify an individual patient other than to define his immune deficiency as primarily cellular, primarily humoral, or combined.

COMBINED IMMUNE DEFICIENCIES (ANLAGE DEFECTS)

Reticular Dysgenesis

DeVaal and Seynhaeve observed twin boys who lacked all types of white blood cells and at autopsy had no lymphoid tissue, apparently owing to a lack of development of the reticular anlage of white cells. Only three such cases have been reported.

Swiss-Type Agammaglobulinemia (Autosomal Recessive Alymphopenic Agammaglobulinemia)

Infants with this disorder fail to grow normally and have serious infections in the first weeks of life. Both sexes are affected, indicating an autosomal recessive type of inheritance. All major immunoglobulin groups (IgG, IgA, and IgM) are severely depressed (total <25 mg/100 ml), and there is a striking deficiency of lymphocytes in the blood (<1000/ml). At autopsy only a few plasma cells and lymphocytes are found, and the thymus is atrophic and lacks Hassall's corpuscles. A deficiency in the reactivity of lymphocytes from patients with this disease can be demonstrated by the lack of in vitro stimulation by phytohemagglutinin.

Thymic Alymphoplasia (Primary Lymphopenic Immunologic Deficiency)

The immune defect in thymic alymphoplasia is similar to that in Swiss-type agammaglobulinemia except that it occurs only in males, indicating a sex-linked recessive mode of inheritance. The thymus is aplastic. Both cellular and antibody responses are grossly diminished, and all immunoglobulin levels are below normal. The site of action appears to be identical to that of the Swiss-type of agammaglobulinemia.

In severe cases of thymic alymphoplasia and Swiss-type agammaglobulinemia (Combined Immune Deficiency Diseases), symptoms may appear within the first few days of life, but in most cases infectious complications do not appear until 4–6 months of age. It must be suspected that maternal transfer of some cellular immune function, as well as immunoglobulin, must occur. Otherwise, death from overwhelming infections due to an absence of cellular immunity would occur earlier in life. Children with severe combined immune deficiencies frequently develop a skin rash consistent with that of a graft-vs-host reaction and believed to be caused by maternal lymphoid cells. Maternal lymphocytes may cross the placenta during gestation (see page 238). Normally such placentally transferred cells are rejected by the immune system of the fetus. However, if the fetus is unable to react to them, the foreign cells may proliferate in the immune-deficient child and produce a graft-vs-host reaction. Such cells may also provide some cellular immunity and protect the child from fulminant viral infections during the first 4–6 months of life.

Some children with combined immune deficiency also have an absence or

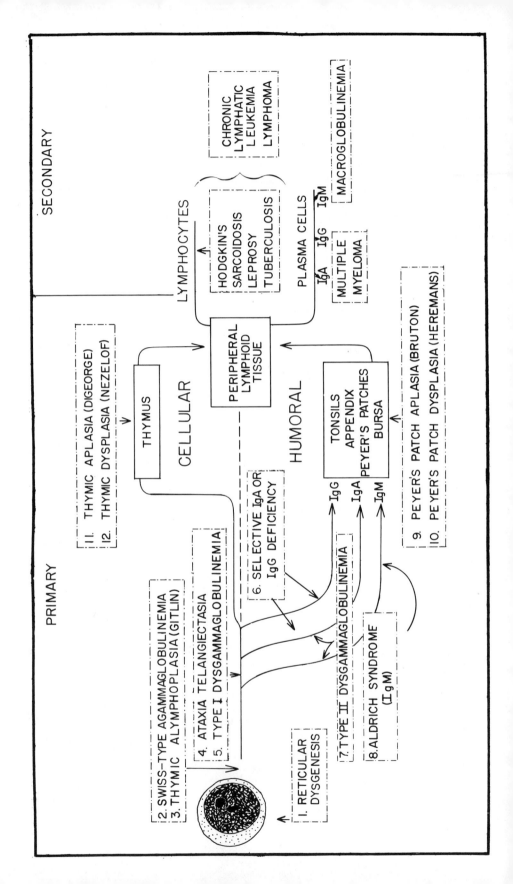

deficiency of an enzyme, adenosine deaminase (40). The relation of this deficiency to the mechanism of immune deficiency is not known. However, if an adenosine deaminase deficiency linked to immune deficiency is suspected during pregnancy because the parents had a previous child with immune deficiency and adenosine deaminase deficiency, testing of the amniotic fluid for adenosine deaminase may permit a prenatal diagnosis. If this diagnosis is made prior to birth, therapeutic abortion would prevent the birth of an immune-deficient child.

Ataxia Telangiectasia

Ataxia telangiectasia is most likely due to a developmental mesenchymal defect inherited as an autosomal recessive. Clinically it presents as progressive cerebellar ataxia, oculocutaneous telangiectasia, and recurrent severe infections. The serum IgA level is usually well below normal, the IgG level may be low or normal, but the IgM level is usually normal. Patients may have a deficient antibody response to some common antigens. Delayed-type reactions are markedly depressed, as indicated by prolonged allograft survival, lack of response to common skin tests, and inability to sensitize with contact-type haptens (dinitrofluorobenzene). The lymphoid tissues are practically devoid of lymphocytes, although plasma cells may be present in some cases. The thymus is atrophic or absent and contains

Fig. 19–1. Immune deficiency diseases. Primary immune deficiencies are genetically controlled abnormalities in development of immune maturity. Deficiency type manifested depends upon level in development that abnormality affects. Blocks 1 through 12 indicate postulated sites of developmental defects in primary immune deficiencies. Names in parentheses indicate eponyms applied to disease. Blocks 1–5 indicate combined immune deficiencies. In 1) reticular dysgenesis, 2) Swiss-type agammaglobulinemia, and 3) thymic alymphoplasia, both cellular and humoral immuno-responses are severely depressed. In 4) ataxia telangiectasia, and 5) type I dysgammaglobulinemia, depression of cellular responses is associated with depressed IgG and IgA production, although IgM production may be normal or elevated. Selective immunoglobulin deficiencies with normal cellular activities include 6) selective IgA or IgG deficiency, 7) type II dysgammaglobulinemia, and 8) selective IgM deficiencies. In 9) Peyer's patch aplasia and 10) Peyer's patch dysplasia, there is absence of all immunoglobulins and plasma cells, with normal cellular reactivity. 11) Thymic aplasia and 12) thymic dysplasia feature loss of cellular reactivity with normal immunoglobulin and humoral antibody production. Secondary immune deficiencies may result from naturally occurring diseases affecting mature immune system. Type of deficiency depends upon location of disease effect. Hodgkin's disease, sarcoidosis, leprosy, and tuberculosis depress cellular or delayed reactivity (anergy). Multiple myeloma and macroglobulinemia are associated with depressed humoral antibody levels, and chronic lymphatic leukemia and lymphomas are associated with depression of both humoral and cellular reactivity. Individuals with other conditions such as uremia, terminal neoplasia, and diabetes mellitus may also demonstrate depressed immune reactivity, but nonspecific defensive mechanisms may also be affected so that a precise analysis of the immune defect is difficult. (From Sell S. Arch Pathol 86:95, 1968)

no Hassall's corpuscles. The associated increased incidence of lymphoreticular malignancies has been blamed on lack of thymic control of the lymphoid system (lack of suppressor T cells). Thymectomized mice may also develop a marked proliferation of the reticuloendothelial system. A fundamental defect in the response of lymphocytes in ataxia telangiectasia is supported by the impaired in vitro phytohemagglutinin stimulation of lymphocytes from patients with this disorder.

Type I Dysgammaglobulinemia

Type I dysgammaglobulinemia occurs predominantly in males and appears at any age, although usually in infancy. There are associated lymphadenopathy, hepatosplenomegaly, and susceptibility to respiratory infections. The serum IgM level is usually elevated while IgG and IgA levels are low or absent. Plasma cells may be normal in tissue sections, but IgM-containing plasma cells predominate. Since a defect in cellular reactivity may be present, the site of action in this syndrome must occur prior to the influence of the thymus. However, since not all patients show a cellular defect, some variation within this syndrome may also occur.

HUMORAL IMMUNE DEFICIENCIES

Dysgammaglobulinemias (Non-Sex-Linked Primary Immunologic Deficiencies with Variable Onset and Expression)

The recognition of the major immunoglobulin subgroups (IgG, IgA, and IgM) and the development of sensitive immunochemical methods of measurement have permitted identification of selective or paired immunoglobulin deficiencies.

Many of these were formerly thought to be primary acquired agammaglobulinemias—idiopathic agammaglobulinemias of late onset and not associated with lymphomas. Now, however, there is evidence for a genetic basis for these disorders, and they probably should be considered late-appearing, genetically controlled defects. The dysgammaglobulinemias that have now been reported include all of the six possible combinations of depressed levels of a major immunoglobulin group or groups associated with normal or elevated levels of the other immunoglobulins: selective IgA or IgG deficiency; selective IgM deficiency (Aldrich's syndrome); deficiencies of IgG and IgA with normal IgM (type I dysgammaglobulinemia, usually associated with cellular immune deficiency); deficiencies of IgM and IgA with normal IgG (type II dysgammaglobulinemia); and deficiency of IgG and IgM associated with normal or elevated levels of IgA. Studies on immunoglobulin-producing myelomas suggest that there are separate linked cistrons coding for the specific parts (H-chains) of the immunoglobulin molecules, i.e., a separate cistron for the H-chains of IgA, IgG, and IgM respectively. It appears likely then that the absence or failure in expression of the genetic material necessary for the production of the specific immunoglobulin would result in a selective deficiency. The development of the capacity to produce IgM is thought to occur before the development of IgA- and IgG-producing ability because IgM has been found to be the most evolutionary primitive immunoglobulin and is usually the first antibody to appear following immunization. IgA-producing ability is though to develop before IgG-producing ability, but there are limited data to support this assumption.

Selective IgA and IgG Deficiencies

A selective deficiency of IgA has been associated with steatorrhea and a malabsorption syndrome believed to be secondary to this antibody deficiency; however, many individuals with selective IgA deficiency have no clinical symptoms (4). The lymphocytes of patients with selective IgA deficiency may be stimulated to produce IgA by treatment in vitro with pokeweed mitogen suggesting a maturation arrest of the IgA-producing cells that can be overcome by appropriate stimulation (94). The potential therapeutic application of this finding is intriguing. Selective IgG deficiency is exceedingly rare, and the clinical findings in patients with this defect have not been well documented, although recurrent pyogenic infections may occur (71).

Type II Dysgammaglobulinemia

Type II dysgammaglobulinema is characterized by low serum levels of IgA and IgM, normal levels of IgG, and normal cellular reactivity. It is most commonly seen in infancy in males only, indicating a sex-linked recessive mode of inheritance. However, since similar syndromes have been reported in adult women, the genetic status of this disorder remains unclear. As with the other deficiencies, increased susceptibility to infection is the most common clinical finding.

Wiskott-Aldrich Syndrome (Immune Deficiency with Thrombocytopenia and Eczema)

This syndrome is a sex-linked, recessive, antibody deficiency manifested by eczema, thrombocytopenia, and increased susceptibility to infection resulting in death in infancy. Serum IgA and IgG levels are usually normal; the characteristic deficiency is in IgM. Because of the thrombocytopenia, bleeding may be the first manifestation of the disease.

Gastrointestinal Tract–Dependent Defects

In the disorders discussed below, the defect appears to be located at the level of central gastrointestinal lymphoid development.

Bruton's Congenital Sex-Linked Agammaglobulinemia (Infantile Sex-Linked Agammaglobulinemia)

This, the first recognized primary immune deficiency disease, occurs only in males. Symptoms appear when transplacentally acquired maternal antibodies disappear from the circulation at the age of 5–6 months. Serious infections develop which can be treated with antibiotics or γ-globulins, but early death is usual. Affected children lack all three of the major immunoglobulins, but can develop reactions of the delayed type. The structure of the thymus is normal, but plasma cells are absent and, there is a striking lack of tonsilar, appendiceal, and Peyer's patch lymphoid tissue, suggesting a relation to bursectomized chicks, which manifest similar deficiencies.

Nodular Lymphoid Hyperplasia

A dysgammaglobulinemia associated with nodular lymphoid hyperplasia of the small intestine has recently been described. The report concerned eight patients with absence of IgA and IgM and a moderate depression of IgG, who had a sprue-like disorder. The lymphoid hyperplasia is extensive enough to be detectable by roentgenologic studies as multiple mucosal nodules. The nodules consist of enlarged lymphoid follicles within the lamina propria which contain large germinal centers and conspicuous mitotic activity. The cells are almost all in the lymphocyte series, and plasma cells are usually absent, although a few may be seen in some patients. This lymphoid hyperplasia may be the result of an overcompensation of the cellular immune system (thymus-dependent system) occurring in the absence of an immunoglobulin-producing (gastrointestinal-dependent) system. Delayed reactions were not tested.

THYMUS-DEPENDENT DEFECTS (CELLULAR DEFICIENCIES)

Thymic Aplasia

Thymic aplasia is characterized by an absence of the thymus, deficiency of cellular reactions, and a normal immunoglobulin-producing system. There is evidence of developmental failure of the third and fourth pharyngeal pouches with absent or rudimentary thymus and absent parathyroids. Peripheral blood lymphocyte counts and serum immunoglobulin levels are normal. Patients with this defect cannot be sensitized with contact sensitivity haptens, are unable to reject allografts, and have an increased susceptibility to fungal infections. This syndrome must be differentiated from thymic alymphoplasia, which features abnormalities of the immunoglobulins as well as depressed cellular immunity.

Thymic Dysplasia (Autosomal Recessive Lymphopenia with Normal Immunoglobulins)

Thymic dysplasia is characterized by vestigial embryonic thymus, diminished cellular immunity, and normal immunoglobulins. No lymphocytes are evident in the lymphoid tissues, although plasma cells are normal. The thymus is small and difficult to identify. It has a disorganized stroma of reticulum cells, no cortical-medullary differentiation, rare lymphocytes, and no Hassall's corpuscles. A wasting disease similar to that observed in neonatally thymectomized mice may be the terminal event in individuals with a deficient thymus-dependent system.

VARIABLE IMMUNODEFICIENCY

Many patients with primary immunodeficiencies remain unclassifiable and are referred to as having a "variable immunodeficiency" (24). This simply means the findings of these patients do not clearly match one of the above syndromes. The identification of different functional lymphocytes in the mouse (T cells and B cells, see page 35) and the development of techniques which tentatively identify such cells in the human (see page 38) has led to studies of lymphocyte populations in patients with primary immune deficiencies (2,21,47). At this writing it is too early to determine the significance of the variety of T and B cell distributions observed, but it is possible that such data will provide a more precise understanding of primary immune deficiency diseases.

Suppressor T Cells

A role of suppressor T cells in the pathogenesis of some cases of common variable immune deficiency has been proposed (88). Many of these patients have normal percentages of circulating B lymphocytes, but are unable to produce normal quantities of immunoglobulins. A similar defect has been found in some patients who have an isolated IgA deficiency (94). The peripheral blood lymphocytes of some patients with common variable immune deficiency suppress the in vitro production of immunoglobulins of lymphocytes from normal individuals; but mixtures of lymphocytes from two normal individuals produce normal amounts of immunoglobulins in vitro (88). The immunoglobulin synthesis by normal lymphocytes is also suppressed when they are co-cultured with purified T cells from a hypogammaglobulemic patient but not when co-cultured with T cells from normals. Thus, an abnormality in numbers or activity of suppressor cells may prevent the normal synthesis and release of immunoglobulins in these patients. The possible therapeutic advantages of limiting this suppressor effect remain to be explored.

REPLACEMENT THERAPY OF IMMUNE
DEFICIENCY DISEASES

Since immunoglobulin deficiencies are caused by the lack of antibody, of immunologically competent cells or both, attempts have been made to correct these deficiencies by replacing the missing defense system (6,12,13,26,28). For many years the antibody deficiency syndromes have been treated with partial success by injections of pooled normal immunoglobulins (27,29,67). While such injections give some protection, they do not provide the high levels of specific antibody that are produced in response to an infectious organism by a normal individual and do not provide any cellularly mediated immunity.

Attempts have been made to treat immunologic deficiencies of the cellular and combined cellular and immunoglobulin types by bone marrow or thymus transplantation, or transfer of cell products (6,12,16,20,26,69,85). Such transplants must be selected carefully to correct the specific immune deficiency with a minimum potential of unwanted effects. Patients with cellular deficiencies only, such as DiGeorge Syndrome, have been successfully treated with thymus transplants (6,16,26,69). Patients with combined immune deficiencies may be reconstituted by transfer of bone marrow cells which contain stem cells (6,20,26,85). Reconstitution of immune reactivity is due to proliferation of donor cells which repopulate the host tissue. Bone marrow transplantation may also provide a longer lasting replacement for patients with immunoglobulin deficiencies only. Transfer factor (42,43), a dialysate of an extract from peripheral blood lymphocytes, may reconstitute certain immune deficient patients (66,74,81,82). However, this factor has been used in diseases such as Wiskott-Aldrich syndrome and mucocutaneous candidiasis, which have a variable course with temporary spontaneous improvement. Therefore, the clinical improvement noted in many cases cannot be unequivocably attributed to the effect of transfer factor. However, the number of cases where a definite clinical response has been seen has now increased to where an effect of transfer factor on some cellularly mediated reactions must be considered valid. Transfer factor therapy is most applicable for patients with a specific infection, such as candidiasis, coccidiomycosis or histoplasmosis. In these cases the administration of transfer factor obtained from the blood lymphocytes of individuals with a positive skin reaction to antigens of the infectious agent may induce a prompt reaction in infected individuals. Transfer factor is only useful in patients with a limited deficiency and not a stem cell deficiency; transfer factor may push arrested cells to limited differentiation, but cannot replace an absent cell type.

Stem cell function may be replaced by transfer bone marrow cells (see page 237). The transplantation of living immunocompetent cells to an immune deficient recipient is possible because the recipient is unable to reject the transplanted cells. However, the transplanted immunocompetent cells may react to the recipient tissues and death may result from a graft-vs-host reaction (see page 236). Therefore, attempts must be made to circumvent this reaction in order to treat immunodeficient patients with living immunocompetent cells. A variety of method have proved at least partially feasible (6):

1. The use of donor cells from an identical twin will not produce a graft-vs-host reaction.
2. The use of donor cells from an HL-A identical sibling will be identical for both serologic- and lymphocyte-defined histocompatibility antigens; such transplants should not produce a graft-vs-host reaction.
3. The use of cells from an HL-A and mixed lymphocyte reaction (MLR) identical unrelated donor may also be used. In these situations a temporary graft-vs-host reaction may occur which passes and results in the establishment of survival of the donor cells in the host environment (chimera). The immune competence is due mainly to donor cells with a variable contribution by recipient cells (6).

4. The use of very low doses of mismatched donor cells may produce a similar effect (akin to the sneaking through phenomenon described for tumor cells (see page 338). That is, a very low dose of allogeneic bone marrow cells may produce a mild graft-vs-host reaction which resolves and results in the establishment of a chimeric state. The practical application of this procedure remains untested.

5. Treatment of the recipient with immunosuppressants (see below) such as cyclophosphomide or antilymphocyte serum may reduce the graft-vs-host reaction and permit survival of the recipient and the donor cells (6).

6. Treatment of donor cells with antilymphocyte serum specific for T cells may also reduce graft-vs-host reactions but permit survival of stem cells that can repopulate the host.

7. Blocking factors (see Enhancement, page 224) including humoral antibody from the donor, which reacts with antigens of the recipient, may interfere with the graft-vs-host reaction (13). Blocking factors have been described in patients who have survived graft-vs-host reactions (36), but immunologic manipulation of the recipient to induce blocking antibody is not yet feasible.

8. Bone marrow cells may be fractionated in an attempt to remove the cells responsible for the graft-vs-host reaction while retaining the stem cells required for reconstitution of the recipient. Such fractionation by density gradient centrifugation has proved feasible in experimental animals but has been disappointing in human trials (6).

9. Specific killing of donor cells that recognize recipient antigens may be accomplished in vitro by mixing donor and recipient cells and treating the cultures with doses of radiolabeled thymidine that will kill cells that are stimulated to synthesize DNA (mixed lymphocyte culture). After the reactive cells have been destroyed, the remaining cells which can react to antigens other than those of the recipient can be transferred, thus eliminating the graft-vs-host reaction. Preliminary trials with this technique are not conclusive (68).

Using a variety of the above techniques a number of successful transplants of bone marrow cells have been made to immune-deficient individuals with some spectacular successes but more disappointing failures (6,69,85). The fact that there are so many methods used to reduce or prevent graft-vs-host reactions indicates that the status of bone marrow transplantation is still less than satisfactory.

Fetal thymus transplants have been reported to restore cellular immunity in a few patients with combined immune deficiencies who have then been maintained with passive gammaglobulin to cover humoral antibody deficiency (3). The responding cells in patients treated with transplantation of the thymus are of donor origin, indicating the presence of T cell precursors in the thymus—but not B cell precursors as humoral antibody production is not restored (3). The thymus must be selected from fetuses before the fourteenth week of gestation. Under these circumstances only minimal graft-vs-host reactivity has been observed. Therefore fetal thymus grafts may be attempted for severe combined immune deficiency when bone marrow grafting is impossible.

NONIMMUNOLOGICALLY SPECIFIC DEFICIENCIES

Immunologically mediated defense against bacterial infections involves 1) the reaction of specific antibody with the bacteria, 2) the activation of complement components resulting in chemotaxis and immune phagocytosis, and 3) the ingestion of the bacteria by phagocytic cells (polymorphonuclear leukocytes or macrophages), resulting, in turn, in the destruction of the ingested bacteria by products of the phagocytic cells. Therefore, increased susceptibility to bacterial infections may be due to 1) a lack of immunoglobulin antibody, 2) a deficiency in certain complement components (See Chapter 11), or 3) an abnormality in phagocytic cells (phagocytic dysfunction).

COMPLEMENT DEFICIENCIES

A number of patients who have low or absent serum complement components have been identified (see page 154). Since complement plays an important accessory role in the effectiveness of the immune response, it would be anticipated that such patients might have a decreased resistance to bacterial infections. In fact, such is the case in some, but not all, patients (Table 19-1). The precise relationship of the individual deficiencies to the clinical manifestations is not clear. A loss of specific complement function, as discussed in Chapter 11, is the most likely explanation. Thus, deficiencies of those components responsible for activation of the opsonin, vascular permeability or chemotactic activity of complement (C1–C5) are associated with recurrent infections; whereas deficiencies of those associated only with cell lysis (C6 and C7) are not.

PHAGOCYTIC DYSFUNCTION

Phagocytic dysfunction (22,30,38,59) occurs when phagocytic cells ingest bacteria normally but cannot kill them. Such a dysfunction may be due either to an abnormality in the digestive vacuole (lysosome) or to a lack

TABLE 19-1
Serum Complement Deficiencies in Man

Deficiency	Clinical manifestations
C1r	Recurrent infections, chronic renal disease, SLE
C1s	SLE
C2	None, SLE, recurrent infections
C3	Recurrent severe infections
C3b	Recurrent severe infections
C4	SLE
C5	Recurrent infections, Leiner's disease
C6	None
C7	None

Modified from Müller-Eberhard H. Scripps Clinic and Research Foundation, La Jolla, California.

of digestive enzymes in the vacuole. These disorders are characterized by increased susceptibility to bacterial infections associated with the accumulation of lipochrome-laden macrophages and granulomas in the affected tissues. The granulomas are caused by a reaction to bacterial products and the debris of the dead and dying phagocytic cells.

Large abnormal lysosomes are found in the Chediak-Higashi syndrome (59). These granules are found in all the peripheral white blood cells, and the digestive capacity of the affected cell is markedly impaired. The disease appears to be transmitted by non-sex-linked inheritance, and partial phagocytic deficiencies are present in heterozygous carriers. Similar findings occur in animals including the beige mouse (8), Aleutian mink (58), and associated with partial albinism in Hereford cattle (58). The human disease is also associated with partial oculocutaneous albinism and a high incidence of lymphoproliferative neoplasia (59).

Deficiencies of lysosome enzyme function are found in chronic granulomatous disease of children (CGD) (30,38,92) and Job's syndrome (19). CGD is a sex-linked inherited disease, and mothers of affected male children demonstrate partial deficiency (30,92). A similar defect found in girls has been termed Job's syndrome, and is apparently inherited as an autosomal recessive as the parents of affected female children have normal leukocyte function (19). It has been suggested that CGD might be called Jonah's syndrome (22). The Biblical character Jonah was phagocytized by a large multicellular organism that was unable to digest him, and he was eventually released. The enzymatic defect in CGD and Job's syndrome can be tested by the inability of isolated polymorphonuclear cells from affected individuals either to kill bacteria in vitro or to reduce the dye nitroblue tetrazolium.

SECONDARY IMMUNE DEFICIENCIES

Secondary immune deficiencies may result from certain naturally occurring disease processes (29) or from the effect, either intentional or unintentional, of the administration of suppressive agents (25). In either case, the process operates upon an already developed immune system and, therefore, either destroys or interferes with the expression of immune reactions (Fig. 19–1).

NATURALLY OCCURRING DISEASES

Diseases affecting cellular reactions include Hodgkin's disease, Boeck's sarcoidosis, leprosy, tuberculosis, and measles. All these processes usually affect lymphoid tissue directly (70). Hodgkin's disease is considered neoplastic; sarcoidosis is an inflammatory process of unknown etiology; and leprosy, tuberculosis, and measles are specific infections. These diseases may have similar effects on immune processes. Depression of cellular reactions may also be found in uremic individuals. Diseases affecting only humoral immunity include multiple myeloma and Waldenström's macroglobulinemia (70). Other lymphoproliferative neoplasias may affect both cellular and humoral immunity.

Hodgkin's Disease

Hodgkin's disease is a lymphogranulomatous neoplastic process not limited to a single cell type (70). The degree of immune abnormality depends upon the extent of the disease. Immunoglobulin levels are usually normal, although hypoalbuminemia is common. Increased serum levels of haptoglobin and C-reactive protein may also be found, and high levels of these proteins indicate a poor prognosis. Antibody responses may be depressed but are usually normal. Responses to delayed hypersensitivity skin tests are usually deficient. Attempts to induce delayed-type hypersensitivity with BCG or dinitrochlorobenzene (contact dermatitis) indicate a depression of cellular reactivity. Nonspecific inflammatory responses are usually normal. The sera from patients with Hodgkin's disease contains a factor which inhibits chemotactic factors for inflammatory cells. This chemotactic inhibitory factor affects complement-derived, complement-independent and lymphocyte-derived leukotactic mediators, and may inhibit the cellular reactivity of affected patients to immune stimuli (90). The infectious viral and mycotic complications of Hodgkin's disease are varied, but much more common than in the other lymphoproliferative diseases, and active tuberculosis is common. Passive transfer studies indicate the lack of reactivity (anergy) may result not only from an abnormality of the cells but also from an inability of normal cells to express sensitivity in the Hodgkin's disease environment. However, lymphocytes obtained from patients with Hodgkin's disease have an impaired ability to transform when stimulated in vitro with phytohemagglutinin.

Boeck's Sarcoid

Boeck's sarcoid is a systemic granulomatous disease of unknown etiology. The failure of most patients to give a positive response to the tuberculin skin test has been known since 1917, and BCG immunization of patients with sarcoidosis is relatively ineffective. Delayed reactions to other test antigens are also depressed. Passive transfer of sensitive cells to sarcoid recipients results in positive reactions in contrast to the findings in Hodgkin's disease. The serum levels of immunoglobulins are normal or increased, and the capacity to form antibody is not affected. A cellular defect is also indicated by a diminished response of lymphocytes from patients with sarcoidosis to phytohemagglutinin.

Lepromatous Leprosy

Patients with active lepromatous leprosy without erythema nodosum leprosum may have a diminished capacity for cellular reactions (14).

Antigen Desensitization

Occasional patients with active systemic tuberculosis may not react to the usual tuberculin skin tests. Such patients may be anergic because of an excess of antigen in other tissues of the body or because the reactive cells have been depressed by the toxic action of tuberculin sensitivity.

Measles

Measles infections result in a transient suppression of expression of delayed hypersensitivity reactions (23). Exacerbation of tuberculosis during measles infection may occur. The mechanism of this suppression is unknown, but interference with the function of lymphocytes is suspected, perhaps due to involvement of the immune system in production of sensitivity and reaction to the virus.

Multiple Myeloma

Multiple myeloma is a neoplastic proliferation of immunoglobulin-producing plasma cells characteristically associated with the synthesis of large quantities of a homogeneous immunoglobulin of one class [monoclonal] (5,70). Some myeloma immunoglobulins have been demonstrated to have antibody activity, and myeloma proteins are structurally representative of immunoglobulin molecules. Although the morphology of the plasma cells in myeloma varies from patient to patient, there is no apparent correlation between the morphologic characteristics and the type of immunoglobulin produced. Immunochemical and physiochemical studies of the myeloma immunoglobulins have allowed considerable insight into the structure and interrelations of normal nonmyeloma immunoglobulins and of antibody (see Chapter 5). Bence Jones proteins are part of the immunoglobulin molecule (L-chains) which appear in the urine of over 50% of individuals with myeloma. About half of the patients with Bence Jones proteins also produce a complete immunoglobulin. Proteinaceous tissue deposits (paramyloid) may be observed in about 20% of myelomas, and these deposits may be associated with the production of Bence Jones protein. The overproduction of the H-chains of immunoglobulins has also been reported with myeloma. A few patients with an elevated myeloma-like serum protein and no demonstrable tumor (monoclonal gammopathies) have subsequently developed overt myelomas, but this is an uncommon event. Myeloma patients have depressed levels of normal immunoglobulins and an impaired capacity to produce antibody. Increased catabolism of normal immunoglobulins may further reduce antibody levels (89). Cellular reactions appear normal, but affected patients are subject to bacterial infections, particularly pneumonia, due to a lack of specific circulating antibody.

Waldenström's Macroglobulinemia

Waldenström's macroglobulinemia is a neoplastic proliferation of lymphocytoid reticulum cells (small round cells with budding, fragile cytoplasm) accompanied by a marked increase in serum concentrations of immunoglobulins of the IgM (macroglobulin) class (monoclonal) and may be considered a variant of multiple myeloma (5). Bone lesions are not a feature of this disease, but there may be transitions between macroglobulinemia, myeloma, lymphatic leukemia, and lymphoma. The serum level of normal immunoglobulins is usually low, and antibody production is impaired. Cellular reactions are normal.

316 IMMUNITY

Hypercatabolic States

A depression of humoral immune mechanisms also occurs in certain hypercatabolic states such as protein-losing enteropathies, the nephrotic syndrome, or exfoliative dermatitis (89).

Lymphoproliferative Neoplasias

Lymphoproliferative neoplasias may affect both humoral and cellular immunity (52,70). Lymphosarcoma and chronic lymphatic leukemia are examples. In lymphoproliferative diseases the immune cell precursors may be considered to bypass the influence of the central lymphoid tissue and pass directly into the peripheral lymphoid tissue. Low immunoglobulin levels are frequently observed, and in many cases low levels of one or two immunoglobulins are associated with normal or high levels of the other immunoglobulin. Antibody responses to usual antigens are poor. Delayed-type reactions may be normal but tend to be depressed when the disease becomes systemic. These patients are particularly susceptible to bacterial pneumonia and skin infections. Chronic lymphatic leukemic cells manifest an impaired ability to be stimulated with phytohemagglutinin in vitro. Acute leukemias are usually associated with a nonimmune depression of the inflammatory response. There may be a deficiency in circulating mature granulocytes, and the inflammatory response may be relatively acellular. Organisms usually considered nonpathogenic may cause infectious disease, and septicemia is a frequent complication. Immunoglobulin levels are usually normal.

Agammaglobulinemia, lymphopenia, deficient antibody, and cellular responses may be associated with neoplasia of the thymus (thymoma) (37). Such deficiencies may be associated with bone marrow aplasia (panhypoplasia). The thymus may show enlargement of epithelioid stromal cells in areas not involved with tumor, and both germinal centers and paracortical areas of lymph nodes are deficient.

IATROGENIC DEFICIENCIES

The mechanism of action of the so-called immunosuppressive agents is extremely varied (Fig. 19–2). These agents may affect 1) the specific induction of the immune response (primary response), 2) the expression of humoral antibody formation only, 3) the expression of cellular immunity only, or 4) the expression of both humoral and cellular immunity. Their effect may be even more varied, e.g., the establishment of specific tolerance, or failure of expression of a primary response to a given antigen with production of memory cells, so that a secondary response occurs upon reexposure to the same antigen, even though a primary response was not detectable (72,73).

All these agents have systemic effects on cells other than those of the lymphoid system. The total effect of these agents in vivo is as yet poorly understood. In high doses most cause derangements of any tissue that is metabolically active, e.g., depression of the bone marrow with subsequent

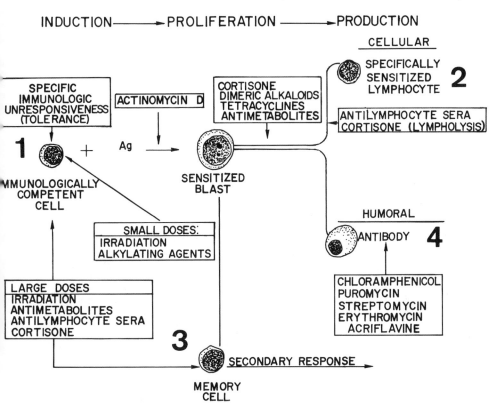

INDUCTION ⟶ PROLIFERATION ⟶ PRODUCTION

Fig. 19–2. Sites of action of immunosuppressive agents.   Agents that affect immune responses include radiation, radiomimetic drugs, antimetabolites, and antilymphocyte serum. Effects include 1) prevention of specific induction of immune response, presumably by action on immunologically competent cell either by interfering with immune recognition of antigen or by prevention of proliferation or differentiation of immunologically competent cell lines; 2) suppression of cellular hypersensitivity reactions by destruction of specifically sensitized lymphocytes or nonspecific effector cells; 3) prevention of expression of immune memory (secondary response) due to direct action on memory cells; 4) prevention of production of circulating antibody by disruption of protein synthesis by plasma cells. Mixed effects upon two or more immune activities with different degrees of effectiveness is the most common result, with secondary response (memory) being most resistant to immunosuppressive action. Most specific immunosuppression is that induced in specific immune tolerance in that only immune reactions to antigen used to induce tolerance are suppressed, while reactions to other antigens are not. (From Sell S. Arch Pathol 86:95, 1968)

loss of peripheral blood cell elements, or denudation of the lining epithelium of the gastrointestinal tract.

The effect of various drugs on the immune response is best considered in relation to the stage of interference in the response. The mechanism of action of many of these agents is unclear (9). Immunosuppressive therapy has become of paramount importance in preventing homograft rejection, especially in regard to organ transplantation (49), and experimental results indicate that such agents may be effective in prevention or suppression of various autoallergic reactions, but the incidence and severity of opportunistic infections and reticular neoplasias are substantially increased (48).

Irradiation

Large doses of radiation (900–1200 r) destroy the host's capacity to muster an immune response by destroying both unstimulated immunologically competent cells and memory cells, so that both the primary and the secondary response may be lost (84). Smaller doses (300–500 r) destroy most of the immunologically competent cells, but the memory cells survive so that secondary responses are less affected. If induction of the antibody response is carried out at a suitable time prior to sublethal irradiation, primary antibody production may actually be greatly enhanced, presumably due to disproportionate proliferation of sensitized cells because depletion of other nonsensitized cells permits more living space.

Radiomimetic Drugs

These drugs are called radiomimetic because the effect of their administration resembles the effect of irradiation (9,25,80,84). They are generally alkylating agents that combine with DNA and interfere with cell division. Included are nitrogen mustard, cyclophosphamide, tetramine, busulfan, and mustard gas. The action of these drugs is only temporary, and immune reactions return when therapy is discontinued.

Antimetabolites

Antimetabolites interfere with the synthesis of RNA, DNA, or protein, and prevent cell division and proliferation (25,72,73,80). 6-Mercaptopurine and thioguanine are purine analogs. Very large doses may not only depress bone marrow function severely, but also antibody production, cellular immunity, and even secondary responses. At lower doses, the secondary response is not affected. Schwartz (72,73) has emphasized that the effects of 6-mercaptopurine on antibody formation are determined by 1) the timing of the drug administration with respect to antigenic stimulus, 2) the dose of the drug, 3) the dose of the antigen, and 4) the nature of the antigenic challenge. By varying these parameters one may obtain 1) suppression of all classes of antibody, 2) selective suppression of IgG antibody, 3) enhancement of IgM synthesis, or 4) enhancement of both IgM and IgG antibody (73). The enhancement of an immune response following the administration of an "immunosuppressive" has now been observed under similar situations by others and is believed to be caused by decreasing the number of "suppressor" cells (see page 114) so that when antigen is given, a greater than normal immune response may be observed. In the guinea pig, 6-mercaptopurine can inhibit cellular reactions with little alteration of antibody production. Azaserine and duazomycin A block the utilization of glutamine and interfere with purine synthesis. The effect of these drugs on immune reactions is slight. Pyrimidine analogs (fluorouracil, thiouracil) appear to have little effect on antibody synthesis except in very large doses. Folic acid antagonists (methotrexate, amethopterin, aminopterin) interfere with the metabolism of folic acid and the formation of DNA and inhibit cell division. In appropriate dose, these agents can temporarily suppress antibody production and cellular reactions without bone marrow suppression. Methotrexate reduces the degree of primary response when injected with antigen, but does not prevent the development of immune memory. Actinomycins inhibit RNA synthesis by combining specifically with the guanine base of the DNA molecule without markedly inhibiting DNA synthesis. This results in a reduction in RNA synthesis at the time of the primary injection of antigen. The capacity of cells to become sensitized to antigen may be diminished by actinomycin, as an anamnestic response does not occur following a second injection of antigen in the absence of actinomycin. Agents that inhibit protein synthesis without preventing RNA synthesis (puromycin, streptomycin, erythromycin, chloramphincol) have very little inhibitory effect on primary immunization unless large doses are given. With doses of chloramphenicol large enough to block protein synthesis and depress antibody formation during the primary response, the development of an anamnestic response on reexposure is not affected, indicating interference not in induction but at a later stage in antibody production. There is an affinity between both RNA and DNA for diaminoacridines (acriflavine), and administration of acriflavine greatly suppresses the primary responses. No apparent interference with cell replication is observed. Dimeric alkaloids (vinblastine, vincristine) completely inhibit antibody formation and cellular reactivity when given at the same time as antigen and appear to inhibit proliferation of lymphoid cells. Vincristine also has a nonspecific antiinflammatory effect. The mechanism of action of these drugs is unknown, although interference with DNA function is most likely.

Antibiotics

Antibiotics may cause an increase in incidence and severity of clinical infections with unusual organisms (*Candida albicans, Asperigillus* spp). The mechanisms by which antibiotics operate to decrease resistance to these organisms include 1) overgrowth of organisms not susceptible to the given antibiotic due to a decrease or absence of competing susceptible organisms, 2) inhibition of immune responses, and 3) inhibition of phagocytosis. Corticosteroids may also increase the incidence and severity of such infections by a nonimmune depression of the inflammatory response (25), perhaps through stabilization of lysosomal membranes with resulting decrease in release of inflammatory agents from the granules of polymorphonuclear leukocytes. The tetracyclines in large doses may have a marked effect on all types of immune reactivity.

Antilymphocyte Serum

Antilymphocyte serum is an antiserum that contains antibody activity directed against lymphocytes (34,77,93). Antilymphocyte globulin is a purified fraction of antilymphocyte serum containing the antibody-active immunoglobulin portion of antilymphocyte serum. Xenogeneic (heterologous) antilymphocyte serum is produced by immunizing an animal of one species (rabbit) with lymphoid cells obtained from another species (thymus or spleen of mouse). With proper selection of the lymphocyte source, and care in preparation, an antiserum can be obtained that reacts specifically with lymphocytes from the donor animal. The reactivity of this antiserum may be demonstrated in vitro by its ability to agglutinate lymphocytes and to lyse lymphocytes in the presence of complement (lymphocytotoxicity). Although there has been considerable interest in the effects of antilymphocyte serum recently because of its possible use for prolonging human allografts, its properties have been studied since the turn of the century (Table 19–2).

In Vivo Effects of Antilymphocyte Serum. The effect of antilymphocyte serum upon in vivo immune reactions is best understood by consideration of the role of the lymphocyte in different stages of the immune response (Fig. 19–2). Antilymphocyte serum blocks cellular reactions, presumably by cytotoxic destruction of the lymphocytes (sensitized cell). This effect appears to be specific, as other tissues are not affected. Antilymphocyte serum may also prevent a primary response to antigen, presumably by an effect on precursor cells, and if administered in large enough doses, may even suppress or eliminate a second-set graft rejection or secondary antibody responses (loss of immune memory). The serum does not reduce reactions mediated by humoral antibody in animals that are already immunized (Arthus reaction) or nonimmune inflammatory reactions such as are induced by cotton wool or turpentine. Antilymphocyte sera specific for different functional lymphocyte populations of the mouse have been developed (39,65,83): antisera to T cells generally kill T cells and inhibit T cell functions in vitro and in vivo, while antisera to B cell antigens may prevent maturation of antibody-forming cell precursors and thus inhibit antibody formation. Such antisera have been used to define further the role of different lymphoid cell populations in immune reactions (see page 41). Preliminary studies indicate that antisera specific for the T and B cells of other species, including man (1,79), will soon be used clinically. The effects of such specific antisera in man remain to be tested but such antisera may be useful in identifying more precisely cellular immunologic abnormalities (21).

Mechanism of Action of Antilymphocyte Serum. The mechanism of action of antilymphocyte serum is poorly understood (77). This is partially due to the difficulty of comparing the results of one investigator with those of another because of differences in source, preparation, and injection of antigen (lymphocytes); in species used for antiserum production; in fractionation or preparation of antiserum; in dosage, route, or duration of treatment; and in differences in the immune responses tested. The possible mechanisms of immunosuppression by antilymphocyte serum include 1) a direct destruction of lymphocytes (lymphocytotoxicity) resulting in

TABLE 19-2
Some Effects of Antilymphocyte Sera

Date	Author	Effect	Significance
1899	Metchnikoff (51)	Leukocyte agglutination and toxicity	Direct effect on lymphocytes
1917	Pappenheimer (60,61)	Species specificity of toxicity in vivo; cytotoxicity of thymus	Direct effect on lymphocytes
1937	Chew and Lawrence (15)	In vivo lymphopenia	Direct effect on lymphocytes
1941	Cruickshank (18)		
1956	Inderbitzin (32,33)	Depression of delayed skin reaction	Suppression of effector cells
1961	Waksman et al. (86)	Suppression of experimental allergic encephalo-myelitis; prolongation of first-set skin allograft survival	Suppression of effector cells; possible inhibition of induction of cellular sensitization
1963	Pincus and Flick (64)	Prevention of vaccination	Inhibition of induction of cellular sensitization
1966	Gray et al. (31,56)	Inhibition of primary and secondary antibody response; prolongation of first- and second-set skin allograft survival	Inhibition of induction of antibody formation and of cellular sensitization; loss of immune memory
	Levey and Medawar (44–46)		
1967	Boak et al. (10)	Inhibition of graft-versus-host reaction	Inhibition of antigen stimulation of immuno-logically reactive cells
	Brent et al. (11)		

Modified from Sell S: Ann Intern Med 71:177, 1969

lymphopenia; 2) a coating of lymphocytes with antibody so that the lymphocytes can no longer react with antigen (blindfolding); 3) a stimulation of proliferation of lymphocytes that do not have the ability to react with antigen (sterile activation); 4) a specific cytotoxic effect upon one class of lymphocytes (long lived) with the ability to recognize antigen, with little or no effect on nonspecific short-lived lymphocytes (selective lymphocytotoxicity); 5) an inactivation of a thymic factor responsible for development of immunologically competent cells (thymus effect); 6) a direction of immunologically reactive cells toward producing an immune response to the injected serum and away from a response to other antigens (antigenic competition); or 7) a coating of the target organ (skin graft) with antibodies so that the antigens of the target organ are not recognized by the recipient (target organ coating). None of the above satisfactorily explains all the immunosuppressive effects of antilymphocyte serum. In spite of the voluminous experimental data indicating that this material may profoundly affect the immune responses of experimental animals, a statistically significant effect of antisera to human lymphocytes upon allograft survival in human recipients has been difficult to demonstrate. However recent results indicate a prolongation of skin and kidney graft survival in recipients treated with antilymphocytic globulin, and of bone marrow grafts treated prior to transplantations to eliminate immunocompetent cells and reduce graft-vs-host reactions.

EVALUATION OF IMMUNE DEFICIENCY

A patient with a history of recurrent infections must be critically examined for a potential defect in defense against infectious agents. The age, condition and clinical history of the patient are vital in establishing the necessity for further laboratory work-up (55). Because of the complexity of findings in primary or secondary immune deficiencies, a systematic series of tests must be performed to permit adequate evaluation (7,57). Some of the tests indicated are presented in Table 19–3. From the type of recurrent infection one can obtain a clue to the type of deficiency. If mainly viral or fungal, a defect in delayed hypersensitivity (T cell function) must be suspected. Recurrent bacterial infections indicate a defect in humoral antibody production. Various nonimmunologic factors can be tested by measuring general inflammatory indexes such as white blood count or serum factors such as complement or various inhibitors. Phagocytic capacity (see page 120) should be determined to rule out a phagocytic defect. Serum complement concentrations should be measured. Humoral antibody capacity can be measured by determining serum immunoglobulin concentrations, by the presence of performed antibody or the number of B lymphocytes (EAC rosettes), by determining the capacity of blood lymphocyte cultures to synthesize Igs, by the response to antigens that elicit antibody, such as immunization to diphtheria, pertussis and tetanus (DPT), or by the response to specifically selected antigens such as keyhole limpet hemocyanin (KLH). Skin tests may also demonstrate anaphylactic or Arthus reactivity. Delayed reactivity can be determined by the transformation response of blood lymphocytes to mitogens such as phytohemag-

TABLE 19-3
Diagnostic Tests For Immune Competence

HISTORY AND PHYSICAL

INFLAMMATION	PHAGOCYTOSIS	HUMORAL ANTIBODY	CELLULAR SENSITIVITY
White blood cell count and differential	Phagocytic index	In Vitro	In Vitro
Sedimentation rate	Bactericidal tests	Serum Ig levels	Lymphocyte transformation by mitogens; antigen
C-Reactive protein	NBT test	Isohemagglutinins	Lymphocyte mediators; MIF
Chemotactic assays	Specific leukocyte enzymes	Secretory IgA	Rosettes with SRBC
Chemotactic inhibitors	Tissue biopsy	Lymphocytes with surface Ig	Serum inhibitors
		EAC rosette forming cells	
		Ig synthesizing capacity by lymphocyte cultures	In Vivo
Complement levels		In Vivo	Delayed skin tests (TB, etc.)
Complement inhibitors		Immediate skin tests	Sensitization to DNCB
Skin window techniques		Shick or Dick test	Skin graft rejection
		Response to immunization DPT, Polio, KLH	X-ray for thymus
			Node biopsy

glutinin, pokeweed extract or concanavalin A, as well as to selected specific antigens. The production of lymphocytic mediators, such as macrophage inhibitory factor, as well as the presence of serum inhibitors of transformation can be measured. In addition, the number of blood lymphocytes that form rosettes with unsensitized sheep red blood cells indicate the percentage of T cells. In vivo tests for delayed hypersensitivity include skin tests to antigens such as the PPD of tubercule bacilli, coccidioidin, etc; the ability to induce contact dimunition to dinitrochlorobenzene (DNCB), or other haptens; skin graft rejection; x-ray examination for the thymic shadow, and lymph node biopsy. From the results of a selection of these tests one can define the nature of defect leading to recurrent or unusual infections and institute appropriate therapy.

SUMMARY

Primary immune deficiency diseases are genetically controlled abnormalities in the maturation of the immune system. The type of deficiency manifested depends upon the level in development that the abnormality affects. Secondary immune deficiencies are the result of naturally occurring diseases or administration of immunosuppressive agents that operate upon a mature immune system. The type of deficiency observed depends upon the location of effect of the given disease or the mechanism of action of the immunosuppressive agent. Since many immunosuppressive agents have effects utilized for the treatment of diseases that also depress immune mechanisms, a complicated clinical picture may result.

REFERENCES

1. Aiuti F, Wigzell H: Function and distribution pattern of human T lymphocytes. I. Production of anti-T lymphocyte-specific sera as estimated by cytotoxicity and elimination of function of lymphocytes. Clin Exp Immunol 13:171, 1973
2. Aiuti F, Wigzell H: Function and distribution pattern of human T lymphocytes. II. Presence of T lymphocytes in normal humans and in humans with various immunodeficiency disorders. Clin Exp Immunol 13:183, 1973
3. Ammann AJ, Wara DW, Salmon S, Perkins H: Thymus transplantation: Permanent reconstitution of cellular immunity in a patient with sex-linked combined immunodeficiency. N Engl J Med 289:5, 1973
4. Ammann AJ: Selective IgA deficiency: Presentation of 30 cases and a review of the literature. Medicine 50:223, 1971
5. Alper CA, Rosen FS, Janeway CA: The gamma globulins. II. Hypergammaglobulinemia. N Engl J Med 275:652, 1966
6. Van Bekkum DW: Use and abuse of hemopoietic cell grafts in immune deficiency disease. In Lymphoid Cell Replacement Therapy. Moller G (ed). Transplant Rev 9:3, 1972
7. Bellanti JA, Schlegel RJ: The diagnosis of immune deficiency diseases. Pediatr Clin North Am 18:49, 1971
8. Bennett JM, Blume JM, Wolff SM: Characterization and significance of abnormal leukocyte granules in the beige mouse: A possible homologue for Chediak-Higashi Aleutian trait. J Lab Clin Med 72:235, 1969
9. Berenbaum MC: Effects of carcinogens on immune processes. Br Med Bull 20:159, 1964
10. Boak JL, Fox M, Wilson RE: Activity of lymphoid tissues from antilymphocyte-serum-treated mice. Lancet 1:750, 1967

11. Brent L, Courtenay T, Gowland G: Immunological reactivity of lymphoid cells after treatment with antilymphocyte serum. Nature 215:1416, 1967
12. Buckley RH: Reconstitution: Grafting of bone marrow and thymus. In Progress in Immunology, Amos B (ed). New York, Academic Press, 1971, p 1061
13. Buckley RH, Amos B, Kremer WB, Stickel DL: Incompatible bone-marrow transplantation in lymphopenic immunologic deficiency. Circumvention of fatal graft-vs-host disease by immunologic enhancement. N Engl J Med 285:1035, 1971
14. Bullock WE: Studies of immune mechanisms in leprosy. I. Depression of delayed allergic response to skin test antigens. N Engl Med 278:298, 1968
15. Chew WB, Lawrence JS: Antilymphocyte serum. J Immunol 33:271, 1937
16. Cleveland WW, Fogel BJ, Brown WT, Kay HE: Foetal thymic transplant in a case of DiGeorge syndrome. Lancet 2:1211, 1968
17. Cooper MC, Peterson RDA, South MA, Good RA: The functions of the thymus system and the bursa system in the chicken. J Exp Med 123:75, 1966
17a. Cooper MD, Lawton AR III: The development of the immune system. Sci Am 231:58, 1974
18. Cruickshank AM: Antilymphocytic serum. Br J Exp Pathol 22:126, 1941
19. Davis SD, Schallar S, Wedgewood RJ: Job's syndrome: Recurrent "cold" staphylococcal abscesses. Lancet 1:1013, 1966
20. DeKoning J, Van Bekkum DW, Dicke KA, Dooren LJ, Van Rood JJ, Radl J: Transplantation of bone marrow cells and fetal thymus in an infant with lymphopenic immunologic deficiency. Lancet 1:1223, 1969
21. Dickler HB, Adkinson NF Jr, Fisher RI, Terry WD: Lymphocytes in patients with variable immunodeficiency and panhypogammaglobulinemia. J Clin Invest 53:834, 1974
22. Douglas SD, Fundenberg HH: Host defense failure: The role of phagocytic dysfunction. Hosp Pract 4:29, 1969
23. Fireman P, Friday G, Kumate J: Effect of measles vaccine on immunologic responses. Pediatrics 43:264, 1969
24. Fundenberg HH, Good KA, Goodman HC, Hitzig W, Kunkel HG, Roitt IM, Rosen FS, Rowe DS, Seligmann M, Soothill JR: Primary immunodeficiencies report of a World Health Organization Committee. Pediatrics 47:927, 1971
25. Gabrielsen AE, Good RA: Chemical suppression of adaptive immunity. Adv Immunol 6:92, 1967
26. Good RA: Progress toward a cellular engineering, JAMA 214:1289, 1970
27. Good RA, Bergsma D (eds). Immunologic Deficiency Diseases in Man. Vol 4. No. 1. New York, National Foundation Press, 1968
28. Good RA, Gabrielsen AE (eds). The thymus in Immunobiology. New York, Harper & Row, 1964
29. Good RA, Kelly WD, Rotstein J, Varco RL: Immunological deficiency diseases. Prog Allergy 6:187, 1962
30. Good RA, Quie PG, Windhorst DB, Page AR, Rodey GE, White J, Wolfson JJ, Holmes BH: Fatal (chronic) granulomatous disease of children: A hereditary defect of leukocyte function. Semin Hematol 5:215, 1968
31. Gray JG, Monaco AP, Wood ML, Russell PS: Studies on heterologous antilymphocytic serum in mice. I. In vivo and in vitro properties. J Immunol 96:217, 1966
32. Inderbitzin T: The relationship of lymphocytes, delayed cutaneous allergic reactions, and histamine. Int Arch Allergy Appl Immunol 8:150, 1956
33. Inderbitzin T: Histamine in Allergic Responses of the Skin. In Henry Ford Hospital Symposium on Mechanisms of Hypersensitivity. Boston, Little, Brown, 1959
34. James K: The preparation and properties of antilymphocytic sera. Prog Surg 7:140, 1969
35. Jankovic BD: The development and function of immunologically reactive tissue in the chicken. Wiss Z Friedrich-Shiller Univ, 17:137, 1968
36. Jeannet M, Rubinstein A, Pelet B: Studies on non-HL-A cytotoxic and blocking factor in a patient with immunological deficiency successfully reconstituted by bone marrow transplantation. Tissue Antigens 3:411, 1973
37. Jeunet F, Good RA: Thymoma: Immunologic Deficiencies and Hematological Abnormalities. In Immunologic Deficiency Diseases in Man. Good RA, Bergsma D (eds). Vol. 4. No. 1 New York, National Foundation Press, 1968

38. Landing BH, Shirkey HS: A syndrome of recurrent infection and infiltration of viscera by pigmented lipid histiocytes. Pediatrics 20:431, 1957
39. Laskov R, Rabinowitz R, Schlesinger M: Antigenic characterization of immune rosette and plaque-forming cells. Immunology 24:939, 1973
40. Knudsen BB, Dissing J: Adenosine deaminase deficiency in a child with severe combined immunodeficiency. Clin Genet 4:344, 1973
41. Law LW: Studies of thymus function with emphasis on the role of the thymus in oncogenesis. Cancer Res 26:551, 1966
42. Lawrence HS: Transfer factor. Adv Immunol 11:195, 1969
43. Lawrence HS: Selective immunotherapy with transfer factor. Bach FH, Good RA (eds). In Clin Immunobiol 2:116, 1974
44. Levey RH, Medawar PB: Nature and mode of action of anti-lymphocytic antiserum. Proc Natl Acad Sci USA 56:1130, 1966
45. Levey RH, Medawar PB: Some experiments on the action of antilymphoid antisera. Ann NY Acad Sci 129:164, 1966
46. Levey RH, Medawar PB: Further studies on the action of antilymphocytic antiserum. Proc Natl Acad Sci USA 58:470, 1967
47. Luckasen JR, Sabad A, Gajl-Peczalska KJ, Kersey JH: Lymphocytes bearing complement receptors, surface immunoglobulins and sheep erythrocyte receptors in primary immunodeficiency diseases. Clin Exp Immunol 16:535, 1974
48. Lurie HI, Duma RS: Opportunistic infections of the lungs. Hum Pathol 1:233, 1970
49. Mannick A: Inhibition of the transplantation immune response. J Surg Res 6:451, 1966
50. McIntire KR, Sell S, Miller JFAP: Pathogenesis of the postneonatal thymectomy wasting syndrome. Nature 204:151, 1964
51. Metchnikoff E: Etudes sur la resportion des cellules. Ann Inst Pasteur 13:737, 1899
52. Miller DG: Patterns of immunological deficiencies in lymphoma and leukemias. Ann Intern Med 57:703, 1962
53. Miller JFAP, Marshall AHE, White RG: The immunological significance of the thymus. Adv Immunol 2:111, 1965
54. Miller JFAP, Osoba D: Current concepts of the immunological function of the thymus. Physiol Rev 47:437, 1967
55. Miller ME: Clinical aids in diagnosis of immunologic disease. Clin Pediatr 8:189, 1969
56. Monaco AP, Wood ML, Gray JG, Russell PS: Studies on heterologous antilymphocyte serum in mice. II. Effect on the immune response. J Immunol 96:229, 1966
57. Moore EC, Meuwissen HJ: Immunologic deficiency disease. Approach to diagnosis. NY State J Med 73:2437, 1973
58. Padgett GA: The Chediak-Higashi syndrome: A review. Adv Vet Sci Comp Med 12:240, 1968
59. Page AR, Berendes H, Warner J, Good RA: The Chediak-Higashi syndrome. Blood 20:339, 1962
60. Pappenheimer AM: Experimental studies on lymphocytes. I. The reactions of lymphocytes under various experimental conditions. J Exp Med 25:635, 1917
61. Pappenheimer AM: Experimental studies upon lymphocytes. II. The action of immune sera upon lymphocytes and small thymus cells. J Exp Med 26:163, 1917
62. Parrott DM, DeSousa MAB, East J: Thymus-dependent areas in lymphoid organs of neonatally thymectomized mice. J Exp Med 123:191, 1966
63. Peterson RDA, Cooper MD, Good RA: The pathogenesis of immunological deficiency diseases. Am J Med 38:579, 1965
64. Pincus WB, Flick JA: Inhibition of the primary vaccinial lesion and of delayed hypersensitivity by an antimononuclear cell serum. J. Infect Dis 113:15, 1963
65. Raff MC: Two distinct populations of peripheral lymphocytes in mice distinguishable by immunofluorescence. Immunology 19:637, 1970
66. Rocklin RE, Chilgren RA, Hong R, David JR: Transfer of cellular hypersensitivity in chronic mucocutaneous candidiasis monitored in vivo and in vitro. Cell Immunol 1:290, 1970
67. Rosen FS, Janeway CA: The gamma globulins. II. The antibody deficiency syndrome. N Engl J Med 275:709, 1966
68. Salmon SE, Mogerman SN, Perkins H, Smith BA, Lehrer RI, Shinefield HR: Trans-

plantation of treated lymphocytes in lymphopenic immunologic deficiency. Am J Dis Child 123:111, 1972

69. Santos GW: Application of marrow grafts in human disease. Am J Pathol 65:653, 1971

70. Scharff, MD, Uhr JW: Immunological deficiency disorders associated with lymphoproliferative diseases. Semin Hematol 2:47, 1965

71. Schur PH, Borel H, Gelfand EW, Alper CA, Rosen FS: Selective gamma-G globulin deficiencies in patients with recurrent pyogenic infections. N Engl J Med 283:631, 1970

72. Schwartz RS: Immunosuppressive drugs. Prog Allergy 9:246, 1965

73. Schwartz RS: Specificity of immunosuppression by antimetabolites. Fed Proc 25:165, 1966

74. Schulkind ML, Adler WH III, Altemeier WA III, Ayoub EM: Transfer factor in the treatment of a case of chronic mucocutaneous candidiasis. Cell Immunol 3:606, 1972

75. Seligman M, Fudenberg HH, Good RA: Editorial: A proposed classification of primary immunologic deficiencies. Am J Med 45:817, 1968

76. Sell S: Immunological deficiency diseases. Arch Pathol 86:95, 1968

77. Sell S: Antilymphocytic antibody: Effects in experimental animals and problems in human use. Ann Intern Med 71:177, 1969

78. Smith RT, Meischer P, Good RA: The Phylogeny of Immunity. Gainesville, Fla, Univ of Florida Press, 1966

79. Smith RW, Terry WD, Buell DN, Sell KW: An antigenic marker for human thymic lymphocytes. J Immunol 110:886, 1973

80. Speirs RS: Examination of the mechanism of antibody formation using nucleic acid and protein inhibitors. Nature 1207:371, 1965

81. Spitler LE, Levin AS, Fudenberg HH: Transfer factor. In Clin Immunobiol, Bach FH, Good RA (eds). 2:154, 1974

82. Spitler LE, Levin AS, Stites DP, Fudenberg HH, Pirofsky B, August CS, Stiehm ER, Hitzig WH, Gatti RA: The Wiscott-Aldrich Syndrome. Results of transfer factor therapy. J Clin Invest 51:3216, 1972

83. Takahashi T, Carswell EA, Thorbecke GJ: Surface antigens of immunocompetent cells. I. Effect of θ and Pc. 1 alloantisera on the ability of spleen cells to transfer immune responses. J Exp Med 132:1181, 1970

84. Taliaferro WH: Modification of the immune response by radiation and cortisone. Ann NY Acad Sci 69:745, 1957

85. Thomas ED: Bone Marrow Transplantation. Bach FH, Good RA (eds). Clin Immunobiol 2:2, 1974

86. Waksman BH, Arbouys S, Arnason BG: The use of specific lymphocyte antisera to inhibit hypersensitive reactions of the delayed type. J Exp Med 114:997, 1961

87. Waksman BH, Arnason BG, Jankovic BD: Role of the thymus in immune reactions in rats. III. Changes in the lymphoid organs of thymectomized rats. J Exp Med 116:187, 1962

88. Waldman TA, Broder S, Durm M, Blackman M, Blaese RM, Strober W: The role of suppressor T cells in the pathogenesis of common variable hypogammaglobulinemia. Lancet 2:609, 1974

89. Waldmann TA, Strober W: Metabolism of immunoglobulins. Prog Allergy 13:1, 1969

90. Ward PA, Berenberg JL: Defective regulation of inflammatory mediators in Hodgkin's disease. Supernormal levels of a chematactic inhibitory factor. N Engl J Med 290:76, 1974

·91. Warner NL, Szenberg A: The immunological function of the bursa of Fabricius in the chicken. Ann Rev Microbiol 18:253, 1964

92. Windhorst DB, Page AR, Holmes B, Quie RG, Good RA: Pattern of genetic transmission of leukocyte defect in fatal granulomatous disease of childhood. J Clin Invest 47:1026, 1968

93. Wolstenholme GEW (ed). Antilymphocytic Serum. Boston, Little Brown, 1967

94. Wu LYF, Lawton AR, Greaves MF, Cooper MD: Evaluation of human B lymphocyte differentiation using Pokeweed mitogen (PWM) stimulation: in vitro studies in various antibody deficiency syndromes. In Seventh Leukocyte Conference. Daguillard F (ed). Academic Press, New York, 1973, p 485

20

Immunology of Cancer

Cancer is not a single disease but a term applied to a large number of diseases which are expressed as the abnormal and continued growth of cells of a given tissue. In some cases growth occurs only at one site while in others the growing cells seed to other sites (metastases). The events which lead to the development, and the factors which control the growth, of cancers are poorly understood. This chapter deals with the role of host immune mechanisms in the development and growth of cancer. In addition, the use of immune mechanisms for treatment of cancer (immunotherapy) will be discussed.

HOST-TUMOR RELATIONS

Although one of the classic characteristics of a cancer is its apparent autonomy, i.e., its ability to grow and metastasize independently of the host, the growth of a tumor is dependent upon host factors. An example is the case reported by Woodruff (142). A 50-year-old woman had a radical mastectomy for carcinoma of the breast. Three years previously she had had a malignant melanoma removed from her right foot with no evidence of local recurrence or metastasis. Following mastectomy, she received deep x-ray therapy and within a few weeks there were thousands of subcutaneous melanomatous nodules in the irradiated area. Metastases developed in other organs and within a few months she was dead. Woodruff concluded that with the trauma of the operation or radiotherapy, or both, the tumor-host relation had been disturbed. There is no way of knowing how much longer the melanoma cells might have remained quiescent in the absence of these stimuli. The host possesses defense mechanisms operating against a given tumor; the growth and spread of cancer are not dependent upon characteristics of the neoplasm alone. Immune responses to tumor antigens may be one of the host's mechanisms for preventing tumors or limiting their growth.

328

TUMOR IMMUNITY

It is now generally accepted that most transplanted tumors of experimental animals have tumor-specific antigens [Tumor-Specific Transplantation Antigens, TSTAs] (80). Tumor tissues contain many different antigenic specificities, including organ-specific antigens and histocompatibility antigens (54,58,61,108). If a given tumor is transplanted from one individual of a species to another, an obvious brisk immune response and rejection are observed. As early as 1910 it was observed that the serum of mice that had recovered from tumors, inhibited growing tumors in other mice, sometimes causing regression and an apparent cure (54,105,125). Attempts were made to treat cancer with immunization methods similar to those that had proved successful with infectious diseases (see Chapter 18), and promising results were obtained in experimental animals. This raised high hopes that tumor-specific immune reactions could cure cancer. However, it soon became apparent that the results obtained were not due to tumor-specific antigens, but to histocompatibility antigens. In other words, normal tissue from the same donor was rejected in a similar manner by the same recipient. Other antigens which must be considered when an immune response to a transplanted tumor occurs are blood group antigens, leukocyte antigens, Forssman-type antigens, and antigens formed due to necrotic tissue alterations (54). In order to establish validity for an immunologic approach to cancer prevention or therapy, it is necessary to identify cancer-specific antigens, i.e., antigens that are present only in the tumor tissue and not in normal nontumor tissue. The inability to demonstrate TSTAs led to a general loss of interest in tumor immunity.

The development of inbred strains of mice led to the discovery that tumors did contain specific antigens. In 1943 Ludmik Gross (48) transplanted tumors (sarcomas) induced by the chemical methylcholantherene in inbred mice. He found that tumor nodules appeared when tumor cells were injected into the skin, grew for a few days and then regressed. After regression, reinjection of cells from the same tumor did not produce a tumor nodule, demonstrating that the animals that had rejected the transplanted tumor were now resistant to this tumor. This interesting observation was not pursued immediately; it was not until ten years later that Foley followed up Gross' observations (39,40). He tested 6-methylcholanthrene-induced sarcomas of C3H/HE mouse origin. Immunization was accomplished by strangulation of the first or second transplant generation of tumor grafts. Following tumor regression, the animals were rechallenged with living cells and the frequency of takes compared with that in untreated controls. Resistance to challenge was noted when the mice were reinjected with the same tumor. Appropriate controls involving skin grafts and immunization with normal tissue ruled out the possibility that rejection was due to antigens not present on the tumor. In 1957 Prehn extended these observations by showing that tumor-specific immunity could be produced by letting a tumor grow then removing it by surgical excision (110). Animals that had been immunized in this way could then suppress the growth of the same transplantable tumor even if greater numbers of tumor cells were injected. He also found that chemically induced tumors possessed individually specific tumor antigens; immunization of an animal to one chemically induced tumor did not protect it from growth of a different chemically induced tumor. These studies clearly demonstrated tumor specific transplantation antigens in chemically induced transplantable tumor of mice.

IMMUNE RESPONSE OF PRIMARY-TUMOR-BEARING HOST

The term autochthonous is used to indicate the relation between a tumor and the individual in which that tumor arose (primary host). In 1960 it was shown that the primary-tumor-bearing host can be immunized against his own tumor (79). The primary tumor was excised and maintained by passage in syngeneic animals. The animal in which the tumor arose was then immunized with x-irradiated tumor cells and subsequently challenged with viable tumor cells (see Fig. 20-1). Transplantation resistance to reimplantation of a methylcholanthrene-induced sarcoma will occur if 3–4 weeks previously the major portion of the primary tumor is ligated (132). An experimental animal may make an immune response to its own tumor and this response may be effective in controlling the growth of the tumor (autochthonous tumor resistance).

Colony inhibition has been used to study the immune response of the tumor-bearing host (57,58,61). The technique involves in vitro culture of recently obtained tumor cells with lymphocytes from the tumor-bearing animal. After approximately 3–4 days the number of tumor cell colonies is counted. This technique has been applied to mice bearing primary methylcholanthrene tumors, mammary tumors, or tumors induced by Moloney virus. The primary-tumor-bearing animal (autochthonous host) has an immune response which can be demonstrated in vitro, but the tumor grows progressively in vivo in spite of this immune response (57,58). Reasons for the failure of an immune response to affect tumor growth are presented below.

TUMOR ANTIGENS

A number of antigenic changes may occur in tissues that undergo malignant change (46). These include 1) the loss of antigenic specificities present in normal tissue (26), 2) the addition of new antigenic specificities not present in normal tissue (54,125), 3) the appearance of antigens present in fetal or embryonic tissue but not present in normal adult tissue (embryonic reversion) (1,42), and 4) combinations of the above.

The primary problem in the study of tumor immunity is the identification of new tumor-specific antigens not present in normal tissues. At least three types of tumor antigens have been identified: 1) those found associated with chemically or physically induced tumors or with many spontaneous tumors of animals and man (108), 2) virus-induced tumor antigens (54) and 3) embryonic reversion antigens (1,42,121).

The first type of tumor antigen includes those found by transplantation in experimental animals [TSTAs] (80) and those identified in some human tumors (see below). These antigens may be divided into two general

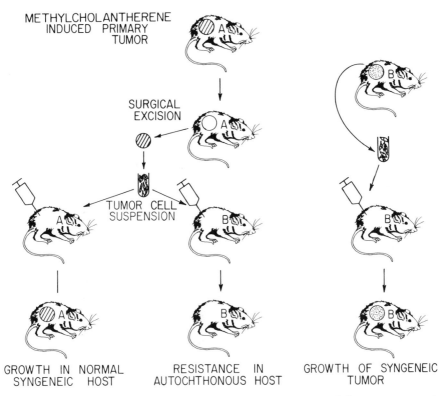

METHYLCHOLANTHERENE
INDUCED PRIMARY
TUMOR

SURGICAL
EXCISION

TUMOR CELL
SUSPENSION

GROWTH IN NORMAL
SYNGENEIC HOST

RESISTANCE IN
AUTOCHTHONOUS HOST

GROWTH OF SYNGENEIC
TUMOR

Fig. 20–1. **Demonstration of specific rejection of an autochthonous tumor.** A chemically induced primary tumor is removed surgically, a suspension of the tumor cells made and a dose of tumor cells that will grow in a normal syngeneic mouse of the same strain as that in which the tumor was induced is injected into the original primary-tumor-bearing animal (autochthonous host). This tumor does not grow in the autochthonous host; the autochthonous host has developed immune resistance to growth of his own tumor. However, a second tumor arising in another individual of the same strain will grow when injected into the host of the first tumor. Thus, the tumor resistance is specific for the first tumor and does not extend to other tumors (Tumor-Specific Transplantation Immunity). This type of experiment demonstrates that an individual can develop immunity to his own tumor.

classes: 1) Those which are specific for a given tumor, and 2) those which are shared by two or more tumors, generally of a particular histologic type. A given tumor may have both unique and shared antigens (9,108,135). For diagnostic and therapeutic purposes in humans antigenic specificities shared by a large number of tumors of a given class are potentially much more valuable than unique antigens. A shared antigen could be used to set up a screening test for tumors in different individuals or used for preventative immunization, whereas a unique antigen would not be detected by a common antigen screening test and would be effective as an immunogen only in the individual with that tumor (20). A tumor induced in a mouse by methylcholanthrene is usually antigenically different from every other tumor induced by methylcholanthrene (9,108). Indeed two tumors induced in the same animal may be antigenically distinct. This demonstration of individually distinct antigenic specificities extends to other chemically induced tumors including sarcomas induced by aromatic hydrocarbons, hepatomas induced by azo dyes, and mammary carcinomas induced by methylcholanthrene, as well as to tumors induced by physical agents such as implantation of cellophane films or millipore filters. Most spontaneous tumors of man have individually specific antigens, but shared antigens occur with some tumors such as melanoma and sarcoma (59).

Attempts have been made to solubilize cell surface TSTAs in order to isolate and characterize the tumor antigen (7,130). The availability of characterized soluble tumor antigens would permit much more sophisticated analysis of the effect of immunization by different forms of antigen on the type of an immune response to a tumor and could provide the means to develop much more sensitive assays for immune responses to TSTAs. Soluble surface antigens may be obtained by a variety of techniques (113). The techniques required for solubilization indicate that TSTAs are protein components of the cell wall. The biochemical nature of soluble tumor antigens is still not well known. Some soluble-tumor-associated antigen extracts have been shown to possess antigenic activity (7,65,93,130) but the purity of such fractions is questionable. In other words, the tumor antigen extract may be contaminated with a variety of nonantigenic or nontumor-specific molecules extracted from the tumor cell surface. TSTAs are protein or glycoprotein in nature (7,113), but as yet have not been adequately characterized.

Tumors induced by a given virus share tumor antigens (54). An animal immunized against polyoma virus resists challenge with any polyoma tumor regardless of the tumor of origin. Group-specific transplantation antigens have now been shown to exist in all other virus-induced tumor systems (54,76). Some virus-induced tumors, in addition to carrying a common group-specific transplantation antigen, have been found to contain individually distinct rejection-inducing antigens (100). The demonstration of the common antigenicity of virus-induced tumors strongly suggests that the neoplastic transformation associated with virus infection represents a direct effect of the virus. The simplest mechanism that can account for this stability is the continuous presence of genetic information derived from the virus genome. This genome information is coded for the antigen and determines the neoplastic phenotype of the cell. An alternative possibility is that the antigenicity is determined by the cell genome which is activated by the virus. The virus itself may be the specific antigen in the virus-induced tumors, or the virus may react with components of the infected cell to produce a specific antigen.

Oncofetal antigens were identified by transplantation as early as 1906, when Schone found that tumor transplants which would kill normal mice would be rejected by mice which had previously been immunized with fetal tissue; immunization with adult tissue was ineffective (117). In the 1930s humoral antibodies that cross reacted with fetal and tumor tissue were identified (64,141). At the present time two major oncofetal antigens have been studied in great detail: carcinoembryonic antigen [CEA] (42,43) and α_1 fetoprotein [α_1F] (1,121).

Carcinoembryonic antigen (*CEA*) is a general term that has been applied to one class of oncofetal antigen. CEA was first found in cancers of the gastrointestinal tract, particularly the colon (42). Specific antisera to CEA was obtained by immunizing rabbits with extracts of colon carcinoma and then absorbing these antisera with extracts of normal tissue (42). Using such antisera an absolute identity between precipitation lines produced by reaction with different colonic tumors and extracts of fetal intestinal tissue was found when tested by double-diffusion-in-agar. Extracts of colonic cancer have been made and the fractions containing CEA characterized (21,81,134). CEA is a component of the cell wall as it requires extraction procedures similar to those required for transplantation antigens (113). However, some CEA is released by cells either through secretion or as a result of cell death as CEA can be detected in the serum of patients with CEA-producing tumors (52,83,88,95). It is a glycoprotein containing approximately 50% carbohydrate with a molecular weight of approximately 200,000 (21,81,134), but may exist in more than one molecular form (21,81). Sensitive and accurate radioimmunoassays for CEA have been developed (52,82,136). At first thought to be specific for colonic or gastrointestinal tumors, CEA has now been detected in the serum of patients with a variety of neoplastic and non-neoplastic diseases (52,83,88,95). CEA is found in the serum of normal individuals and an upper limit of 2.5 ng/ml has been established. Serum concentrations greater than 2.5 μg/ml are not only found with colonic cancers but also with tumors of the lung, pancreas, stomach, breast and others, as well as in non-neoplastic diseases, such as emphysema, ulcerative colitis, pancreatitis and alcoholism and in heavy smokers (52,82,83,88,95). Therefore an elevated serum CEA concentration is not diagnostic for colonic carcinoma and is not even specific for cancer. Elevated CEA serum concentrations can only be considered along with other clinical parameters in the diagnosis of carcinoma. On the other hand if a pathologically proven carcinoma associated with an elevated serum CEA is removed surgically or otherwise treated, decreasing serum CEA concentration may indicate a good result while increasing concentrations suggest recurrence or growth of metastases.

Alpha$_1$ fetoprotein (*α_1F*), in contrast to CEA, is a serum protein not attached to the cell surface, but rapidly secreted from the cell (1,121). α_1F is found in high concentrations in fetal sera, maternal sera and in sera of adults with tumors of the liver [hepatomas] (1,121) or certain germinal tumors with blastic elements such as testicular teratoblastomas (1,31). α_1F is a glycoprotein containing approximately 4% carbohydrate (115), has a molecular weight of about 60,000 (115,121), and crosses the placenta from fetus to mother (121). Radioimmunoassays for α_1F have been developed (114,119). There is a normal adult serum concentration of 0.03 μg/ml (114,119) but concentrations as high as 5–10 mg/ml may be detected in fetal rat serum (121) or serum of rats bearing transplantable hepatomas (120). In the human, high α_1F concentrations in maternal serum during pregnancy may indicate fetal distress or fetal death (118). Normally the sera α_1F concentration of pregnant women rises during the second and third trimester to as high as 0.5 μg/ml, but may reach much higher levels–up to 10 μg/m, if intrauterine fetal death occurs (118). High amniotic fluid concentrations of α_1F may also indicate fetal abnormalities (122).

The serum concentration of α_1F may be used as a diagnostic aid for liver or germinal tumors (1,121). The serum concentration of rats with transplantable hepatomas varies considerably (120), but with humans as many as 90% or more of patients with hepatomas have elevated serum α_1F concentrations (121). Because it is so infrequently found in other conditions, an elevated serum α_1F does have diagnostic significance. Non-neoplastic conditions such as hepatitis or cirrhosis, which may produce an elevated serum α_1F, do not cause as high a rise as tumors and the non-neoplastic elevation is usually a temporary one. Therefore a sustained elevation of α_1F almost always indicates the presence of an α_1F-producing tumor (121).

Both CEA and α_1F may be used to aid in the diagnosis of human cancer, but a role for either as an antigen which might be used by the host for an immune reaction to the tumor has not been convincingly documented. Perhaps the most interesting finding related to α_1F production is the appearance of a sustained elevation in the serum concentration of α_1F in rats fed low doses of hepatocarcinogens [less than 1/1000 of the oncogenic dose (10)], suggestive that α_1F production may be the earliest event now recognized as a response of an hepatocyte upon contact with a carcinogen.

MECHANISM OF TUMOR CELL DESTRUCTION

It is generally believed that the immune mechanism responsible for the rejection of solid tumors in experimental animals is the same as that responsible for homograft rejection, i.e., *delayed hypersensitivity* (54,125). However, through the use of diffusion chambers (permeable to antibody and complement, but not permeable to cells) it has been demonstrated that antibody and complement may cause the death of some kinds of tumor cells. Lymphomas and leukemias are very sensitive to antibody in vivo and in vitro, while sarcoma and carcinoma cells are usually, but not always, resistant to the effect of antibody and complement. Thus, the cytotoxic reaction may be responsible for the death of tumor cells that grow primarily in suspension and the delayed-type reaction responsible for the rejection of solid tumors (54).

The mechanism of tumor cell destruction by specifically sensitized cells has been studied in vitro. These mechanisms are presented in detail on page 209. The major mechanism of destruction is the interaction of sensitized lymphocytes with tumor cell surface antigens. Following this the sensitized cell may be activated to become a killer cell or may synthesize and/or release mediators (lymphokines) that activate other cells such as macrophages to participate in target cell killing.

Studies of hepatomas in syngeneic guinea pigs have shown destruction of tumor cells in vivo by a two-step mechanism similar to other cell-mediated immune responses. Sensitized cells are necessary to initiate the reaction with tumor cells, but macrophages accumulate at the site of the reaction with tumor cells and are responsible for the final cell destruction. If macrophages are mixed with tumor cells, or if they are brought to the site of tumor cell inoculation by nonspecific means, tumor cell destruction may still occur (12,146,147). Thus the mechanism of tumor cell killing in vivo is similar to that of the delayed skin reaction depicted in Fig. 14–4.

IMMUNE SURVEILLANCE

If tumors have specific antigens that are recognizable by the autochthonous host, then it is possible that such antigens may be used by the host to eliminate developing cancer cells. A currently popular thesis is that the major survival role of delayed hypersensitivity (homograft rejection) is to prevent the development of tumors, the immune system providing an anticancer screening system (immune surveillance) (109). Burnet postulates that if it were not for the graft rejection mechanism, vertebrates would die at an early stage of development from tumor growth (18). Potential malignant cells that develop new antigenic determinants are recognized as foreign by the individual's immune system and eliminated by a specific immune response (18). The existence of surveillance has been suggested experimentally by the increased incidence of virus-induced and chemically induced tumors in neonatally thymectomized animals, in antilymphocyte-serum-treated animals, or after exposure of animals to whole body irradiation. It has not been demonstrated that immune surveillance is significant in preventing the development of tumors in man, although tumors appear more frequently in individuals with depressed immune reactivity [see Chapter 19] (41,44). However, the tumors found in immunosuppressed patients are not the types more frequently found in non-immunosuppressed patients, i.e., adenocarcinomas of the breast, colon or lung; but are of the reticuloendothelial system, in particular, reticular cell sarcomas. Therefore, it has been suggested that immunosuppression produces an effect on suppressor T cells so that control of lymphoid cell proliferation is deranged leading to lymphoproliferative neoplasms because of overgrowth of B cell lines.

If tumor immunity is to operate as a surveillance mechanism a number of requirements must be met (109).

1. The developing tumor cells must be antigenic and this tumor antigen must appear early in the development of the tumor.
2. The tumor antigen must be able to initiate an immune response in the host (i.e., be immunogenic).
3. The host must be immunologically competent to respond to the tumor antigen.
4. The host response must not result in tolerance or enhancement (see below).
5. The expression of the antigen must be constant and each tumor cell must have a recognizable antigen.
6. The immune reaction to the tumor antigen must affect the viability (cytotoxic), or otherwise inhibit growth, of the tumor cells (cytostatic).

FAILURE OF AN IMMUNE RESPONSE TO AFFECT TUMOR GROWTH

If progressive growth of a tumor implies breakdown of an immune surveillance mechanism, then malignancy may represent a failure of the host's immune defense. There are at least 8 explanations for the failure of the immune response in the tumor-bearing host: 1) A lack of a specific tumor antigen on the tumor cells that can be recognized by the host, 2) specific immune tolerance, 3) immunosuppression or a decrease in the overall immune status of the primary host, 4) immune enhancement, 5) antigenic modulation or immunoselection of a varying tumor antigenicity, 6) imbalance between tumor growth and host response so that there is either insufficient antigenic stimulation or insufficient host destruction of tumor cells, 7) production of suppressor cells which may prevent an effective immune response, and 8) tumor growth in immunologically privileged sites.

Nonantigenic Tumors

Antigenicity is not necessarily a constant feature of all tumors and in some instances tumor-specific antigens are undetectable even when extensively tested for (5). Clearly if a given tumor does not have an antigen that can be recognized by the autochlonous host an immune response to the tumor will not take place.

Immune Tolerance (see Chapter 7)

The increasing evidence which shows that the primary host responds immunologically even in the face of tumor growth suggests that tolerance does not usually exist in the tumor-bearing animal. However, full tolerance was found to prevail in animal systems where a viral oncogen was introduced into a fetal or newborn host capable of supporting virus proliferation and maturation (123). This included the RNA viruses such as mouse mammary tumor agent, murine leukemia agents of Gross, and other mouse leukemia agents. A role for tolerance in human cancer victims cannot be ruled out.

Immunosuppression (see Chapter 19)

Increased tumor incidence has been observed in patients who have been treated with immunosuppressive drugs (92) or who have congenital immunologic deficiency diseases (41). Surveys have generally concluded that while patients with solid tumors may have normal ability to form antibodies, they often have an impaired delayed cutaneous hypersensitivity. Even if impaired cellular immune mechanisms have no effect upon the growth and or development of the tumor, they have clinical importance in response to the infectious disease complications of cancer.

Immune Enhancement

Immune enhancement was described by Kaliss in 1956 as the progressive growth of normally rejected strain-specific tumors in foreign recipients who had been pretreated either with antiserum directed against the tumor (passive enhancement) or with repeated injections of antigenic material of the tumor [active enhancement] (68–70). Although first seen in allogeneic systems, enhancement has been demonstrated to occur in syngeneic transplantation models with methylcholanthrene sarcomas, mammary adenocarcinomas derived from mammary-tumor-virus-carrying mice, and possibly Moloney-virus-induced lymphomas. Most of these later studies involved immunization of animals with tumor-derived materials in such a way as to induce the formation of humoral antibody. Transfer of tumors to such immunized recipients or to recipients injected with serum from immunized animals results in a more rapid growth than occurred in untreated tumor recipients. Growth of the tumor is enhanced in the presence of humoral antibody, and such enhancement has been attributed to the presence of "blocking antibodies" (59,68,69,70) [see Fig. 20–2]. Mechanisms of enhancement in relation to the immune response may be afferent, efferent, or central. Afferent inhibition implies that the recipient did not become immunized by graft antigens because of the simultaneous presence of antibody. Central inhibition would occur if the host lymphoid cells failed to be stimulated despite being presented with the antigen in a suitable immunogenic form. Efferent inhibition would apply if the recipient became immunized, but

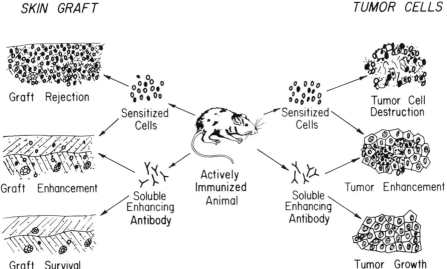

SKIN GRAFT   TUMOR CELLS

Graft   Rejection

Sensitized Cells   Sensitized Cells

Tumor Cell Destruction

Graft   Enhancement

Soluble Enhancing Antibody

Actively Immunized Animal

Soluble Enhancing Antibody

Tumor Enhancement

Graft   Survival   Tumor Growth

Fig. 20–2. **Immune responses to tissue grafts and to tumors.** An individual may produce two general types of immune reaction to tissue antigens, humoral antibody or delayed hypersensitivity. The eventual outcome of a tissue graft (survival or rejection) or a tumor graft (growth or rejection) depends upon the relative response. If delayed hypersensitivity is predominant, then sensitized cells will destroy the graft or kill the tumor cells. If humoral antibody is predominant, a foreign graft may survive and tumor cells grow. If a mixture of sensitized cells and humoral antibody are produced, the eventual outcome will depend upon their relative strength. Attempts to manipulate the immune response of an individual to prolong graft survival or to promote tumor rejection must be guided by the possibility of inducing an effect opposite that desired. Enhancing antibody is desirable for survival of a normal tissue graft, but is undesirable for growth of a malignant tumor. The effects of humoral enhancing antibody may be mediated by antibody–antigen complexes in some situations.

the response which resulted was ineffective against the tumor (69,70). Recent studies using the colony-inhibition technique show that sera from some humans and animals bearing tumors are occasionally effective in blocking tumor cell destruction by lymphocytes in vitro (56,59) [efferent effect]. In some instances both cellular sensitivity and humoral factors are present in the autochthonous host, but the humoral factor blocks the colony-inhibiting effect of the sensitized cells (blocking factor). Although the term "blocking antibody" has been used to identify this factor, the antibody or immunoglobulin nature of the blocking factor has not been clearly established (59). It is possible that "blocking factor" is a complex of tumor antigen and antibody that inhibits the reaction of sensitized lymphocytes with antigen on the tumor cell or it may be free antigen (6, 124). In addition, a serum factor which can decrease the effects of blocking factor has been described and is called unblocking factor (8,58,60). Humoral factors may also cause enhanced tumor growth either through physiologic changes in the tumor cells (69,70) or through stimulation of a substance produced by tumor cells that produces unresponsiveness in lymphoid cells (4).

Antigenic Modulation

Complete loss of antigenicity or a significant antigenic change with selective overgrowth of the changed variant is a possible mechanism of escape from the immune mechanism. Theoretically this escape mechanism is possible but it has been difficult to demonstrate. Loss of the H2 antigens of one parental strain can be induced by passage of a tumor arising in an F_1 animal in the other parental strain (14), and cell surface antigens of mouse leukemic cells, the TL antigen, may disappear after treatment of the cells with antiserum to the TL antigen, but reappear after removal of the antiserum (105,106). Attempts to produce antigenic modulation by serial passage of tumor cells in preimmunized syngeneic hosts have been unsuccessful (123). A stable subline of a Moloney tumor which is immunoresistant to Moloney-specific cytotoxicity antiserum was produced by combining incubating tumor cells in cytotoxic antiserum in the presence of complement and then inoculating these samples into preimmunized mice (37). These observations support the concept that tumor cells under immunologic attack may be able to survive by not expressing the tumor-specific antigen to which the immune response is directed and thus thwart immune surveillance.

Imbalance of Immunity and Tumor Mass

The ability of an immune response to protect against the continued growth of a tumor depends upon the mass of the tumor that is being contained. Old and Boyse (104) postulated that "sneaking through" of tumor cells might occur, i.e., with a low cell dose of tumor cells, insufficient antigenic stimulation may be unable to provide effective immunization but at the higher cell dose antigenic stimulation is sufficient to provide effective immunization which in turn prevents tumor growth. However, the presence of a large tumor mass may exhaust the supply of lymphocytes produced by the host (a form of desensitization) (94,139). Most forms of immunotherapy effective in experimental animals may be overcome by a tumor of sufficient size, immunotherapy being effective only for relatively small tumors or in preventing growth of small numbers of injected tumor cells.

Suppressor Cells

Specific suppressor cells for immunologic reactions have been identified and characterized (see page 114), and some evidence exists that suppressor cells may depress the effect of an immune response to a tumor antigen (45). Thus an immune response to a tumor not only might result in the production of killer cells to the tumor but also in suppressor cells which protect the tumor from the killing effector cells. The mechanism of the suppressor effect is unknown but appears to be nonantigen specific (45).

Immunologically Privileged Site

A tumor may arise in an immunologically sheltered site where surveillance functions play no role in antagonizing tumor development. Such a site is known to occur in the hamster cheek pouch (13). The hamster cheek pouch is frequently used to transplant tumors in a way that will avoid an immune reaction to the tumor. In fact, propagation of human colonic tumors that produce CEA has been carried out using the hamster cheek pouch. (43). It is not clear just why the hamster cheek pouch is a privileged site for transplantation but it is possible that such sites may serve as a locus for the development of primary tumors that avoid immune surveillance until growth of the tumor cannot be reversed by the immune mechanism.

ALLOGENEIC INHIBITION

Possible nonimmunologically mediated processes that might control tumor cell growth involve interactions of other cell types that might inhibit growth. For instance, normal nonimmune cells may inhibit the growth of tumor cells in vitro (128). As a rule homozygous tumors of syngeneic origin take more frequently and grow after a shorter latency period when small numbers of tumor cells are transferred than do tumors transplanted to semisyngeneic F_1 hybrid recipients. Since the F_1 hybrid hosts should not recognize as foreign a tumor from a parental strain due to histocompatibility antigens, but should have the same ability to recognize a TSTA as the syngeneic host, the effect must be due to some mechanism other than immune rejection. This phenomenon has been designated "syngeneic preference" in relation to the parental syngeneic host and "allogeneic inhibition" with reference to the F_1 hybrid host (55). F_1 hybrid recipients may also reject normal bone marrow grafts of parental origin, a phenomenon termed hybrid resistance (22). These phenomena are poorly understood but may represent a nonimmunologic surveillance mechanism for eliminating arising neoplastic cells.

TUMOR IMMUNITY IN HUMANS

Although tumor immunity has now been repeatedly demonstrated in animal systems, significant immunity to tumor antigens in humans is more difficult to demonstrate because of the lack of inbred strains and the ethical limits on human experimentation. However there are a number of findings that support the conclusion that immune reactivity to tumors is important in humans.

1. Spontaneous remissions of different human tumors have been recognized. Although many claims of spontaneous remission of human cancer do not hold up to critical review, Emerson (32), after an extensive survey, accepted 130 cases of spontaneous regression of malignant tumors. Of these, 10% were chorionepitheliomas in which there is a known distribution of paternal antigen foreign to the maternal host.

2. Tumor tissue is often infiltrated by large numbers of lymphocytes perhaps due to a cellular immunologic reaction to tumor antigens and it has been suggested that tumor growth is less rapid when tumor tissue is so infiltrated (11,17).

3. An increased incidence of cancer is found in patients with primary or secondary immune deficiency states (41). A tabulation on the occurrence of primary cancer in transplant patients during immunosuppressive therapy showed that the overall occurrence for all cancers was far greater (13/2000) than in the general population [8.2/100,000] (92); most of these are lymphoreticular.

4. Some cancer patients have decreased cell-mediated immune responses to a variety of antigens (53) and these patients appear to have more rapid tumor growth than cancer patients whose cell-mediated immunity is not decreased (29). In addition, cellular immune deficiency is more marked in patients with disseminated tumor growth (66) or those who respond poorly to therapy (63).

5. Tumor-specific antigens have been identified by a variety of in vitro assays, both serologic (105,125) and cellular (62), including immunofluorescence (74,75,76,84,99,101), colony inhibition (56,57) immunodiffusion (42), and complement fixation (30). The presence of tumor-associated antigens has been shown in a variety of human neoplasma. These include Burkitt's lymphoma (74,75,76), malignant melanoma (84,99,101), neuroblastoma, osteosarcoma (30), colonic carcinomas (42), and other tumors (56,57). This increasing evidence from studies with human cancer suggests that, as in animal neoplasms, tumor-specific antigens exist and are immunogenic in the autochthonous (primary) host. Most of these antigens are class specific (i.e., not unique to a single tumor but present in most tumors of the same histologic type) and therefore are potentially useful in the diagnosis and treatment of human cancer.

6. A tumor-bearing patient may produce a delayed hypersensitivity skin reaction against a membrane extract of his own tumor cells, but the significance of such a reaction is difficult to evaluate (35,62). In addition immediate (2 min) skin reactions to tumor extracts preincubated

with the patients serum [Makari test (89)] may serve as an indicator of the presence of tumors (133). The immunologic significance of this reaction is unknown.

The evidence is now convincing that an immune response occurs to human tumors and that this response may in some cases be responsible for regression of inoperable primary tumors. It is also possible that potential new tumors arise frequently in the life span of any single individual but are eliminated by an immune surveillance mechanism. The important question remains: Can tumor immunity be stimulated in humans to cure (Immunoprophylaxis) or prevent (Immunotherapy) tumor growth?

IMMUNOPROPHYLAXIS OF CANCER

The dream of many scientists, some of whom were eminently successful in producing vaccines for infectious diseases, has been to produce a "cancer vaccine" that could prevent tumors in man (97,116). Popularization of a possible viral origin of cancer in man (16,64a,138) because of the documented role of viruses in causation of tumors of animals (49) has led to increasing enthusiasm that a prophylactic tumor vaccine could be produced. This enthusiasm arises because tumors caused by viruses share common antigens (54,76) so that proper immunization might produce an immune response that would prevent development of primary tumors caused by oncogenic viruses. However an unequivocal demonstration of an human oncogenic virus has not occurred. Perhaps the closest approximation is the identification of a virus associated with Burkitts lymphoma (77,78), but for other human tumors there is little evidence for a common viral origin. Therefore the practicality of prophylactic immunization against human tumors remains in limbo until a common tumor antigen can be identified, isolated and tested.

Nonspecific prophylaxis may also prove feasible, but the effect of this type of prophylaxis is also subject to doubt. As will be described in detail below, certain agents serve to stimulate nonspecifically the reticuloendothelial system and in particular the phagocytic capacity of macrophages. One of the agents is BCG (Bacillus-Calmette-Guarin), a strain of Myocobacterium bovis. This is an attenuated organism that has been used as a vaccine for the prevention of human tuberculosis (see Chapter 18). It has been claimed that death from leukemia is half as common among BCG vaccinated as among non-vaccinated children (27). However this exciting result remains to be confirmed and extended to other human tumors. Until clarified this must be considered an isolated report of great interest.

IMMUNOTHERAPY OF CANCER

Immunotherapy of cancer is defined as any immune procedure which adversely affects the growth of an established tumor (20). Such immune procedures may be specific or nonspecific (97,112). Specific immunotherapy involves the use of tumor specific antigens for immunization while nonspecific therapy involves procedures which increase the activity of the effector arm of the rejection response in a manner that does not involve the use of specific antigen. Specific immunotherapy may be accomplished by active or passive immunization.

Active Immunization

Several requirements exist: 1) the tumor must possess tumor-specific transplantation antigen(s) or tumor-associated antigen(s), 2) the host must be able to recognize these antigens, 3) there must be an effective means of immunizing the host against the tumor to produce an immune response that results in tumor cell destruction, and 4) a small tumor mass must be treated, as failure of the immune reactions to affect a large tumor is to be expected. Autogenous human tumor vaccines using cells prepared from the tumor to be treated have generally been unsatisfactory. (23–25,47,71,86,129). A variety of methods to accomplish immunization against the tumor have been attempted, including injection of living (47,86) or killed (71,129) tumor cells and coupling cell extracts with chemical haptens or foreign proteins, in the hope that some postulated cancer specific antigen may be rendered more immunogenic (23–25,107). Attempts have also been made to immunize a patient with tumors from other patients. This therapy rests on the assumption that specific tumor antigens might be common to the cancers of other individuals (67), as is the case for virus-induced animal tumors. In humans these approaches have generally been unsuccessful, but in animal models, where experimental conditions and the time of immunization can be modified, better results have been observed (33,34,50,51,143). Caution must be emphasized in attempts to immunize actively human patients as the effects may be the opposite of that desired if blocking factors, tolerance and/or suppressor cells are produced which might cause increased growth of the tumor (Tumor Enhancement, see above).

Passive Immunization

Requirements for passive immunization include a donor of serum or cells that recognize tumor antigens of the recipient but not the recipient's normal tissue, and a donor immune response that is effective in destroying tumor cells but does not affect normal tissue when products of the immune response are transferred to the recipient. Attempts to treat tumor-bearing animal hosts with specifically sensitized lymphocytes or with antisera prepared against cancer tissue in another species have had limited success (3,28,38,143), and the results of such procedures in humans have been even less satisfactory (102,103). One major difficulty which is encountered in human passive immunotherapy is that of obtaining immunologically reactive cells in numbers sufficient to effect an anti-tumor response (102,103). Moore has attempted passive immunotherapy using large numbers of cultured "lymphocytes," but the immune potential of such cells has not been documented and his results are equivocal (96). Other transfer experiments with leukemia patients have not been encouraging (91). However since immune cells may have marked specificity for tumor cells and be active against a small tumor load while chemotherapy and radiotherapy can destroy a large tumor load but are limited because of nonspecificity, the combination of passive immunotherapy combined with radiation or chemotherapy might prove effective in some instances (36). In addition the use of antochthonous lymphoid cells nonspecifically activated in vitro has been proposed (19) as has been the use of transfer factor (87) and "immune RNA" (111).

Nonspecific Stimulation

Stimulation of the reticuloendothelial system may result in a more effective resistance to tumor growth. Stimulation of animals with BCG may permit the animal to mount a more effective immune response against a tumor (90). A number of studies, including trials in man, indicate that under certain circumstances inoculation of BCG may be effective in reducing tumor growth (15,112). Morton has injected BCG directly into melanoma nodules of patients with tuberculin sensitivity, and the tumor nodules occasionally regressed (98). Similar results have been obtained with metastatic breast tumors, basal cell tumors of the skin, and other solid tumor nodules (15). BCG vaccine may either act as an adjuvant, inducing a heightened delayed response to tumor antigens, or induce a local reaction to antigens in the vaccine. Tumor cells may then be destroyed as "innocent bystanders" (72). [For further discussion of the activated macrophage, see page 273.]

Other agents which may nonspecifically activate or potentiate a host response to a tumor includes a variety of microorganisms or subcellular fractions as well as nonbacterial macromolecules (i.e. polynucleotides) (144). More extensive clinical use of BCG does not appear justified at this time because of lack of a demonstrable inhibitory effect on noncutaneous solid tumors, the occasional increased tumor growth related to BCG inoculation, and adverse side effects of BCG such as fever and hepatitis (126).

Attempts have also been made to modify the local response of the host to the presence of the tumor. Klein has treated basal cell and squamous cell skin carcinomas by painting the skin lesions with contact sensitivity haptens such as dinitrochlorobenzene (DNCB) after the patients have been sensitized to DNCB (73,140). A delayed hypersensitivity reaction occurs to the sensitizing chemical, and the tumor tissue appears to be destroyed by the accumulation of macrophages which are influenced by the reaction of sensitized lymphocytes to the DNCB (85,127). The possibility exists that the sensitizing agent may couple with the tumor cell making the cells more antigenic.

Evaluation of Cancer Immunotherapy

The variable course of cancer as a disease makes therapeutic assessment extremely difficult. Experience with chemotherapeutic agents over the last 10 years demonstrates the problems involved. Although there are many reports to the contrary and exceptional cases where complete cure is documented, it is now generally accepted that the effect of chemotherapy on

TABLE 20–1
Some Reasons for Failure of Tumor Immunotherapy

1. Tumor does not have antigen
2. Tumor antigen is not immunogenic
3. Tumor antigen is not expressed sufficiently on cells to permit effect of immune response
4. Tumor antigen may be removed from cells by immune reaction (modulation)
5. Tumor may achieve too large a size to be significantly affected by the time the immune response takes place (imbalance)
6. Humoral antibody may block the effect of a cellular or antibody–antigen complex response (enhancement)
7. The host may become unresponsive to the tumor antigen (tolerance)
8. Products of an immune response may not be able to reach the tumor (privileged site)
9. Suppressor cells may interfere with effector cells

most solid nonlymphoid tumors may be useful for individual patients but is clinically unsatisfactory in most cases. The biologic problems involved in evaluating the effects of therapy are even more complicated for immunotherapy than for chemotherapy. For instance, there are a number of mechanisms whereby an otherwise immunologically adequate individual is unable to make an effective response to a tumor (Table 20–1). These must be considered in evaluating the results of a given immune therapeutic procedure. It is possible that by attempting to immunize an individual to his own tumor, the physician may actually cause the tumor to grow more rapidly by influencing the immune response in such a way as to inhibit or block the rejection mechanism.

SUMMARY

There is documented evidence in experimental animals and convincing, but somewhat circumstantial, observations in humans that tumors contain specific antigens and that immune responses occur to these antigens. The identification of cancer-associated antigens in the serum of affected patients has resulted in diagnostic tests for a few human tumors (hepatoma, colonic cancers). Immune recognition of new tumor antigens may be important in preventing growth of newly mutated cancer cells (immune surveillance). Active or passive immunity to tumor antigens may restrict the growth of an established tumor under appropriate circumstances, but a number of coexisting phenomena may interfere with this effect. Understanding and control of these phenomena may result in effective immunotherapy of cancer in humans.

REFERENCES

1. Abelev GI: Production of embryonal serum α-globulin by hepatomas: Review of experimental and clinical data. Cancer Res 28:1344, 1968
2. Alexander P: Fetal antigens in cancer. Nature 235:137, 1972

3. Alexander P, Delorme EJ, Hall JG: The effect of lymphoid cells from the lymph of specifically immunized sheep on the growth of primary sarcomata in rats. Lancet 1:1186, 1966
4. Amos DB, Cohen I, Klein WS: Mechanisms of immunologic enhancement. Transplant Proc 2:68, 1970
5. Baldwin RW: Tumor-specific antigens associated with chemically induced tumors. Rev Eur Etud Clin Biol 15:593, 1970
6. Baldwin RW, Bowen JG, Price MR: Detection of circulating hepatoma D23 antigen and immune complexes in tumor serum. B J Cancer 28:16, 1973
7. Baldwin RW, Harris JR, Price MR: Fractionation of plasma membrane-associated tumor specific antigen from an aminoazo dye–induced rat hepatoma. Int J Cancer 11:385, 1973
8. Bansal SC, Sjogren HO: Counteraction of the blocking of cell-mediated tumor immunity by inoculation of unblocking sera and splenectomy: Immunotherapeutic effects on primary polyoma tumors in rats. Int J Cancer 9:490, 1972
9. Basombrio MA: Search for common antigenicities among twenty five sarcomas induced by methylchalantharene. Cancer Res 20:2458, 1970
10. Becker FF, Sell S: Early elevation of α_1-fetoprotein in N-2-fluorenylacetamide hepatocarcinogenesis. Cancer Res 34:2489, 1974
11. Berg JW: Morphologic evidence for immune response to breast cancer. Cancer 28:1453, 1971
12. Bernstein ID, Thor DE, Zbar B, Rapp HJ: Tumor immunity: Tumor Suppression in vivo initiated by soluble products of specifically stimulated lymphocytes. Science 172:729, 1971
13. Billingham RE, Ferrigan LF, Silvers WK: Cheek pouch of the Syrian hamster and tissue transplantation immunity. Science 132:1488, 1960
14. Bjaring B, Klein G: Antigenic characterization of heterozygous mouse lymphomas after immunoselection in vivo. J Natl Cancer Inst 41:1411, 1968
15. Borsos T, Rapp H (eds): Conference on the use of BCG in therapy of cancer. National Cancer Institute Monograph 39, Bethesda, 1973
16. Bryan WR: The search for causative viruses in human cancer: A discussion of the problem. J Natl Cancer Inst 29:1027, 1962
17. Black MM: Human breast cancer. A model for cancer immunology. Isr J Med Sci 9:284, 1973
18. Burnet FM: The concept of immunological surveillance. Prog Exp Tumor Res 13:1, 1970
19. Cheema AR, Hersh EM: Local tumor immunotherapy with in vitro activated autochthonous lymphocytes. Cancer 29:982, 1972
20. Cinader B: The future of tumor immunology. Med Clin North Am 56:801, 1972
21. Colligan JE, Lautenschleger JT, Egan ML, Todd CW: Isolation and characterization of carcinoembryonic antigen. Immunochemistry 9:377, 1972
22. Cudkowicz G, Bennett M: Peculiar immunobiology of bone marrow allografts. II. Rejection of parental grafts by resistant F_1 hybrid mice. J Exp Med 134:1513, 1971
23. Cunningham TJ, Olson KB, Laffin R, Horton J, Sullivan J: Treatment of advanced cancer with active immunization. Cancer 24:932, 1969
24. Czajkowski NP, Rosenblatt M, Cushing FR, Vasquez J, Wolf PL: Production of active immunity to malignant neoplastic tissue. Cancer 19:739, 1966
25. Czajkowski NP, Rosenblatt M, Wolf PL, Vasquez J: A new method of active immunization to autologous human tumor tissue. Lancet 2:905, 1967
26. Davidsohn I, Louisa YN: Loss of isoantigens A, B, and H in carcinoma of the lung. J Pathol 57:307, 1969
27. Davignon L, Lemonde P, Robillard P, Frappier A: BCG vaccination and leukemia mortality. Lancet 2:638, 1970
28. Delorme ES, Alexander P: Treatment of primary fibrosarcoma in the rat with immune lymphocytes. Lancet 2:117, 1964
29. Eilber FR, Morton DL: Impaired immunologic reactivity and recurrence following cancer surgery. Cancer 25:362, 1970
30. Eilber FR, Morton DL: Sarcoma-specific antigens: Detection by complement fixation with serum from sarcoma patients. J Natl Cancer Inst 44:651, 1970
31. Elgort DA, Abelev GI, Levina DM, Marienbach EV, Martochkina GA, Laskina

AV, Solovjeva EA: Immunoradioautography test for alpha fetoprotein in the differential diagnosis of germinogenic tumors of the testis and in the evaluation of the effectiveness of their treatment. Int J Cancer 11:586, 1973

32. Emerson TC: Spontaneous regression of cancer. Ann NY Acad Sci 114:721, 1964
33. Evans GA, Gorman LR, Ito Y, Weiser RS: Antitumor immunity in the Shope papilloma carcinoma complex in man. I. Papilloma regression induced by homologous and autologous tissue vaccine. J Natl Cancer Inst 29:277, 1962
34. Evans GA, Gorman LR, Ito Y, Weiser RS: Antitumor immunity in Shope papilloma carcinoma complex of rabbits. II. Suppression of a transplanted carcinoma, Vx7 by homologous papilloma vaccine. J Natl Cancer Inst 29:287, 1962
35. Fass L, Herberman RB, Ziegler JL, Kiryabwire JWM: Cutaneous hypersensitivity reactions to autologous extracts of malignant melanoma cells. Lancet 1:116, 1970
36. Fefer A: Adaptive tumor immunotherapy in mice as an adjunct to whole body irradiation and chemotherapy. A review. Isr J Med Sci 9:350, 1973
37. Fenyo EM, Klein E, Klein G, Sweich K: Selection of an immunoresistant Moloney lymphoma subline with decreased concentration of tumor-specific surface antigens. J Natl Cancer Inst 40:69, 1968
38. Fisher JC, Hammond WG: Inhibition of tumor cell growth by syngeneic spleen cell transfer. Surg Forum 17:102, 1966
39. Foley EJ: Attempts to induce immunity against mammary adenocarcinoma in inbred mice. Cancer Res 13:578, 1953
40. Foley EJ: Antigenic properties of methylcholanthrene-induced tumors in mice of strain of origin. Cancer Res 13:853, 1953
41. Gatti RA, Good RA: Occurrence of malignancy in immunodeficiency diseases: A literature review. Cancer 28:89, 1971
42. Gold P, Freedman SO: Specific carcinoembryonic antigens of the human digestive system. J Exp Med 122:467, 1965
43. Goldenberg DM, Hansen HJ: Carcinoembryonic antigen present in human colonic neoplasms serially propagated in hamsters. Science 175:1117, 1972
44. Good RA, Finstad J: Essential relationship between the lymphoid system, immunity and malignancy. Natl Cancer Inst Monogr 31:41–58, 1969
45. Gorczynski RM: Immunity to murine sarcoma virus induced tumors. II. Suppression of T cell-mediated immunity by cells from progressor animals. J Immunol 112:1826, 1974
46. Gorer PA: The antigenic structure of tumors. Adv Immunol 1:345, 1961
47. Graham JB, Graham RM: Autogenous vaccine in cancer patients. Surg Gynecol Obstet 114:1, 1962
48. Gross L: Intradermal immunization of CSH mice against a sarcoma that originated in an animal of the same line. Cancer Res 3:326, 1943
49. Gross L: Oncogenic Viruses. New York, Pergamon Press, 1970
50. Haddow A: Immunology of the cancer cell. Br Med Bull 21:133, 1965
51. Haddow A, Alexander P: An immunological method of increasing the sensitivity of primary sarcomas to local irradiation with X-rays. Lancet 1:452, 1964
52. Hansen HJ: Carcinoembryonic antigen (CEA) assay. Hum Pathol 5:139, 1974
53. Harris J, Copeland D: Impaired immunoresponsiveness in tumor patients. Ann NY Acad Sci 230:56, 1974
54. Hattler B, Amos B: The immunology of cancer: Tumor antigens and the responsiveness of the host. Monogr Surg Sci 3:1, 1966
55. Hellstrom KE, Hellstrom I: Allogeneic inhibition of transplanted tumor cells. Prog Exp Tumor Res 9:40, 1967
56. Hellstrom KE, Hellstrom I: Immunologic enhancement as studied by cell culture techniques. Annu Rev Microbiol 24:373, 1970
57. Hellstrom KE, Hellstrom I: Cellular immunity against tumor antigens. Adv Cancer Res 12:167, 1969
58. Hellstrom KE, Hellstrom I: Immunological defenses against cancer. Hosp Pract 5:45, 1970
59. Hellstrom KE, Hellstrom T: Lymphocyte-mediated cytotoxicity and blocking serum activity to tumor antigens. Adv Immunol 18:209, 1974
60. Hellstrom I, Hellstrom KE, Sjogren HO, Warner GA: Serum factors in tumor-free patients cancelling the blocking of cell mediated tumor immunity. Int J Cancer 8:185, 1971

61. Hellstrom KE, Moller G: Immunological and immunogenetic aspects of tumor transplantation. Prog Allergy 9:158, 1965
62. Herberman RB: Cellular immunity to human tumor-associated antigens. Isr J Med Sci. 9:300, 1973
63. Hersh EM, Whitecar PJ Jr, McCredie KB, Bodey CP, Freireich EJ: Chemotherapy, immunocompetence, immunosuppression and prognosis in acute leukemia. N Engl J Med 285:1211, 1971
64. Hirszfeld L, Halber W, Laskowski J: Undersuchungen Uber Serohogische Eigenschaften der Gewebe. II. Mitteilung uber serologische eigenschaften der neubildungen. Ztschr Immunitats 64:81, 1929
64a. Holland JF, Spiegelman S: Leukemia-specific DNA sequences in leukocytes of the leukemic member of identical twins. Proc Nat Acad Sci USA 70:2629, 1973
65. Holmes EC, Kahan BD, Morton DL: Soluble tumor-specific transplantation antigens from methylcholontherene-induced guinea pig sarcomas. Cancer 25:373, 1970
66. Hughes LE, Mackay WD: Suppression of the tuberculin response in malignant disease. Br Med J 2:1346, 1965
67. Humphrey LJ, Boehm B, Jewell WR, Boehm OR: Immunologic response of cancer patients modified by immunization with tumor vaccine. Am Surg 176:554, 1972
68. Kaliss N: Immunological enhancement of tumor homografts in mice: A review. Cancer Res 18:992, 1958
69. Kaliss N: Immunological enhancement. Int Rev Exp Pathol 8:241, 1969
70. Kaliss N: Dynamics of immunologic enhancement. Transplant Proc 2:59, 1970
71. Kellock TH, Chambers H, Russ S: An attempt to procure immunity to malignant disease in man. Lancet 202:217, 1922
72. Keller R: Cytostatic elimination of syngeneic rat tumor cells in vitro by non-specifically activated macrophage. J Exp Med 138:625, 1973
73. Klein E: Immunotherapy of cutaneous and mucosal neoplasms. NY State J Med 68:900, 1968
74. Klein G: Tumor antigens. Annu Rev Microbiol 20:223, 1966
75. Klein G: Tumor specific transplantation antigens. GHA Clowes Memorial Lecture. Cancer Res 28:625, 1968
76. Klein G: Experimental studies in tumor immunology. Fed Proc 23:1739, 1969
77. Klein G: Immunological studies on a human tumor. Dilemmas of the experimentalist. Isr J Med Sci 7:111, 1971
78. Klein G, Clifford P, Klein E, Smith RT, Minowada J, Kourilsky FM, Burchenal JH: Membrane immunofluorescence reaction of Burkitt lymphoma cells from biopsy specimens and tissue cultures. J Natl Cancer Inst 39:1027, 1967
79. Klein G, Sjogren HO, Klein E, Hellstrom K: Demonstration of resistance against methylcholanthrene-induced sarcomas in the primary autochthonous host. Cancer Res 20:1561, 1960
80. Koldovsky P: Tumor specific transplantation antigen. In Recent Results in Cancer Research. Rentchnick P (ed). Vol 22. New York, Springer-Verlag, 1969
81. Krupey J, Gold P, Freedman SO: Physiochemical studies of the carcinoembryonic antigens of the human digestive tract. J Exp Med 128:387, 1968
82. Kupchik HZ, Zamcheck N, Savaris CA: Editorial: Immunologic studies of carcinoembryonic antigens: Methodologic considerations and some clinical implications. J Natl Cancer Inst 51:1741, 1973
83. Lebel JS, Deodhar SD, Brown CH: Newer concepts of cancer of the colon and rectum: Clinical evaluation of a radioimmunoassay for CEA. Dis Colon Rectum 15:111, 1972
84. Lewis MG, Ikonopisu RL, Navin RC, Phillips TM, Fairley HG, Bodenham PC, Alexander P: Tumor-specific antibodies in human malignant melanoma and their relationship to the extent of the disease. Br J Med 1:547, 1969
85. Lewis WR, Kraemer KH, Klinger WG, Peck GL, Terry WD: Topical immunotherapy of basal cell carcinomas with dinitrochlorobenzene. Cancer Res 33:3036, 1973
86. Leyden E, Blumenthal F: Vorlaufige mittheilungen über einige ergebnisse der Krebsforshung auf der I. Medizinischek Klinik. Dtsch Med Wochenschr 28:637, 1902
87. LoBuglio AF, Neidhart JA, Hilberg RW, Metz EN, Balcerzak SP: The effect of transfer factor therapy on tumor immunity in alveolar soft part sarcoma. Cell Immunol 7:159, 1973

88. Logerfo P, Krupey J, Hansen PJ: Demonstration of an antigen common to several varieties of neoplasia. Assay using zirconyl phosphate gel. N Engl J Med 285:138, 1971
89. Makari JG: The intradermal cancer test (ICT). J Am Geriatr Soc 17:755, 1969
90. Mathe G, Amiel JL, Schwarzenberg L, Schneider M, Cattan A, Schlumberger JR, Hapat M, DeVassal F: Active immunotherapy for acute lymphoblastic leukemia. Lancet 1:697, 1969
91. Mathe G, Amiel JL, Schwarzenberg L, Cattan A, Schneider M: Adaptive immunotherapy of acute leukemia: Experimental and clinical results. Cancer Res 25:1525, 1965
92. McKhann CF: Primary malignancy in patients undergoing immunosuppression for renal transplantation. Transplantation 8:209, 1969
93. Meltzer MS, Leonard EJ, Rapp HJ, Borsos T: Tumor-specific antigen solubilized by hypertoxic potassium chloride. J Natl Cancer Inst 47:703, 1971
94. Mikulska ZB, Smith C, Alexander P: Evidence for an immunological reaction of the host directed against its own actively growing primary tumor. J Natl Cancer Inst 36:29, 1966
95. Moore TL, Kantrowitz PA, Zamcheck N: Carcinoembryonic antigen (CEA) in bowel diseases. JAMA 8:944, 1972
96. Moore GE, Moore MB: Auto-inoculation of cultured lymphocytes in malignant melanoma. NY State J Med 69:460, 1969
97. Morton DL: Immunotherapy of cancer, present status and future potential. Cancer 30:1647, 1972
98. Morton DL, Eilber FR, Malmgren RA, Wood WC: Immunological factors which influence response to immunotherapy in malignant melanoma. Surgery 68:158, 1970
99. Morton DL, Malmgren RA, Holmes EL, Hetcham AS: Demonstration of antibodies against human malignant melanoma by immunofluorescence. Surgery 64:223, 1968
100. Morton DL, Miller GF, Wood DA: Demonstration of tumor-specific immunity against antigens unrelated to the mammary tumor virus in spontaneous mammary adrenocarcinomas. J Natl Cancer Inst 42:289, 1969
101. Muna NM, Marcus S, Smart C: Detection of immunofluorescence of antibodies specific for human malignant melanoma cells. Cancer 23:88, 1969
102. Nadler SH, Moore GE: Clinical immunological study of malignant disease: Response to tumor transplants and transfer of leukocytes. Ann Surg 164:482, 1966
103. Nadler SH, Moore GE: Immunotherapy of malignant disease. Arch Surg 99:376, 1969
104. Old J, Boyse EA: Immunology of experimental tumors. Annu Rev Med 15:167, 1964
105. Old LJ, Boyse EA, Geering G, Oettgen HF: Serologic approaches to the study of cancer in animals and in man. Cancer Res 28:1288, 1968
106. Old LJ, Stockert E, Boyse EA, Kim JH: Antigenic modulation. Loss of TL antigen from cells exposed to TL antibody. Study of the phenomenon in vitro. J Exp Med 127:523, 1968
107. Prager MD: Immunologic stimulation with modified cancer cells. Biomed 18:261, 1973
108. Prehn RT: Tumor-specific antigens of nonviral tumors. Cancer Res 28:1326, 1968
109. Prehn RT: Immunosurveillance, regeneration and oncogenesis. Prog Exp Tumor Res 14:1, 1970
110. Prehn RT, Main JM: Immunity to methylcholantherene induced sarcomas. J Natl Cancer Inst 18:769, 1957
111. Ramming KP, Pilch YH: Transfer of tumor-specific immunity with RNA: Inhibition of growth of murine tumor isografts. J Natl Cancer Inst 46:735, 1971
112. Rapp HJ: Immunotherapy of cancer. In Current Research in Oncology. Anfinsen CB, Potter M, Schechter AN (eds). Academic Press, 1972, p 143
113. Reisfeld RA, Ferrone S, Pellegrino MA: Isolation and serological evaluation of HL-A antigens solubilized from cultured human lymphoid cells. In Methods in Membrane Biology. Korn ED (ed). Vol 1. New York, Plenum Press, 1974, p 143
114. Ruoslahti E, Seppala M: Studies of carcino-fetal proteins. III. Development of a radioimmunoassay for α-fetoprotein. Demonstration in serum of healthy human adults. Int J Cancer 8:374, 1971

115. Ruoslahti E, Seppala M, Pihko H, Vuopio P: Studies of Carcinofetal proteins. II. Biochemical comparison of α-fetoprotein from human fetuses and patients with hepatocellular cancer. Int J Cancer 8:283, 1971

116. Schein PS: Cancer chemotherapy: Current concepts and results. In Current Research in Oncology. Anfinsen CB, Potter M, Schechter AN (eds). Academic Press, 1973

117. Schone G: Untersuchngen Uber Kakzinomimmunitat Bei Mausen. Munch Med Wochenschr 53:2517, 1906

118. Seppala M, Ruoslahti E: Alpha fetoprotein in maternal serum: A new marker for detection of fetal and intrauterine death. Am J Obstet Gynecol 115:48, 1973

119. Sell S, Gord D: Rat alpha fetoprotein. III. Refinement of radioimmunoassay for detection of 1 μg rat α₁ F. Immunochemistry 10:439, 1973

120. Sell S, Morris HP: Rat alpha 1 fetoprotein: Relationship to growth rate and chromosome composition of Morris hepatomas. Cancer Res 34:1413, 1974

121. Sell S, Wepsic HT: Alpha fetoprotein. In The Liver—The Molecular Biology of Its Diseases. Becker FF (ed). New York, Marcel Dekker Inc., 1974

122. Seller MJ, Coltart TM, Campbell S, Singer JD: Early termination of anencephalic pregnancy after detection by raised alpha fetoprotein levels. Lancet 2:73, 1973

123. Sjogren HO: Studies on specific transplantation resistance to polyoma-virus-induced tumors. IV. Stability of the polyoma cell antigen. J Natl Cancer Inst 32:661, 1964

124. Sjogren HO, Hellstrom I, Bansal SC, Warner GA, Hellstrom KE: Elution of "Blocking Factors" from human tumors, capable of abrogating tumor cell destruction by specifically immune lymphocytes. Int J Cancer 9:274, 1972

125. Smith RT: Tumor specific immune mechanisms. New Engl J Med 278:1027, 1268, 1326, 1968

126. Sparks FC, Silverstein MJ, Hunt JS, Haskell CM, Pilch YH, Morton DL: Complications of BCG immunotherapy in patients with cancer. N Engl J Med 289:827, 1973

127. Stjernsward J, Levin A: Delayed hypersensitivity-induced regression of human neoplasma. Cancer 28:628, 1971

128. Stoker M: Regulation of growth and orientation in hamster cells transformed by polyoma virus. Virology 24:165, 1964

129. Stone HB, Curtis RM, Brewer JH: Can resistance to cancer be induced? Ann Surg 134:519, 1951

130. Tacker JR, Hyde RM: Partial characterization of an antigen in spontaneous murine mammary tumors. Int J Cancer 4:21, 1969

131. Takeda K: Immunology of cancer with special reference to tumor immunity in the primary autochthonous host. Vol. 2. Sapporo, Japan, Hokkaido Univ. Medical Library Series, 1969

132. Takeda K, Aizawa M, Kikuchi Y, Yamawaki S, Nakamura K: Tumor autoimmunity against methylchonanthrene-induced sarcomas of the rat. Gann 57:211, 1966

133. Tee DEH: Clinical evaluation of the Makari tumor skin test. Br J Cancer 28:187, 1973

134. Terry WD, Henkart PA, Coligan JE, Todd CW: Structural studies of the major glycoprotein in preparations with carcinoembryonic antigen activity. J Exp Med 136:200, 1972

135. Thompson DMP, Alexander P: A cross-reacting embryonic antigen in the membrane of rat sarcoma cells which is immunogenic in the syngeneic host. Br J Cancer 27:35, 1973

136. Thompson DM, Krupey J, Freedman SO, Gold P: The radioimmunoassay of circulating carcinoembryonic antigens of the human digestive system. Proc Natl Acad Sci USA 64:161, 1969

137. Thomas L: Discussion. In Cellular and Humoral Aspects of the Hypersensitive State. Lawrence HS (ed). New York, Harper & Row, 1959

138. Todaro GJ, Heubner RJ: The viral oncogene hypothesis: New evidence. Proc Natl Acad Sci USA 69:1009, 1972

139. Wepsic HT, Bernstein IB, Zbar B, Borsos T, Rapp HJ: Abrogation of passively transferred tumor immunity in vitro by antigenically related tumor cells. J Natl Cancer Inst 46:195, 1971

140. Williams AC, Klein E: Experiences with local chemotherapy and immunotherapy in pre-malignant and malignant skin lesions. Cancer 25:450, 1970

141. Witebsky E: Sur serologischen spezifitat des carcinomgewebes Klin Wochenschr 9:58, 1930
142. Woodruff MFA: Immunological aspects of cancer. Lancet 2:265, 1964
143. Woodruff MFA, Boak JL: Inhibitory effect of pre-immunized CBA spleen cells on transplants of A-strain mouse mammary carcinoma in (CBA XA) F₁ hybrid recipients. Br J Cancer 14:411, 1965
144. Yasphe DJ: Immunological factors in nonspecific stimulation of host resistance to syngeneic tumors. A Review. Isr J Med Sci 7:90, 1971
146. Zbar B, Wepsic HT, Borsos T, Rapp HJ: Tumor-graft rejection in syngeneic guinea pigs: Evidence for a two-step mechanism. J Natl Cancer Inst 44:473, 1970
147. Zbar B, Wepsic HT, Rapp HJ, Steward LC, Borsos T: Two-step mechanisms of tumor graft rejection in syngeneic guinea pigs. II. Initiation of reaction by a cell reaction containing lymphocytes and neutrophils. J Natl Cancer Inst 44:701, 1970

21

Shwartzman Reaction

The Shwartzman reaction (4) is not an immune reaction, but an alteration in factors affecting intravascular coagulation (2).

THE LOCAL REACTION

The local Shwartzman reaction is a lesion confined to a prepared tissue site (usually skin) and is a two-stage reaction (2). The tissue site is *prepared* by the local injection of an agent (gram-negative endotoxin) that causes accumulation of polymorphonuclear leukocytes. It is believed that the granulocytes then condition the site by releasing lysosomal acid hydrolases which damage small vessels, setting up the site for reaction to a provoking agent. A mild Arthus reaction may serve as a preparative event. *Provocation* is accomplished by injection into the prepared site of agents that initiate intravascular coagulation (gram-negative endotoxins, antigen–antibody complexes, serum, starch). The main lesion is intravascular clotting with localization of platelets, granulocytes, and fibrin, forming white cell thrombi that lead to necrosis of vessel walls and hemorrhage. The administration of nitrogen mustard (decreased granulocytes) or vasodilators inhibits the reaction, while agents that block the reticuloendothelial system (carbon) increase the intensity of the reaction. Specific immunization is not necessary. Although immune reactions may serve as either a preparatory or provocative event, nonimmune reactions are also effective.

THE GENERALIZED REACTION

The classic generalized Shwartzman reaction (1,2) is elicited by giving a young rabbit two intravascular injections of endotoxin 24 hours apart (Fig. 21-1). After the first injection, few fibrin thrombi are found in vessels of liver, lungs, kidney, and spleen capillaries. Following the second injection, many more thrombi are found. Bilateral renal cortical necrosis and splenic hemorrhage and necrosis are prominent. The fibrin thrombi do

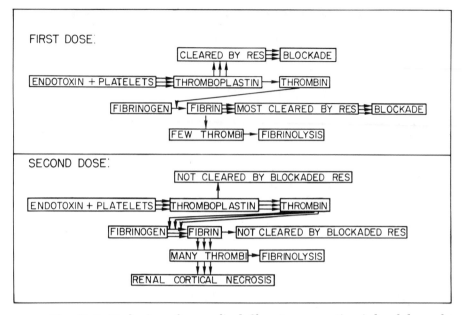

Fig. 21–1. **Mechanism of generalized Shwartzman reaction induced by endotoxin.** Classic generalized Shwartzman reaction is elicited by giving rabbits two doses of endotoxin 24 hours apart. Primary effect of first (preparatory) dose of endotoxin is to cause release of platelet thromboplastin. Most of this thromboplastin is cleared by reticuloendothelial system (RES). Some thrombin triggers conversion of fibrinogen to fibrin, but again most of this fibrin is cleared by reticuloendothelial system. If animal is examined after one dose of endotoxin (preparative dose), a few fibrin thrombi are found in vessels of liver, lungs, and spleen. These thrombi appear to be quickly removed by fibrinolysis with no damage to treated rabbit. However, because of action of reticuloendothelial system in clearing thromboplastin and fibrin, blockade of reticuloendothelial system occurs. This blockade permits second dose of endotoxin to produce severe intravascular coagulation. Second dose (provocative dose) initiates same release of platelet thromboplastin as first dose, but with reticuloendothelial system blockaded, this thromboplastin is not cleared; most goes on to form thrombin and initiate conversion of fibrinogen to fibrin. This fibrin cannot be cleared by blockaded reticuloendothelial system, and most become lodged in capillaries, capillaries of renal glomeruli in particular. Fibrinolytic system may not be capable of overcoming large amounts of fibrin formed in a short period of time. End result may be fatal renal cortical necrosis.

not contain clumps of platelets or leukocytes. In human disease, the generalized Shwartzman reaction develops as an acute and frequently fatal complication of an underlying disease, such as infection. It is triggered by one or more episodes of intravascular clotting leading to the formation of multiple fibrin or fibrin-like thrombi that lodge in small vessels. Such thrombi are prominent in the kidney or adrenal glands and cause necrosis and/or hemorrhage (3). Three steps appear to be necessary (2):

1. Intravascular clotting with fibrin formation.
2. Deposition of fibrin in small vessels. In order for this to happen at

least one, and usually all, of the following conditions must appear: depression of reticuloendothelial clearance of altered fibrinogen, decrease in blood flow through affected organs and liberation of enzymes by granulocytes, which help precipitate fibrin.

3. Once deposited, the fibrin is not removed by fibrinolysis.

Administration of agents that cause blockade of reticuloendothelial clearance (thorotrast, carbon, endotoxin, cortisone) serve as priming agents, and agents that activate intravascular clotting (endotoxin, antigen–antibody complexes, synthetic acid polysaccharide) serve as provoking agents.

ENDOTOXIN SHOCK

Endotoxin shock is different from Shwartzman reaction in that 1) no preparative injection is necessary; 2) shock can be induced in any species (the Shwartzman reaction occurs only in man and rabbit); 3) shock occurs with equal intensity at any age (young rabbits are much more sensitive than old rabbits to the Shwartzman reaction); 4) thrombi are not a prominent feature of endotoxin shock, which features hemorrhage and necrosis, and 5) cortisone enhances the Shwartzman reaction but does not affect endotoxin shock.

There is increasing evidence that endotoxin may function by activation of complement components.

THE SHWARTZMAN REACTION AND PREGNANCY

A single injection of endotoxin in pregnant rabbits produces a generalized Shwartzman reaction (1). Bilateral renal cortical necrosis has been reported in septicemia following induced abortion in humans. Clinical evidence indicates that bilateral renal cortical necrosis in this circumstance represents a human equivalent of the generalized Shwartzman reaction due to endotoxemia and pregnancy. Pregnancy serves as the preparative step, as fibrinolytic activity and reticuloendothelial clearance and decreased during pregnancy. The occurrence of gram-negative septicemia during delivery or abortion serves as the provocative step, leading to hypotension and intravascular clotting. This may be followed by thrombocytopenia and hemorrhage or a typical generalized Shwartzman reaction with bilateral renal cortical necrosis. Fibrin occurs within glomerular capillary loops within 48 hours of the provocation. Hemorrhagic necrosis of the adrenals and/or renal cortical necrosis may occur 60 hours–40 days later.

REFERENCES

1. Apitz KA: Study of the generalized Shwartzman phenomena. J Immunol 29:255, 1935
2. Hjort PF, Rapaport SI: The Shwartzman reaction: Pathologic mechanisms and clinical manifestations. Annu Rev Med 16:135, 1965
3. Rodriguez-Erdmann F: Bleeding due to increased intravascular blood coagulation. N Engl J Med 273:1370, 1966
4. Shwartzman G: Phenomena of Local Tissue Reactivity. New York, Hoeber, 1937

Appendix: Resumé of Immune Mechanisms in Disease

Certain characteristics are ideally demonstrable in an immune response. These include:

1. A well-defined immunizing event (infection, immunization, vaccination).
2. A latent period (usually 6–14 days).
3. A secondary response (a more rapid and more intense reaction on second exposure to the antigen).
4. Passive transfer of the disease state with cells or serum from an affected individual.
5. Specific depression of the disease by large amounts of antigen (desensitization).
6. Identification and chemical characterization of the antigen.

All, or even a few, of these criteria can rarely, if ever, be established for human diseases. The criteria are most closely approximated in certain blood dyscrasias, acute disseminated encephalomyelitis, some atopic or anaphylactic reactions, and neutralization reactions following replacement of biologically active molecules such as exogenous insulin in diabetes.

Presumptive findings consistent with, but only suggestive for, an allergic basis for a disease state include:

1. A morphologic picture consistent with known allergic reactions.
2. The demonstration of antibody or a positive skin reaction.

3. A depression of complement during some stage of the disease.
4. A beneficial effect of agents known to inhibit some portion of an allergic reaction (steroids, radiation, nitrogen mustard, aminopterin).
5. Identification of a reasonable experimental (animal) model that mimics the human disease.
6. An association with other possibly allergic diseases.
7. An increased familial susceptibility to the same disease or other allergic diseases.

The tissue alterations caused by allergic reactions may be considered as variations of the inflammatory reaction. Since more than one organ system may be involved with the same allergic process and because the alterations in different organ systems caused by the same process have pathologic similarities, the lesions caused by allergic reactions are best classified by the type of allergic mechanisms involved. The six immunopathologic mechanisms recognized and discussed here are:

1. Neutralization or inactivation of biologically reactive molecules.
2. Cytotoxic or cytolytic reactions.
3. Atopic or anaphylactic reactions.
4. Arthus or toxic complex reactions.
5. Cellular or delayed hypersensitivity reactions.
6. Granulomatous reactions.

Few immune reactions in humans are the result of the operation of only one of these mechanisms. The complex clinical picture found in many human diseases may be caused by the simultaneous occurrence of two or more immunopathologic mechanisms.

Index

Page numbers in italics represent illustrations; page numbers followed by the letter *t* refer to tables.

Chain specificity of immunoglobulins, 74

Chediak-Higashi syndrome, lysosomes in, 313

Cheese-washer's lung, antigen and source for, 272

Cholera, immunization against, 295

Cholinergic effects, 175

Cholinergic urticaria, 172

Chorea, and rheumatic fever, 196

Chromatin, of plasma cells, 14

Chromic phosphate, clearance by RES, 124

Chromosomal markers, of T cells, 37

Chromosome, definition of, 79

Cigaret smoke, effect on pulmonary clearing mechanisms, 300

Cirrhosis, primary biliary, allergic aspects of, 252

Cistron(s), 79–80

  controlling Gm specificities, 80

  definition of, 79, 230

  distribution within family, 231

  duplication of, 81

  in humoral immune deficiencies, 306

Class specificity, of immunoglobulins, 74

Classic delayed sensitivity, 277

Clonal elimination theory of immune tolerance, 112, 113, 114

  in autoallergic diseases, 257

Clotting. See Blood clotting

Codon

  defined, 79

  sequences, 80–81

Coeliac disease, adult, and HL-A antigens, 235

Cogan's syndrome, and Wegener's granulomatosis, 271

Colchicine, and mediator release, 162

Cold, and histamine release, 172

Cold agglutinin disease, 144

Cold antibody hemolytic disease, 144

Cold urticaria, 164

Colitis, ulcerative, 252

Collagen diseases, 189–190

  and allergic interstitial nephritis, 189

  and amyloidosis, 202

  and immunopathology of NZB mice, 190–191

  pathologic features of, 189

  polyarteritis nodosa, 191

  rheumatoid arthritis, 197–200

  rheumatic fever, 196–197

  systemic lupus erythematosus, 192–195

Colloidal carbon, and blockade of reticuloendothelial system, 123

Complement

  activation, 153–154

  in autoallergic disease, 256

  deficiencies, and immune deficiency, 312

  description of system of, 151–155

  and endotoxin shock, 353

  and glomerulonephritis, 185

  in Goodpasture's disease, 187

  in interactivation of allergic mechanism, 279

  in liver disease, 252–253

  measurement, 322

  in pemphigus and pemphigoid, 201

  role in human diseases, 154

  in systemic lupus erythematosus, 192

Complement chemotactic factor, production of, 183

Complement-fixing antibody, in multiple sclerosis, 247

Complex, toxic. See Arthus reaction

Complex specificity of immunoglobulins, 76

Computer analysis, and tissue matching, 229

Concanavalin A, blood lymphocyte response to, 324

Conjunctivitis, and route of access of antigen, 164

Contact allergy, immunopathology of, 3, 217, 219, *220*, 221

Coombs' test

  and cytotoxic antibodies, 149–150

  in systemic lupus erythematosus, 192

  in warm antibody disease, 144

Copolymers, of amino acids, 3–4

Cork dust, as antigen in suberosis, 272

Corn, Forssman antigen in, 149

Cortex, of thymus, 25

Corticosteroids

  in asthma, 167

  in dermatomyositis, 195–196

  effects on immune response, 319

  and hemolytic anemia, 144

  in pemphigus and pemphigoid, 201

  in polyarteritis nodosa, 191

  in rheumatoid arthritis, 199–200

  in systemic lupus erythematosus, 195

Cosmetics, atopic allergies to, 169

Crossover, definition of, 79

Cryoimmunoglobulins

  in rheumatoid arthritis, 198

  and urticaria, 164

Polymorphonuclear leukocytes (PMNs)
(continued)
basophils, 17–18
eosinophils, 17, *18*
neutrophils, 17
Polypeptide chains
of antibodies, 70, 72
in immunoglobulins, 65, 67, 72–73
Polyps, nasal, in allergic rhinitis, 167, 168
Population studies, of IgG allotypes, 81
Posttransfusion thrombocytopenic purpura, 147
Potatoes, allergy to, 169
PPD (purified protein derivative), delayed skin reaction from, 216–271, *218*
Prausnitz-Kustner test, for reagin, 159–160
Precipitin reaction, 90, 91, *92*, 93
in agar, 95–98
antigen concentration effects on, 93
quantitative, 93, *94*, 95
Precipitinogen, definition of, 91
Pregnancy
graft-vs-host reactions in, 238–240
Shwartzman reaction in, 353
Preplasma cells, 19
Primary familial amyloidosis, 202
Primary immune deficiencies, 302–303, *304*, 305–306
Primary lymphopenic immunologic deficiency. See Thymic alymphoplasia
Primary lysosomes, 120
Primary sporadic amyloidosis, 202
Private specificities, 230–231
Procainamide
and antibodies to DNA, 194
induction of systemic lupus erythematosus by, 194
Progressive multifocal leukoencephalopathy, 242
Progressive systemic sclerosis, 196
Proliferative-inhibitory factor, as lymphocyte mediator, 216
Properdin, and complement activation, 155
Prophylactic immunization, 294–296
Protein(s)
denaturation of, 4
myelomas producing, 81, 83
Proteolipil, as antigen in allergic encephalomyelitis, 255
Proteus OX-19, in Weil-Felix test, 9
Protozoal infections, specific immunity to, 290
Psoriasis, possible allergic origin of, 252

Psychological factors
and asthma, 172
and hay fever, 167
Psychotherapy
in asthma, 166
in atopic reactions, 177

Quarternary structure of immunoglobulins, 72–73
Quinidine, hemolytic reaction to, 145
Quinine (Sedormid) purpura, immunopathology, 148

Rabbits
anaphylactic shock in, 162
serum sickness in, 182
Rabies virus
immune response to, 242
immunization against, 295
infection by, relation to acute disseminated encephalomyelitis, 246–247
Race, and allotypes, 77, 80, 81
Radiation chimera, in bone marrow transplants, 237
Radioallergosorbent test (RAST), for reagin, 160, 161
Radioimmunoassays, 101–102
of insulin, 133
use of antigen-antibody reactions in, 101–102
Radiomimetic drugs, effects on immune response, 318
Ragweed, allergy to, 161
Rat, anaphylactic shock in, 163
Reagin
in atopic reactions, 159–161
clinical test for, 160
in serum sickness, 182
tests for, 160–161
Recognition cells, and immune tolerance, 112
Red blood cells. See Erythrocytes
Red pulp of spleen, 22
Regional enteritis, as granulomatous-like disease, 273
Reiter's disease, and HL-A antigens, 235
Renal disease, and complement deficiency, 312
Renal failure, in scleroderma, 196
Renal transplants
and anti-basement membrane glomerulonephritis, 185

Sympathetic nervous system, 176
  and ophthalmia, 249
  stimulation of, in treatment of atopic reactions, 177
Synografts, defined, 221
Syphilis
  false positive tests for, and collagen diseases, 189–190
  TPI test for, 104
  tertiary, granulomas from, 271
  Wasserman antigen in, 159, 254
Systemic lupus erythematosus, 192–195
  and complement deficiency, 312
  and cytotoxic antibodies, 148–149
  drug induced, 194
  and HL-A antigens, 234
  treatment of, 194–195

Tangerines, allergy to, 169
Tapeworms, 291
T cell(s)
  in antibody formation, 41–50
  antigen receptors of, 40, 54
  and antilymphocyte serum, 320–322
  B cell interactions with, 45, 47
  "carrier primed," 41
  defect of, in low responders, 54–55
  and histocompatibility system, 235
  and immune tolerance, 112, *113*
  and immunity, 209–214
  killing effects of lymphocytes on, 209, *210–211*, 212, *213*, 214
  in mixed lymphocyte reactions test, 228–229
  of NZB mice, 39, 190–191
  origin of, 35
  subpopulations of, 37–38
  suppressor activity, 114–115
  transfer of receptors from, 45, 47
  in variable immune deficiency diseases, 309
Temperature, effect on atopic reactions, 157
Terasaki system of tissue matching, 232–233
Tertiary structure
  of antibody, 55
  of antigens, 4
Testes, inflammation of. See Orchitis
Tetanus, prophylactic immunization for, 295
Tetracyclines, effects on immune response, 319
Thatch, as antigen in New Guinea lung, 272
Theophylline, effects on cellular level of cyclic AMP, 173

Thermoactinomyces vulgaris, as antigen in allergic alveolitis, 272
Thioguanine, 318
Third-man test, for histocompatibility antigens, 228
Thrombocytopenia, in Wiskott-Aldrich syndrome, 307
Thrombocytopenic purpura
  acute idiopathic, 147–148
  chronic idiopathic, 148
  neonatal, 147
  posttransfusion, 147
  thrombotic, 196
Thrombosis, and polyarteritis nodosa, 191
Thy antigen, 37
Thymectomy, 306
  and antibody production to thymus-independent antigens, 114
  and immune maturity, 301–302
  and myasthenia gravis, 135–136
  of neonatal animals, 22
Thymic alymphoplasia, as immune deficiency disease, 303, 305, 308
Thymic aplasia, as immune deficiency disease, 308
Thymic humoral factors, and T cell maturation, 38
Thymitis, experimental, 136
Thymocytes, in thymus, 25
Thymosin, 25
  and T cell maturation, 38
Thymus
  and humoral immune deficiencies, 308–309
  in lymphoproliferative neoplasias, 316
  of NZB mice, 190
  role in development of immune maturity, 301–302
  structure of, 25, *26*
  and T-cell maturation, 38
  transplantation of, in immune deficiency therapy, 310–311
Thymus-leukemia antigen, 39
Thyroglobulin
  antibody to, 250
  as antigen in thyroiditis, 250–251
Thyroid colloid antigen, antibody to, 250–251
Thyroid stimulator, long acting, of Graves' disease, 135
Thyroiditis
  antigens in, 183
  as autoallergic disease, 250–251
  autoantibodies in, 254, 255

75 76 77 78 79 80   10 9 8 7 6 5 4 3 2